Imaging of Brain Tumors

Editor

RIVKA R. COLEN

MAGNETIC RESONANCE IMAGING CLINICS OF NORTH AMERICA

www.mri.theclinics.com

Consulting Editors
SURESH K. MUKHERJI
LYNNE S. STEINBACH

November 2016 • Volume 24 • Number 4

ELSEVIER

1600 John F. Kennedy Boulevard • Suite 1800 • Philadelphia, Pennsylvania, 19103-2899

http://www.mri.theclinics.com

MRI CLINICS OF NORTH AMERICA Volume 24, Number 4
November 2016 ISSN 1064-9689, ISBN 13: 978-0-323-45975-4

Editor: John Vassallo (j.vassallo@elsevier.com)
Developmental Editor: Meredith Clinton

Magnetic Resonance Imaging Clinics of North America (ISSN 1064-9689) is published quarterly by Elsevier Inc., 360 Park Avenue South, New York, NY 10010-1710. Months of issue are February, May, August, and November. Business and Editorial Offices: 1600 John F. Kennedy Blvd., Ste. 1800, Philadelphia, PA 19103-2899. Customer Service Office: 3251 Riverport Lane, Maryland Heights, MO 63043. Periodicals postage paid at New York, NY and additional mailing offices. Subscription prices are $380.00 per year (domestic individuals), $636.00 per year (domestic institutions), $100.00 per year (domestic students/residents), $420.00 per year (Canadian individuals), $828.00 per year (Canadian institutions), $545.00 per year (international individuals), $828.00 per year (international institutions), and $275.00 per year (international and Canadian students/residents). International air speed delivery is included in all *Clinics* subscription prices. All prices are subject to change without notice. **POSTMASTER:** Send address changes to *Magnetic Resonance Imaging Clinics*, Elsevier Health Sciences Division, Subscription Customer Service, 3251 Riverport Lane, Maryland Heights, MO 63043. Customer Service (orders, claims, online, change of address): Elsevier Health Sciences Division, Subscription **Customer Service, 3251 Riverport Lane, Maryland Heights, MO 63043. Tel:1-800-654-2452 (U.S. and Canada); 314-447-8871 (outside U.S. and Canada). Fax: 314-447-8029. E-mail: journalscustomer service-usa@elsevier.com (for print support); journalsonlinesupport-usa@elsevier.com (for online support).**

Reprints. For copies of 100 or more of articles in this publication, please contact the Commercial Reprints Department, Elsevier Inc., 360 Park Avenue South, New York, NY 10010-1710. Tel.: 212-633-3874; Fax: 212-633-3820; E-mail: reprints@elsevier.com.

Magnetic Resonance Imaging Clinics of North America is covered in the *RSNA Index of Imaging Literature, MEDLINE/PubMed (Index Medicus),* and *EMBASE/Excerpta Medica.*

Contributors

CONSULTING EDITOR

SURESH K. MUKHERJI, MD, MBA, FACR
Department of Radiology, Michigan State
University, East Lansing, Michigan

EDITOR

RIVKA R. COLEN, MD
Assistant Professor, Departments of Cancer
Systems Imaging and Diagnostic Radiology,
Division of Diagnostic Imaging, Section of
Neuroradiology, The University of Texas MD
Anderson Cancer Center, Houston, Texas

AUTHORS

RAHUL ANIL, MBBS
Research Intern, Department of
Neuroradiology, The University of Texas MD
Anderson Cancer Center, Houston, Texas

PRATIP K. BHATTACHARYA, PhD
Associate Professor, Department of Cancer
Systems Imaging, The University of Texas MD
Anderson Cancer Center; The University of
Texas Health Science Center at Houston,
Houston, Texas

JERROLD L. BOXERMAN, MD, PhD, FACR
Associate Professor of Diagnostic Imaging,
Department of Diagnostic Imaging, Rhode
Island Hospital, Alpert Medical School of
Brown University, Providence, Rhode Island

LARA A. BRANDÃO, MD
Chief of Neuroradiology, Clínica Felippe
Mattoso, Barra da Tijuca; Neuroradiologist,
Clínica IRM- Ressonância Magnética,
Rio De Janeiro, Brazil

MAURICIO CASTILLO, MD
Professor of Radiology; Chief of
Neuroradiology, Division of Neuroradiology,
Department of Radiology, University of North
Carolina School of Medicine, Chapel Hill, North
Carolina

ASIM F. CHOUDHRI, MD
Departments of Radiology, Neurosurgery
and Ophthalmology, University of Tennessee
Health Science Center; Le Bonheur
Neuroscience Institute, Le Bonheur
Children's Hospital, Memphis,
Tennessee

RIVKA R. COLEN, MD
Assistant Professor, Departments of Cancer
Systems Imaging and Diagnostic Radiology,
Division of Diagnostic Imaging, Section of
Neuroradiology, The University of Texas MD
Anderson Cancer Center, Houston,
Texas

PRASANTA DUTTA, PhD
Department of Cancer Systems Imaging,
The University of Texas MD Anderson Cancer
Center, Houston, Texas

BENJAMIN M. ELLINGSON, PhD
Associate Professor of Radiology, Psychiatry,
Bioengineering, and Biomedical Physics,
Department of Radiological Sciences, David
Geffen School of Medicine at University of
California Los Angeles, Los Angeles, California

NABIL ELSHAFEEY, MD
Postdoctoral Fellow, Department of Diagnostic
Radiology, The University of Texas MD
Anderson Cancer Center, Houston, Texas

SETH T. GAMMON, PhD
Assistant Professor, Department of Cancer
Systems Imaging, The University of Texas
MD Anderson Cancer Center, Houston, Texas

KETAN GHAGHADA, PhD
Edward B. Singleton Department of Pediatric
Radiology, Texas Children's Hospital;
Department of Radiology, Baylor College of
Medicine, Houston, Texas

BRENT GRIFFITH, MD
Department of Radiology, Henry Ford Health
System, Detroit, Michigan

ISLAM HASSAN, MD
Postdoctoral Fellow, Department of Diagnostic
Radiology, The University of Texas MD
Anderson Cancer Center, Houston, Texas

AMY B. HEIMBERGER, MD
Professor, Department of Neurosurgery,
The University of Texas MD Anderson Cancer
Center, Houston, Texas

JINGZHE HU, BS
Department of Cancer Systems Imaging,
The University of Texas MD Anderson Cancer
Center; Department of Bioengineering, Rice
University, Houston, Texas

RAYMOND Y. HUANG, MD, PhD
Division of Neuroradiology, Department of
Radiology, Brigham and Women's Hospital,
Harvard Medical School, Boston,
Massachusetts

RAJAN JAIN, MD
Associate Professor of Radiology, New York
University School of Medicine, New York
University Langone Medical Center,
New York, New York

PAUL KLIMO Jr, MD, MPH
Department of Neurosurgery, University of
Tennessee Health Science Center; Le Bonheur
Neuroscience Institute, Le Bonheur Children's
Hospital; Division of Neurosurgery, St. Jude's
Children's Hospital; Semmes Murphey

Neurologic & Spine Institute, Memphis,
Tennessee

AIKATERINI KOTROTSOU, PhD
Department of Diagnostic Radiology,
The University of Texas MD Anderson Cancer
Center, Houston, Texas

FREDERICK F. LANG, MD
Professor, Department of Neurosurgery,
The University of Texas MD Anderson Cancer
Center, Houston, Texas

JAEHYUK LEE, PhD
Department of Cancer Systems Imaging,
The University of Texas MD Anderson Cancer
Center, Texas

ARNAV MEHTA, PhD
Medical Scientist Training Program, David
Geffen School of Medicine at University of
California Los Angeles, Los Angeles, California;
Division of Biology and Biologic Engineering,
California Institute of Technology, Pasadena,
California

NIKI ZACHARIAS MILLWARD, PhD
Assistant Professor, Department of Cancer
Systems Imaging, The University of Texas MD
Anderson Cancer Center, Houston, Texas

SRINIVASAN MUKUNDAN Jr, MD, PhD
Division of Neuroradiology, Department of
Radiology, Brigham and Woman's Hospital,
Harvard Medical School, Boston,
Massachusetts

LINDA NGUYEN, BS
The University of Texas Health Science Center
at Houston, Houston, Texas

WHITNEY B. POPE, MD, PhD
Professor-in-Residence, Department of
Radiological Sciences, and Director, University
of California Los Angeles Brain Tumor Imaging,
David Geffen School of Medicine at University
of California Los Angeles, Los Angeles,
California

SHIVANAND PUDAKALAKATTI, PhD
Department of Cancer Systems Imaging,
The University of Texas MD Anderson Cancer
Center, Houston, Texas

O. RAPALINO, MD
Neuroradiology Division, Department of
Radiology, Massachusetts General Hospital,
Boston, Massachusetts

E.M. RATAI, PhD
Neuroradiology Division, Department of
Radiology, Massachusetts General Hospital,
Boston, Massachusetts; MGH/HST Athinoula
A. Martinos Center for Biomedical Imaging,
Charlestown, Massachusetts

TRAVIS C. SALZILLO, BS
Department of Cancer Systems Imaging,
The University of Texas MD Anderson Cancer
Center; The University of Texas Health Science
Center at Houston, Houston, Texas

MARK S. SHIROISHI, MD
Assistant Professor, Division of
Neuroradiology, Department of Radiology,
Keck School of Medicine, University of
Southern California, Los Angeles, California

ADEEL SIDDIQUI, MD
Department of Radiology, University of
Tennessee Health Science Center; Le Bonheur
Neuroscience Institute, Le Bonheur Children's
Hospital, Memphis, Tennessee

PATRICK Y. WEN, MD
Division of Neuro-Oncology, Department of
Neurology, Center For Neuro-Oncology,
Dana-Farber/Brigham and Women's Cancer
Center, Brigham and Women's Hospital,
Harvard Medical School, Boston,
Massachusetts

JOSEPH WEYGAND, BS
Department of Cancer Systems Imaging,
The University of Texas MD Anderson Cancer
Center; The University of Texas Health Science
Center at Houston, Houston,
Texas

NICHOLAS WHITING, PhD
Department of Cancer Systems Imaging,
The University of Texas MD Anderson Cancer
Center, Houston, Texas

PASCAL O. ZINN, MD, PhD
Neurosurgery Resident, Department of
Neurosurgery, Baylor College of Medicine,
Houston, Texas

Contributors

O. RAPALINO, MD
Neuroradiology Division, Department of
Radiology, Massachusetts General Hospital,
Boston, Massachusetts

E.M. RATAI, PhD
Neuroradiology Division, Department of
Radiology, Massachusetts General Hospital,
Boston, Massachusetts; MGH/HST Athinoula
A. Martinos Center for Biomedical Imaging,
Charlestown, Massachusetts

TRAVIS C. SALZILLO, BS
Department of Cancer Systems Imaging,
The University of Texas MD Anderson Cancer
Center, The University of Texas Health Science
Center at Houston, Houston, Texas

MARK S. SHIROISHI, MD
Assistant Professor, Division of
Neuroradiology, Department of Radiology,
Keck School of Medicine, University of
Southern California, Los Angeles, California

ADEEL SIDDIQUI, MD
Department of Radiology, University of
Tennessee Health Science Center; Le Bonheur
Neuroscience Institute, Le Bonheur Children's
Hospital, Memphis, Tennessee

PATRICK Y. WEN, MD
Division of Neuro-Oncology, Department of
Neurology, Center For Neuro-Oncology,
Dana-Farber/Brigham and Women's Cancer
Center, Brigham and Women's Hospital,
Harvard Medical School, Boston,
Massachusetts

JOSEPH WEYGAND, BS
Department of Cancer Systems Imaging,
The University of Texas MD Anderson Cancer
Center, The University of Texas Health Science
Center at Houston, Houston,
Texas

NICHOLAS WHITING, PhD
Department of Cancer Systems Imaging,
The University of Texas MD Anderson Cancer
Center, Houston, Texas

PASCAL O. ZINN, MD, PhD
Neurosurgery Resident, Department of
Neurosurgery, Baylor College of Medicine,
Houston, Texas

Contents

Dynamic susceptibility contrast (DSC) MR imaging, a perfusion-weighted MR imaging technique typically used in neuro-oncologic applications for estimating the relative cerebral blood volume within brain tumors, has demonstrated much potential for determining prognosis, predicting therapeutic response, and assessing early treatment response of gliomas. This review highlights recent developments using DSC-MR imaging and emphasizes the need for technical standardization and validation in prospective studies in order for this technique to become incorporated into standard-of-care imaging for patients with brain tumors.

Magnetic resonance spectroscopy (MRS) is a magnetic resonance–based imaging modality that allows noninvasive sampling of metabolic changes in normal and abnormal brain parenchyma. MRS is particularly useful in the differentiation of developmental or non-neoplastic disorders from neoplastic processes. MRS is also useful during routine imaging follow-up after radiation treatment or during antiangiogenic treatment and for predicting outcomes and treatment response. The objective of this article is to provide a concise but thorough review of the basic physical principles, important applications of MRS in brain tumor imaging, and future directions.

This article reviews existing and emerging techniques of interrogating metabolism in brain cancer from well-established proton magnetic resonance spectroscopy to the promising hyperpolarized metabolic imaging and chemical exchange saturation transfer and emerging techniques of imaging inflammation. Some of these techniques are at an early stage of development and clinical trials are in progress in patients to establish the clinical efficacy. It is likely that in vivo metabolomics and metabolic imaging is the next frontier in brain cancer diagnosis and assessing therapeutic efficacy; with the combined knowledge of genomics and proteomics a complete understanding of tumorigenesis in brain might be achieved.

The Response Assessment in Neuro-Oncology (RANO) Working Group is an international multidisciplinary group whose goal is to improve response criteria and define endpoints for neuro-oncology trials. The RANO criteria for high-grade gliomas attempt to address the issues of pseudoprogression, pseudoresponse, and nonenhancing tumor progression. Incorporation of advanced MR imaging may eventually help improve the ability of these criteria to better define enhancing and nonenhancing disease. The RANO group has also developed criteria for neurologic response and evaluation of patients receiving immunologic therapies. RANO criteria have been developed for brain metastases and are in progress for meningiomas, leptomeningeal disease, spinal tumors, and pediatric tumors.

The role of radiomics in the diagnosis, monitoring, and therapy planning of brain tumors is becoming increasingly clear. Incorporation of quantitative approaches in radiology, in combination with increased computer power, offers unique insights into macroscopic tumor characteristics and their direct association with the underlying pathophysiology. This article presents the most recent findings in radiomics and radiogenomics with respect to identifying potential imaging biomarkers with prognostic value that can lead to individualized therapy. In addition, a brief introduction to the concept of big data and its significance in medicine is presented.

The integration of imaging characteristics and genomic data has started a new trend in approach toward management of glioblastoma (GBM). Many ongoing studies are investigating imaging phenotypical signatures that could explain more about the behavior of GBM and its outcome. The discovery of biomarkers has played an adjuvant role in treating and predicting the outcome of patients with GBM. Discovering these imaging phenotypical signatures and dysregulated pathways/genes is needed and required to engineer treatment based on specific GBM manifestations. Characterizing these parameters will establish well-defined criteria so researchers can build on the treatment of GBM through personal medicine.

The new World Health Organization classification of brain tumors depends on combining the histologic light microscopy features of central nervous system (CNS) tumors with canonical genetic alterations. This integrated diagnosis is redrawing the pedigree chart of brain tumors with rearrangement of tumor groups on the basis of geno-phenotypical behaviors into meaningful groups. Multiple radiogenomic studies provide a bridge between imaging features and tumor microenvironment. An overlap that can be integrated within the genophenotypical classification of CNS tumors for a better understanding of different clinically relevant entities.

The first generation of cross-sectional brain imaging using computed tomography
(CT), ultrasonography, and eventually MR imaging focused on determining structural
or anatomic changes associated with brain disorders. The current state-of-the-art
imaging, functional imaging, uses techniques such as CT and MR perfusion that
allow determination of physiologic parameters in vivo. In parallel, tissue-based
genomic, transcriptomic, and proteomic profiling of brain tumors has created
several novel and exciting possibilities for molecular targeting of brain tumors. The
next generation of imaging translates these molecular in vitro techniques to
in vivo, noninvasive, targeted reconstruction of tumors and their microenvironments.

Perfusion imaging is a method for assessing the flow of blood occurring at the tissue
level and can be accomplished by both CT and MR perfusion techniques. The use of
perfusion imaging has increased substantially in the past decade, particularly in
neuro-oncologic imaging, where it is has been used for brain tumor grading and
directing biopsies or targeted therapy, as well as for the evaluation of treatment
response and disease progression. This article discusses the basic principles and
techniques of perfusion imaging, as well as its applications in neuro-oncology.

Proton magnetic resonance spectroscopy (H-MRS) may be helpful in suggesting
tumor histology and tumor grade and may better define tumor extension and the
ideal site for biopsy compared with conventional magnetic resonance (MR) imaging.
A multifunctional approach with diffusion-weighted imaging, perfusion-weighted
imaging, and permeability maps, along with H-MRS, may enhance the accuracy
of the diagnosis and characterization of brain tumors and estimation of therapeutic
response. Integration of advanced imaging techniques with conventional MR imaging and the clinical history help to improve the accuracy, sensitivity, and specificity in
differentiating tumors and nonneoplastic lesions.

Cerebellar tumors are the most common group of solid tumors in children. MR
imaging provides an important role in characterization of these lesions, surgical
planning, and postsurgical surveillance. Preoperative imaging can help predict the
histologic subtype of tumors, which can provide guidance for surgical planning.
Beyond histology, pediatric brain tumors are undergoing new classification schemes
based on genetic features. Intraoperative MR imaging has emerged as an important
tool in the surgical management of pediatric brain tumors. Effective understanding of
the imaging features of pediatric cerebellar tumors can benefit communication with
neurosurgeons and neuro-oncologists and can improve patient management.

MAGNETIC RESONANCE IMAGING CLINICS OF NORTH AMERICA

VISIT THE CLINICS ONLINE!
Access your subscription at:
www.theclinics.com

PROGRAM OBJECTIVE

The goal of *Magnetic Resonance Imaging Clinics of North America* is to keep practicing physicians up to date with current clinical practice by providing timely articles reviewing the state of the art in patient care.

TARGET AUDIENCE

All practicing physicians and healthcare professionals who provide patient care utilizing findings from Magnetic Resonance Imaging.

LEARNING OBJECTIVES

Upon completion of this activity, participants will be able to:
1. Review current clinical practice techniques in brain tumor imaging.
2. Discuss the 2016 World Health organization classification of tumors of the central nervous system.
3. Recognize the use of brain tumor imaging in predicting patient outcome.

ACCREDITATION

The Elsevier Office of Continuing Medical Education (EOCME) is accredited by the Accreditation Council for Continuing Medical Education (ACCME) to provide continuing medical education for physicians.

The EOCME designates this enduring material for a maximum of 15 *AMA PRA Category 1 Credit*(s)™. Physicians should claim only the credit commensurate with the extent of their participation in the activity.

All other health care professionals requesting continuing education credit for this enduring material will be issued a certificate of participation.

DISCLOSURE OF CONFLICTS OF INTEREST

The EOCME assesses conflict of interest with its instructors, faculty, planners, and other individuals who are in a position to control the content of CME activities. All relevant conflicts of interest that are identified are thoroughly vetted by EOCME for fair balance, scientific objectivity, and patient care recommendations. EOCME is committed to providing its learners with CME activities that promote improvements or quality in healthcare and not a specific proprietary business or a commercial interest.

The planning committee, staff, authors and editors listed below have identified no financial relationships or relationships to products or devices they or their spouse/life partner have with commercial interest related to the content of this CME activity:
Rahul Anil, MBBS; Pratip K. Bhattacharya, PhD; Jerrold L. Boxerman, MD, PhD, FACR; Lara A. Brandão, MD; Mauricio Castillo, MD; Assim F. Choudhri, MD; Rivka R. Colen, MD; Prasanta Dutta, PhD; Benjamin M. Ellingson, PhD; Nabil Elshafeey, MD; Anjali Fortna; Seth T. Gammon, PhD; Ketan Ghaghada, PhD; Brent Griffith, MD; Islam Hassan, MD; Amy B. Heimberger, MD; Rajan Jain, MD; Jingzhe Hu, BS; Raymond Y. Huang, MD, PhD; Paul Klimo Jr, MD, MPH; Aikaterini Kotrotsou, PhD; Frederick F. Lang, MD; Jaehyuk Lee, PhD; Arnav Mehta, PhD; Niki Zacharias Millward, PhD; Suresh K. Mukherji, MD, MBA, FACR; Srinivasan Mukundan Jr, MD, PhD; Linda Nguyen, BS; Whitney B. Pope, MD, PhD; Shivanand Pudakalakatti, PhD; O. Rapalino, MD; E.M. Ratai, PhD; Travis C. Salzillo, BS; Erin Scheckenbach; Adeel Siddiqui, MD; Mark S. Shiroishi, MD; Lynne S. Steinbach; Karthik Subramaniam; John Vassallo; Patrick Y. Wen, MD; Joseph Weygand, BS; Nicholas Whiting, PhD; Pascal O. Zinn, MD, PhD.

UNAPPROVED/OFF-LABEL USE DISCLOSURE

The EOCME requires CME faculty to disclose to the participants:
1. When products or procedures being discussed are off-label, unlabelled, experimental, and/or investigational (not US Food and Drug Administration [FDA] approved); and
2. Any limitations on the information presented, such as data that are preliminary or that represent ongoing research, interim analyses, and/or unsupported opinions. Faculty may discuss information about pharmaceutical agents that is outside of FDA-approved labelling. This information is intended solely for CME and is not intended to promote off-label use of these medications. If you have any questions, contact the medical affairs department of the manufacturer for the most recent prescribing information.

TO ENROLL

To enroll in the *Magnetic Resonance Imaging Clinics of North America* Continuing Medical Education program, call customer service at 1-800-654-2452 or sign up online at http://www.theclinics.com/home/cme. The CME program is available to subscribers for an additional annual fee of USD 250.

METHOD OF PARTICIPATION

In order to claim credit, participants must complete the following:
1. Complete enrolment as indicated above.
2. Read the activity.

3. Complete the CME Test and Evaluation. Participants must achieve a score of 70% on the test. All CME Tests and Evaluations must be completed online.

CME INQUIRIES/SPECIAL NEEDS

For all CME inquiries or special needs, please contact elsevierCME@elsevier.com.

Foreword

CrossMark

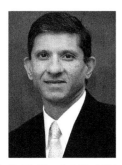

Suresh K. Mukherji, MD, MBA, FACR
Consulting Editor

The term "multiparametric" imaging has become part of our radiology lexicon and is now clinically used to evaluate a variety brain tumors and prostate carcinomas. Multiparametric imaging typically combines information available on standard sequences with other sequences such as diffusion, perfusion, and spectroscopy to increase the diagnostic accuracy of the study. The "Holy Grail" of imaging would be the ability to automatically extract (pixel by pixel) and combine all of the diagnostic imaging information (Radiomics) with genetic information (Radiogenomics) and ultimately pathologic information (Radioproteogenomics) to improve diagnosis, access prognosis, and improve outcome. This would certainly be a logical goal of the promise of "Big Data."

This exciting field is the topic of the current issue of *Magnetic Resonance Imaging Clinics of North America*. Dr Rivka Colen is one the world's experts in this evolving field, and she has done an excellent job in presenting this exciting area in a concise and understandable manner. The timing of this issue could not be better as it coincides with the update of the WHO classification of brain tumors and the AJCC 8th edition. Both of these important documents are integrating imaging and molecular and genetic markers into classification and staging.

I would like to thank Dr Colen and all of the article authors for their outstanding contributions. I especially would like to thank Dr Colen for accepting our invitation and somehow finding the time to guest-edit this visionary issue. Rivka, I am not sure how you did it, but all of us are very thankful for your wonderful contribution!

Suresh K. Mukherji, MD, MBA, FACR
Department of Radiology
Michigan State University
846 Service Road
East Lansing, MI 48824, USA

E-mail address:
mukherji@rad.msu.edu

Magn Reson Imaging Clin N Am 24 (2016) xiii
http://dx.doi.org/10.1016/j.mric.2016.09.002
1064-9689/16/© 2016 Published by Elsevier Inc.

Preface

New State-of-the-Art and Cutting-Edge Advances in Brain Tumor Imaging

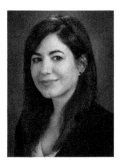

Rivka R. Colen, MD
Editor

Imaging has transformed the way medicine is practiced and has become the cornerstone for assessment of most, if not all, types of diseases. Since the discovery of radiographs by Roentgen and the landmark image demonstrating the hand bones, imaging has undergone tremendous advances with the development of computed tomography and subsequently MR imaging; exquisite tissue characterization and functional imaging of the tissue or tumor microenvironment are now possible. However, there is much more to an image than the visualized qualitative or gross quantitative assessments routinely performed. Toward this end, imaging is witnessing another revolution: focusing on methods to harness the information within an existing acquired image by way of imaging feature extraction through quantitative methods, high-level imaging analysis and analytics, deep learning techniques, and artificial intelligence.

Advances in high-computational power and software analytics have provided the capabilities to develop increasingly more complex quantitative imaging analytics and postprocessing techniques such as can be provided by radiomics. Radiomics is defined as the automated high-throughput extraction of imaging features from standard medical images. Given its ability to analyze the image on a pixel or voxel level, we are able to extract imaging features otherwise not visible to the naked human eye. Similarly, these same advances have provided us the ability to extract large-scale genomic, proteomic, and metabolic information at light speed and at much less cost to the patient; genomics has allowed for a greater understanding in the genomic underpinnings and biological processes of disease. Recently, multiple studies have shown that imaging characteristics are reflective of the underlying biological process, tumor microenvironment, and genomic composition. Imaging genomics (also termed radiogenomics) is the linkage of imaging characteristics with the underlying genomic processes of the tissue or tumor. The ability to noninvasively assess the entire tumor and get a greater spatial understanding the tumor, its imaging genomic landscape, and its response to treatment would be tremendous progress. This issue is dedicated to providing the reader with an in-depth view of these new fields of genomics, radiomics, and imaging genomics, in particular, to how it related to the neuroimaging community. We take the reader through a series of steps in this issue of *Magnetic Resonance Imaging Clinics of North America* from advanced cutting-edge imaging and techniques, imaging tumor metrics for use in the clinical setting and clinical trials, high-level imaging analytics and postprocessing, radiomics, and imaging genomics. The new WHO classification of brain tumors, which is now based on the molecular markers, is reviewed. Other novel applications of imaging such as nanoparticles are also included. Finally, a review of more well-known

Magn Reson Imaging Clin N Am 24 (2016) xv–xvi
http://dx.doi.org/10.1016/j.mric.2016.09.001
1064-9689/16/© 2016 Published by Elsevier Inc.

clinical applications of existing advanced techniques is included.

The issue kicks off with an in-depth discussion on numerous articles related to multiparametric advanced imaging techniques (three articles), quantitative cancer imaging metrics and imaging genomics (four articles), and reviews of novel neuroimaging agents and of basic clinical multiparametric techniques and clinical applications (four articles). I would like to express my gratitude and thanks to all the assembled authors who, as experts in their respective field, have given their invaluable contribution to make this issue a success. I hope the reader enjoys the diverse and cutting-edge topics provided.

I would like to thank Suresh Mukherji, MD, MBA, FACR, the Consulting Editor, for the honor of being selected to lead this important issue. It was a pleasure to work with the team, and I extend my immeasurable gratitude to the series editors, Meredith Clinton and John Vassallo, for their understanding, support, and patience throughout the entire course of this publication.

Finally, I would like to dedicate this issue to my lovely daughter, Mila Rayne Alondra Zinn, who was born during the writing process and production of this issue, and my husband, Pascal Zinn, for their steadfast love and support during this journey; and to my parents, Leila Roger and Joseph Colen, who throughout my upbringing have given me all the love, encouragement, and dedication possible to a daughter.

Rivka R. Colen, MD
Departments of Cancer Systems Imaging
and Diagnostic Radiology
Division of Diagnostic Imaging
Section of Neuroradiology
The University of Texas
MD Anderson Cancer Center
1400 Pressler Street, Unit 1482
Room # FCT 16.5037
Houston, TX 77030, USA

E-mail address:
rcolen@mdanderson.org

Dynamic Susceptibility Contrast MR Imaging in Glioma
Review of Current Clinical Practice

Jerrold L. Boxerman, MD, PhD[a],*, Mark S. Shiroishi, MD[b],
Benjamin M. Ellingson, PhD[c], Whitney B. Pope, MD, PhD[d]

KEYWORDS

- Dynamic susceptibility contrast MR imaging (DSC-MR imaging) • Cerebral blood volume (CBV)
- High-grade glioma • Glioblastoma • Response assessment • Pseudoprogression
- Pseudoresponse • Prognosis

KEY POINTS

- The most common parameter measured with dynamic susceptibility contrast (DSC) MR imaging is relative cerebral blood volume (rCBV), a measure of microvascular density that augments conventional contrast-enhanced MR imaging in the initial evaluation and posttreatment monitoring of brain tumors.
- Lesions with high rCBV tend to distinguish tumor from nontumor, correspond with higher rather than lower tumor grade with worse prognosis, and designate biopsy sites with an increased likelihood of capturing the highest-grade portion of tumor.
- The rCBV values at or compared with baseline may help with response assessment for cytotoxic (progression vs pseudoprogression) and antiangiogenic (response vs pseudoresponse) therapies.
- Preliminary studies suggest that DSC-MR imaging may also have applicability to immunotherapies.
- DSC-MR imaging protocols and postprocessing techniques vary widely in the literature, and validation with standardization of methods providing clinically reliable measurements is needed, particularly in the setting of multicenter clinical brain tumor trials.

BASIC PRINCIPLES OF DYNAMIC SUSCEPTIBILITY CONTRAST–MR IMAGING

As contrast-enhanced MR imaging is the standard of care for assessing brain tumors, perfusion-weighted MR imaging (PWI) techniques using gadolinium-based contrast agents (GBCA) are commonly used for neuro-oncology applications, which include DSC and dynamic contrast-enhanced MR imaging. DSC-MR imaging has been the most prevalent PWI methodology for

Disclosure Statement: Dr Boxerman has nothing to disclose. Dr Shiroishi is a consultant to Bayer and Guerbet. Dr Ellingson is a consultant for Roche/Genentech, Agios, Celegene, Natvis, Tocagen, Northwest Biopharmaceuticals, Amgen, and Excelixis; he serves on the administration board for Roche and Agios and has a grant from the National Brain Tumor Society. Dr Pope is a consultant for Roche, Amgen, Tocagen and Celldex Therapeutics.

[a] Department of Diagnostic Imaging, Rhode Island Hospital, Alpert Medical School of Brown University, 593 Eddy Street, Providence, RI 02903, USA; [b] Department of Radiology, Keck School of Medicine, University of Southern California, 1520 San Pablo Street, Lower Level Imaging L1600, Los Angeles, CA 90033, USA; [c] UCLA Brain Tumor Imaging Laboratory, Department of Radiological Sciences, Center for Computer Vision and Imaging Biomarkers, David Geffen School of Medicine at UCLA, 924 Westwood Boulevard, Suite 615, Los Angeles, CA 90024, USA; [d] Department of Radiological Sciences, David Geffen School of Medicine at UCLA, 757 Westwood Plaza, 1621 East, Los Angeles, CA 90095, USA
* Corresponding author.
E-mail address: jboxerman@lifespan.org

Magn Reson Imaging Clin N Am 24 (2016) 649–670
http://dx.doi.org/10.1016/j.mric.2016.06.005

measuring brain tumor perfusion and is the focus of this article.[1,2]

DSC-MR imaging is a bolus tracking technique that rapidly acquires gradient echo (GRE) or spin echo (SE) echo planar images before (baseline), during, and after (tail) first-pass transit through the brain of an exogenous paramagnetic GBCA that transiently decreases signal intensity.[3] Voxel-wise changes in contrast agent concentration are determined by converting the signal intensity-time curves into relaxivity-time curves assuming that transient signal loss is due solely to changes in T2* (GRE) or T2 (SE) relaxivity. Because relaxivity change is assumed to be directly proportional to contrast agent concentration, the relaxivity-time curves are processed using tracer kinetic modeling and indicator dilution theory to estimate cerebral hemodynamic parameters, such as cerebral blood volume (CBV), cerebral blood flow (CBF), and mean transit time.[4,5] rCBV compared with normal-appearing white matter is the most common DSC-MR imaging metric for evaluating brain tumors[6] because it obviates measurement of an arterial input function, which can be prone to error. Nonetheless, absolute CBV can be determined if the arterial input function is quantified, which is commonly done in a semiautomated fashion by identifying signal-time curves that have arterylike morphology, usually from voxels in the middle cerebral artery or anterior cerebral artery. It should be noted that differences in contrast agent bolus delay and dispersion can introduce systematic error in hemodynamic parameter estimation across the brain.

DSC-MR imaging is based on the classic indicator dilution theory, a methodology used by physiologists to quantitate hemodynamics of whole-organ systems using nondiffusible tracers, such as dyes and radiotracers. The indicator dilution technique assumes intravascular compartmentalization of a nondiffusible tracer, which is violated for GBCA tracers in high-grade gliomas (HGGs) with blood-brain barrier (BBB) disruption and avid contrast enhancement. GBCA extravasation yields T1 shortening, opposing the susceptibility contrast-induced T2 or T2* relaxivity change from intravascular GBCA that forms the basis for CBV estimation. Methods for minimizing the T1 contamination from GBCA extravasation have been developed, although no standardized technique has been universally accepted.[7,8] For single-echo (GRE or SE) DSC-MR imaging acquisitions, low flip angles (ie, 35°–60°) with longer repetition time and echo time (TE) can reduce T1 contamination, and gamma-variate fitting of the relaxivity-time curve can eliminate negative relaxivity changes due to contrast extravasation. However, these techniques

may reduce the signal-to-noise ratio of the computed CBV maps.[9] A preload dose of GBCA administered before the bolus dose of GBCA during dynamic imaging can help mitigate T1 contamination[10] by saturating baseline T1-weighted signal contribution, thereby diminishing dynamic-injection T1-induced increased signal. Preload contrast administration combined with model-based postprocessing leakage correction that diminishes both T1 and T2* extravasation-induced contamination effects[7] improves the accuracy of rCBV estimates in HGGs.[7,11,12] Consensus recommendations for leakage-corrected, single-echo DSC-MR imaging are emerging and seem to be directed toward a technique combining a preload of GBCA with model-based leakage correction.[13] Dual-echo DSC-MR imaging uses 2 GRE acquisitions with different TEs to estimate T2* relaxivity directly, thereby eliminating the T1 contamination effects entirely, but requires special pulse sequences that are less widely available.[14,15] Contrast agent recirculation can introduce smaller periodic decreases in signal intensity after the primary bolus passage. These decreases are either assumed to be negligible or eliminated by using either abbreviated numerical integration or gamma-variate fitting applied to the associated relaxivity-time curve.

APPLICATIONS OF DYNAMIC SUSCEPTIBILITY CONTRAST–MR IMAGING TO BRAIN TUMORS

DSC-MR imaging can augment conventional MR imaging in the initial evaluation and posttreatment monitoring of brain tumors. Although there are many potential neuro-oncologic applications, most fall within 2 distinct categories: (1) improving accuracy in diagnosis, prognosis, and predicting efficacy of a specific therapy before treatment initiation and (2) assessing response to therapy.

Initial Diagnosis, Prognosis, and Predicting Efficacy of Therapy Before Treatment

Distinguishing tumor from nontumor
Differentiating neoplastic from non-neoplastic lesions can be difficult using conventional MR imaging, and often biopsy or follow-up imaging is needed. Multiple studies have shown that the rCBV of infectious lesions is significantly lower than that of metastases or glioblastoma multiformes (GBMs).[16–18] This difference likely reflects the lower microvascular density found in infectious lesions like abscesses relative to that of high-grade tumors.[18] In patients with AIDS, lower rCBV has been reported in toxoplasmosis compared with lymphoma (**Fig. 1**).[19] It should be kept in mind, however, that some infectious lesions like tuberculomas can have elevated rCBV values because of

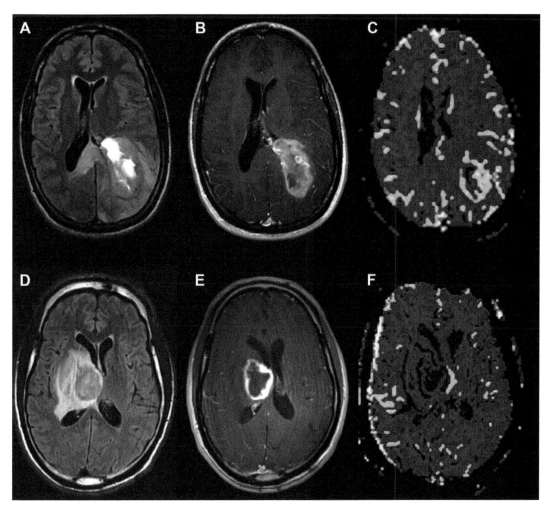

Fig. 1. DSC-MR imaging can help differentiate primary central nervous system (CNS) lymphoma from toxoplasmosis. (A–C): 39-year-old man with human immunodeficiency virus, on highly active antiretroviral therapy, presenting with headache. Fluid-attenuated inversion recovery (FLAIR) (A), postcontrast T1-weighted (B) and rCBV maps (C) demonstrate a peripherally enhancing, FLAIR hyperintense periventricular mass with notably elevated rCBV within lesion enhancement. Biopsy-proven primary CNS lymphoma. (D–F): A 38-year-old man with AIDS (CD4 = 7) presenting with left-sided weakness. FLAIR (D), postcontrast T1-weighted (E) and rCBV (F) images demonstrate a peripherally enhancing mass and surrounding edema in the right basal ganglia with absence of substantial rCBV elevation. The lesion improved on repeat imaging after antitoxoplasmosis therapy.

reactive neovascularization; but rCBV is still typically less than that for HGGs (Fig. 2).[17] In a recent report of 100 consecutive patients with neoplastic (54) and infectious (46) noncortical lesions, a mean rCBV value of 1.3 had 97.8% sensitivity and 92.6% specificity for distinguishing tumor from infection, with a positive predictive value of 91.8%, a negative predictive value of 98.0%, and an accuracy of 95.0%.

With regard to tumefactive demyelinating lesions, rCBV is found to be generally lower than in neoplasms[20,21]; however, very high rCBV is rarely reported in these lesions, possibly because of the consequence of inflammatory angiogenesis.[22] An important caveat to keep in mind is

the potential for overlap of rCBV values between low-grade tumors and non-neoplastic lesions.[23]

The systematic incorporation of DSC-MR imaging as part of a multiparametric advanced MR imaging approach also uses magnetic resonance spectroscopy (MRS) and diffusion-weighted imaging (DWI), which have been proposed as a means for better differentiation between neoplastic and non-neoplastic lesions.[24]

Glioma grading and prognosis

Glioma grade is established histopathologically following biopsy or resection. Sampling error can compromise the accuracy of tumor grading.

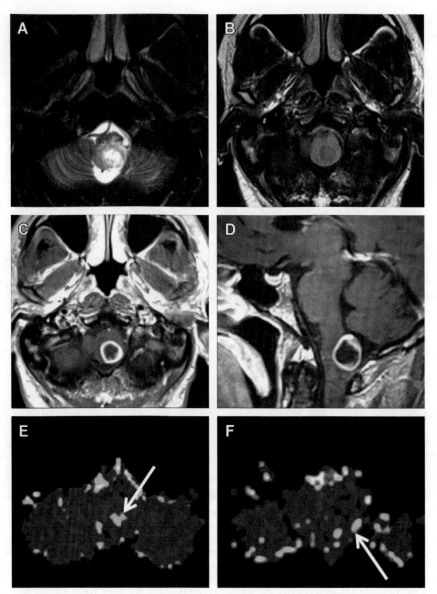

Fig. 2. A 39-year-old man with vasogenic edema on axial T2 (*A*) and fluid-attenuated inversion recovery (*B*) images and a ring-enhancing lesion (*C, D*) at left dorsal-lateral medulla. Differential considerations included neoplasm and infection (demographics and travel history raised the possibility of a tuberculoma). rCBV (*E, F*) was notably elevated (*white arrows;* up to 5–6 times that of normal-appearing cerebellum), favoring high-grade neoplasm. Subsequent biopsy revealed a high-grade glioma (anaplastic ependymoma, World Health Organization III).

Furthermore, low-grade tumors may evolve into high-grade lesions. Imaging has the advantages of noninvasiveness, global assessment of the tumor, and repeatability for longitudinal monitoring of tumor behavior.

Compared with low-grade gliomas (LGGs), HGGs grow more rapidly because of the higher cellular proliferation and tend to develop hypoxic regions, resulting in necrosis and increased angiogenesis. HGGs usually exhibit highly dense, albeit disorganized, microvasculature with increased capillary permeability. Thus, higher rCBV correlates with higher tumor grade (**Fig. 3**).[7,25] Unfortunately, substantial overlap of perfusion markers between tumor grades and histologies limits the ability of perfusion imaging to identify specific tumors. For instance, DSC-MR imaging cannot reliably differentiate between grade III and IV tumors. Furthermore, low-grade oligodendrogliomas can have elevated rCBV mimicking

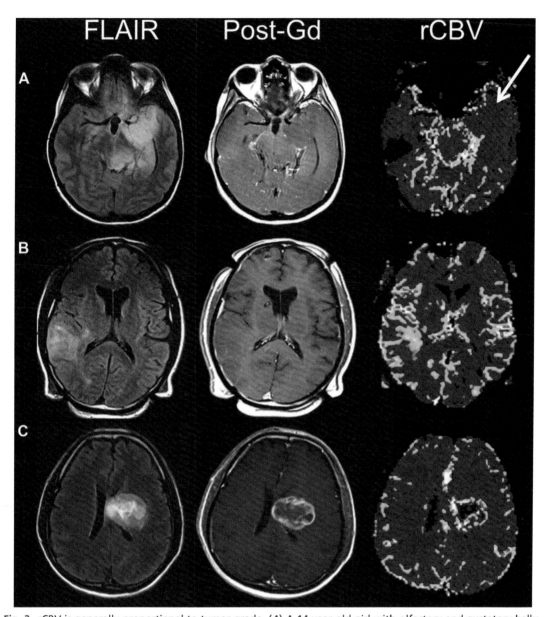

Fig. 3. rCBV is generally proportional to tumor grade. (*A*) A 14-year-old girl with olfactory and gustatory hallucinations. Fluid-attenuated inversion recovery (FLAIR) hyperintense, nonenhancing lesion in mesial left temporal lobe and brainstem has rCBV equivocally higher than normal white matter (*white arrow*). Low-grade astrocytoma (World Health Organization [WHO] II). (*B*) A 69-year-old man with headache and confusion. Ill-defined FLAIR hyperintense lesion in right parieto-temporal region has a paucity of enhancement and moderately elevated rCBV. Anaplastic astrocytoma (WHO III). (*C*) A 49-year-old man with right-sided weakness. Peripherally enhancing mass with central necrosis in the left corona radiata/basal ganglia has substantially elevated rCBV within the enhancing periphery. GBM (WHO IV). Gd, gadolinium.

high-grade astrocytomas.[26,27] Conversely, GBMs with oligodendroglial components have lower rCBV compared with GBMs with no oligodendroglial components.[28] Although no standardized multimodal methodology has been developed thus far, the combination of other markers with DSC-MR imaging, such as MRS and DWI, may improve the accuracy of tumor grade designations.[29,30]

MR imaging may generate prognostic information beyond tumor grade. For instance, grade III gliomas with necrosis reportedly have overall survival (OS) rates comparable with GBMs,[31] possibly because of undergrading of grade III tumors secondary to sampling error. Contrast enhancement is generally a marker for high-grade tumor: it is found in up to 30% of grade II tumors and in more than 50% of grade III tumors, whereas almost all GBMs showed contrast enhancement.[31,32] Enhancement, even within grade II tumors, is associated with poorer outcomes.[33]

DSC-MR imaging may extend prognostic models for HGGs. As with LGGs, higher rCBV has been shown to correlate with poor outcomes.[34] Specifically, maximum rCBV stratifies OS,[35,36] and gliomas with mean rCBV greater than 1.75 progress earlier than those with rCBV less than 1.75.[37]

Prognostic models may be improved by linking imaging features to molecular subtypes of GBM. Hierarchical clustering and random forest analyses have identified clusters of GBMs with high rCBV and gene expression associated with vasculogenesis and endothelial permeability; these patients have worse OS.[38] Similarly, machine learning paradigms have analyzed 60 features from preoperative GBM MR imaging, including perfusion data and stratified survival, and predicted molecular subtype (classic, mesenchymal, neural, proneural) with an overall accuracy of 76%.[39] Links between perfusion metrics and expression of molecular features of GBM, including vascular endothelial growth factor A (primary inducer of angiogenesis and a vasodilator that increases microvascular permeability), which are thought to impact survival, have also been demonstrated.[40] Thus researchers are beginning to extract the molecular underpinnings of elevated perfusion, improving our understanding of tumor biology, and drawing connections to malignant phenotypes that are associated with increased aggressiveness and shorter survival.

Guiding biopsy

Stereotactic biopsy is commonly used for histologic diagnosis in patients with brain masses. However, because of the common heterogeneity in brain tumors and reliance on contrast enhancement to guide biopsy targeting, sampling error remains a significant concern.[41,42] BBB disruption responsible for contrast enhancement may not necessarily correspond to the highest-grade portion of a tumor (Fig. 4). Undergrading is thought to occur in approximately 30% of cases because 30% of HGGs may not enhance and up to 30% of LGGs may enhance.[41,43] Of particular concern are nonenhancing gliomas, which have a greater tendency to be malignant in older patients.[44,45] Furthermore, despite the use of sophisticated methods to identify a brain lesion during stereotactic biopsy, neurosurgeons still have limited ability to visually confirm the position of their needle.[46]

Given the well-known association between rCBV and glioma grade,[7] DSC-MR imaging may provide improved guidance for biopsy target selection. Recent studies have proposed that regions of increased rCBV, serving as a marker of angiogenesis, may better indicate suitable targets for biopsy in patients with gliomas.[41,42]

Predicting therapeutic efficacy

DSC-MR imaging may help predict the response to specific therapies before treatment initiation. For instance, rCBV has been investigated as a predictive marker for GBM in the setting of antiangiogenic therapy. Although patients with bevacizumab-treated GBM generally show little improvement in survival,[47,48] bevacizumab therapy could have a substantial positive impact on a subset of patients.

Two small studies found that baseline rCBV correlates with OS in patients with bevacizumab-treated HGG.[49,50] Another study that examined 2 sizable cohorts of patients with recurrent GBM, only one of which received bevacizumab, found that baseline rCBV stratified progression-free survival (PFS) and OS in the bevacizumab-treated cohort only, with predictive accuracies of 82% for 6-month PFS and 79% for OS.[51] High baseline rCBV (>3.92) was associated with a halving of the median survival in comparison with low baseline rCBV ($\leq$3.92), indicating that rCBV may be a predictive, rather than prognostic, marker of outcome for patients with bevacizumab-treated GBM. Biomarker accuracy for selecting GBM therapy is critical given the extremely limited treatment options in patients with progressive or recurrent disease. These results may improve the selection of targeted therapy before treatment initiation.

Assessing Response to Therapy

Very early response assessment

Cytotoxic therapies DSC-MR imaging may also provide an early response marker of treatment efficacy. For instance, rCBV may be more valuable than enhancing tumor volume for evaluating patients after initiation of cytotoxic therapy,[52,53] as a greater than 5% increase in rCBV reportedly portends poor OS when acquired 4 weeks after chemoradiation, whereas no such relationship between enhancing tumor volume and OS could be demonstrated.[54]

Parametric response maps (PRM) reflecting voxelwise changes in rCBV 1 to 3 weeks after treatment seemed to successfully stratify survival in HGGs following standard chemoradiation

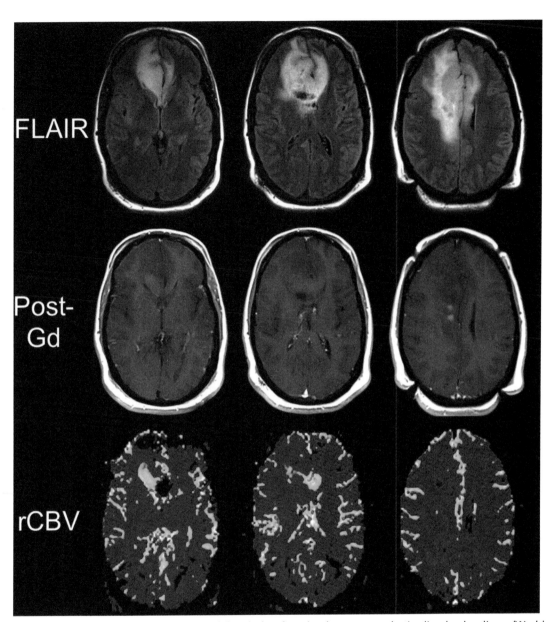

Fig. 4. A 37-year-old woman presenting with headaches found to have an anaplastic oligodendroglioma (World Health Organization III) has a bifrontal, fluid-attenuated inversion recovery (FLAIR) hyperintense mass with surrounding vasogenic edema in the right frontal region. There is a paucity of enhancement, with 2 small discrete enhancing foci in the right frontal posteromedial aspect of the mass. rCBV maps demonstrate heterogeneous elevation, notably corresponding to the nonenhancing portions of the tumor. rCBV (microvascular density) should be distinguished from contrast enhancement (vascular permeability) as an imaging biomarker and considered before stereotactic biopsy.

therapy. Conversely, neither mean rCBV nor rCBF were found to be prognostic of survival.[55] In fact, neither the percentage change of whole-tumor rCBV nor the segmentation into low, medium, and high rCBV generated statistically significant correlates of survival, whereas PRM applied to serial rCBV measurements at baseline and after 1 and 3 weeks of chemoradiation in GBM were predictive of 1-year survival.[56]

Antiangiogenic therapies Perfusion imaging, reflecting normalization of the vasculature, has also provided early markers of response to antiangiogenic therapy. However, linking these changes to patient outcomes has proved challenging, likely because the impact of antiangiogenic therapy on OS in patients with recurrent GBM is modest at best and patients, although initially responsive, may subsequently develop resistance to antiangiogenic therapy. A recent study did find an association between rCBV measured both 60 days before as well as 20 to 60 days after bevacizumab therapy and both PFS and OS in recurrent HGGs (Fig. 5).[50] Conversely, no such association could be demonstrated for volumes of either abnormal fluid-attenuated inversion recovery (FLAIR) signal or contrast enhancement. Another study found that when bias resulting from rCBV variability is

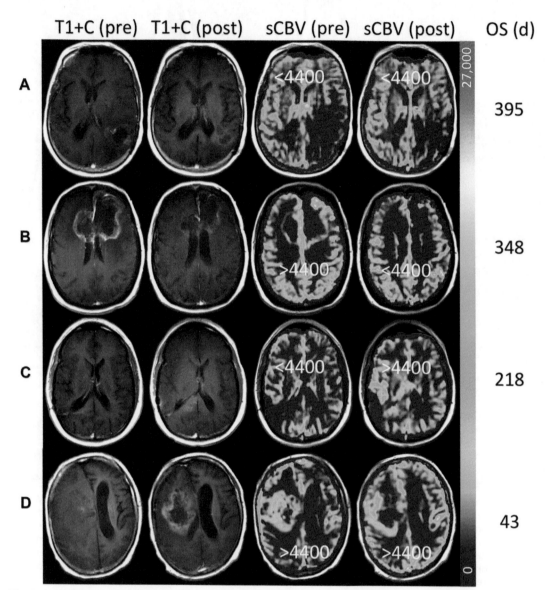

Fig. 5. Use of standardized CBV (sCBV) to prognosticate recurrent GBM treated with bevacizumab. Postcontrast T1-weighted images and corresponding standardized CBV maps acquired before (0–41 days) and after (32–41 days) initiation of bevacizumab in 4 different patients, each demonstrating a different permutation of pre-bevacizumab and postbevacizumab mean sCBV in enhancing lesion with respect to a threshold of 4400. Patient in (A) with low prebevacizumab and postbevacizumab sCBV had longest OS, whereas patient in (D) with high prebevacizumab and postbevacizumab sCBV had the shortest, with intermediate results for patients in (B, C) with mixed prebevacizumab and postbevacizumab sCBV. In general, pretreatment sCBV correlated with OS, with modulation by posttreatment sCBV. (*Courtesy of* Melissa Prah, BS, and Kathleen Schmainda, PhD, Milwaukee, WI; and *Data from* Schmainda KM, Prah M, Connelly J, et al. Dynamic-susceptibility contrast agent MRI measures of relative cerebral blood volume predict response to bevacizumab in recurrent high-grade glioma. Neuro Oncol 2014;16(6):880–8.)

minimized using a population-based rCBV atlas, volumes of both pre–bevacizumab and post–bevacizumab hypervascular rCBV can stratify PFS and OS in GBM, whereas traditional perfusion metrics including mean and maximum rCBV do not.[57] Large decreases in rCBV on DSC-MR imaging acquired within 1 to 2 months of bevacizumab initiation were found to predict longer OS in patients with recurrent GBM (**Fig. 6**).[58] And a multicenter, randomized, phase II trial of bevacizumab with irinotecan or TMZ in GBM (American College of Radiology Imaging Network [ACRIN] 6677/Radiation Therapy Oncology Group [RTOG] 0625) found an association between increasing rCBV from baseline at 2 or 16 weeks after bevacizumab initiation and worse OS (**Fig. 7**).[59] Thus, perfusion may serve as an early marker of response to antiangiogenic agents, but this hypothesis awaits confirmation in prospectively designed well-controlled studies.

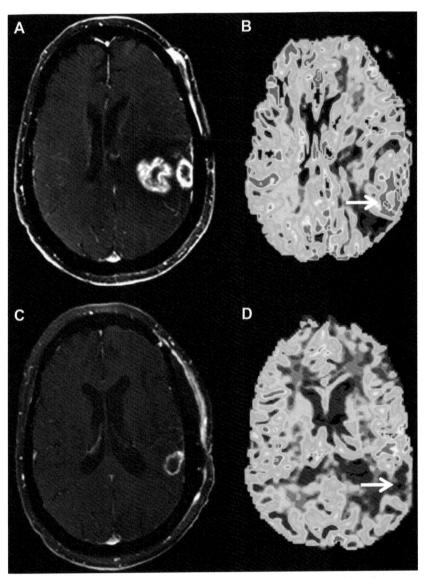

Fig. 6. A 57-year-old woman with recurrent GBM. Postcontrast T1-weighted image (*A*) and rCBV map (*B*) demonstrate 2 adjacent necrotic, peripherally enhancing lesions with elevated rCBV (*white arrow*) consistent with recurrent GBM. After subtotal reresection of the peripheral lesion and 2 weeks of treatment with TMZ and bevacizumab, postcontrast T1-weighted image (*C*) and rCBV map (*D*) show reduced size and decreased intensity of enhancement of the residual medial necrotic rim-enhancing lesion with no significant rCBV elevation (*white arrow*). Findings consistent with response to treatment. The patient had a relatively long OS (>17 months) after bevacizumab initiation.

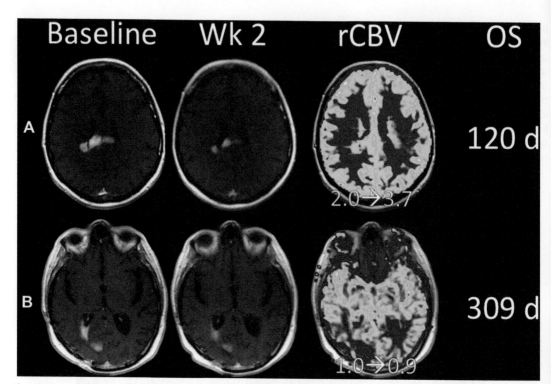

Fig. 7. Two patients with bevacizumab-treated recurrent GBM, both demonstrating decreased enhancement 2 weeks after bevacizumab initiation. Patient in (*A*) had increasing mean enhancement CBV and worse OS compared with patient in (*B*) with stable mean enhancement CBV. (*Courtesy of* Melissa Prah, BS, and Kathleen Schmainda, PhD, Milwaukee, WI; and *Data from* Schmainda KM, Zhang Z, Prah M, et al. Dynamic susceptibility contrast MRI measures of relative cerebral blood volume as a prognostic marker for overall survival in recurrent glioblastoma: results from the ACRIN 6677/RTOG 0625 multicenter trial. Neuro Oncol 2015;17(8):1148–56.)

Distinguishing response from pseudoresponse and identifying nonenhancing tumor

Antiangiogenic therapy normalizes the BBB, diminishing GBCA extravasation and contrast enhancement. This can yield pseudoresponse, defined as decreased contrast enhancement independent of antitumor effect, which likely contributes to reported discordance between high response rates and prolonged PFS without improved OS in bevacizumab-treated GBM.[60] Recent results[61] have shown that patients with progressive enhancement of recurrent GBM after 2 or 4 antiangiogenic therapy cycles had significantly shorter OS than nonprogressives. However, no survival benefit was found for improved versus stable enhancement, likely because of pseudoresponse. Other studies have demonstrated similar shortcomings of conventional imaging,[62,63] posing limitations for early response assessment and leading to inclusion of FLAIR-based measurement of nonenhancing tumor in modified response assessment criteria.[64] Although progressive postbevacizumab FLAIR hyperintensity often represents nonenhancing tumor, persistent edema,

postchemoradiation effects, and leukoaraiosis can have a similar appearance, reducing specificity. The ability of FLAIR to identify nonenhancing tumor and predict OS has been debated. Whereas some studies have found no survival prognostication with FLAIR,[61] others have found the converse to be true.[65]

Emerging evidence suggests that DSC-MR imaging may help predict relative treatment success shortly after initiation of antiangiogenic therapy. Significant differences in OS between patients with recurrent GBM with positive versus negative changes in tumor rCBV at 2, 4, or 16 weeks post-treatment initiation compared with baseline have been found (see **Fig. 7**; **Fig. 8**).[58,59] However, several studies[50,51,59] found that 8-week changes in rCBV were nonpredictive of OS. Therefore, the ability of post-therapy rCBV changes to predict OS may depend on the time at which posttreatment imaging is performed.

It has been suggested that pretreatment rCBV measures alone can predict response to bevacizumab.[50,51] However, although low baseline rCBV predicts longer OS, subsequent change in

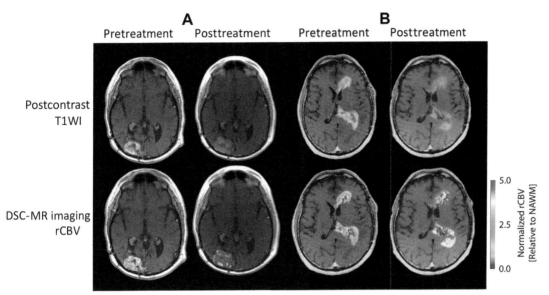

Fig. 8. Prebevacizumab and postbevacizumab (4–6 weeks after initiation) postcontrast T1-weighted images (T1WI) and rCBV maps (normalized to contralateral normal-appearing white matter) in 2 patients with recurrent GBM. (A) Postcontrast T1WI show decreased intensity of enhancement with no change in the enhancing tumor volume; however, median normalized rCBV within the enhancing lesion decreased from 2.66 to 0.70. OS = 168 days. (B) Postcontrast T1WI show decreased intensity of enhancement with no substantial change in the enhancing tumor volume; however, median rCBV in the enhancing lesion increased from 2.07 to 3.52. OS = 93 days. NAWM, normal-appearing white matter.

posttreatment rCBV may further substratify patients.[59] Patients with high baseline rCBV may have shorter OS than patients with low rCBV but may still relatively benefit from bevacizumab, and rCBV change potentially identifies those patients for whom this is true. Patients without progressive contrast enhancement have been found to be substratified into relatively short and long OS based on rCBV change from baseline at 2 weeks after bevacizumab initiation, whereas there was no survival difference between T1 responders and patients with stable enhancement.[66] Therefore, evidence suggests that baseline rCBV can prognosticate OS, and early posttreatment change in rCBV may provide additional response prediction and substratification. A larger multicenter trial exploring both baseline rCBV and early posttreatment change in rCBV is merited.

DSC-MR imaging may also improve identification of nonenhancing tumor by diminishing the nonspecificity of FLAIR signal changes. Decreased rCBV in bevacizumab-treated GBM has helped distinguish vasogenic edema from infiltrative tumor and correlated with PFS.[67] Principal component analysis of temporal DSC-MR imaging data in GBM has identified peritumoral regions likely to be infiltrated with tumor and correlated with OS,[68] and increasing rCBV in nonenhancing peritumoral and transcallosal regions has been shown to be associated with poor OS.[69]

Refinements to traditional DSC-MR imaging may yield promising biomarkers for response to antiangiogenic therapies. For example, vessel size indices derived from combined GRE and SE DSC-MR imaging can potentially identify vascular normalization windows following antiangiogenic therapy that facilitate improved delivery of additional chemotherapies.[70] Independent component analysis of DSC-MR imaging signal data has isolated arterial and venous perfusion signals, with decreased tumor voxels containing significant overlap of these signals after successful therapy.[71] Although most DSC-MR imaging studies have used rCBV to assess response to bevacizumab, increased CBF has been found to occur after therapy in a subset of patients with recurrent GBM with improved tumor oxygenation status and relatively favorable survival.[72,73]

Distinguishing progression from pseudoprogression

PsP represents transient increased contrast enhancement mimicking tumor progression and complicates response criteria for radiological progression. Differentiation from progressive disease (PD) is important for avoiding premature trial failures in the setting of PsP and selecting timely alternative therapies in the setting of PD. PsP, with peak incidence 1 to 6 months after chemoradiation (early delayed effect), commonly follows radiotherapy and TMZ, and is associated with O(6)-methylguanine-DNA methyltransferase (MGMT) promoter methylation and improved survival.[74,75] Its mechanism is incompletely understood,[76] but it is characterized by increased vascular permeability with proinflammatory mediators and cytokines with a mix of quiescent tumor and nonhyalinized necrosis, which yield edema and contrast enhancement difficult to distinguish from PD with conventional MR imaging.[77]

Radiation necrosis, occurring months to years after radiation (late-delayed effect), and PsP are distinct entities on a spectrum of posttreatment enhancement. DSC-MR imaging can readily distinguish tumor (significantly higher mean rCBV) and radiation necrosis (Fig. 9), albeit with different optimal rCBV thresholds (0.7–1.8) depending on the specific DSC-MR imaging protocol.[78,79] However, the distinction of PsP from PD in the setting of progressive enhancement following TMZ chemoradiation of GBMs is more uncertain. Whereas some studies found significantly different median rCBV within enhancing lesion between PsP and PD with optimal thresholds of 1.3[80] and 1.8,[81] another study only found significantly different mean rCBV

between PsP and PD in GBMs with unmethylated (0.87 vs 3.25, $P = .009$) rather than methylated (1.56 vs 2.34, $P = .258$) MGMT.[82] Another study found much better separation of mean rCBV between PD and PsP with ferumoxytol, an intravascular iron-based contrast agent not susceptible to contrast agent leakage effects, than with GBCA.[83] Conversely, a retrospective study of HGGs treated with paclitaxel poliglumex, a powerful radiation sensitizer, found no significant difference in mean rCBV at initial progressive enhancement between lesions destined for PsP and PD.[84]

These inconsistent results may be explained by coexistence of tumor and necrosis yielding a spectrum of chemoradiation-induced vascular morphologies and a wide range of corresponding vascular volumes.[85] Mean rCBV may, therefore, be inadequate early in lesion evolution for capturing the dominant behavior. Conversely, rCBV trends or histograms identifying temporal and spatial variations, respectively, may be more predictive. For example, temporal changes in rCBV predicted lesion destiny in the paclitaxel study, with rCBV stabilizing or trending downward for PsP (Fig. 10) and upward for PD (Fig. 11).[84] Changes in rCBV histogram skewness and

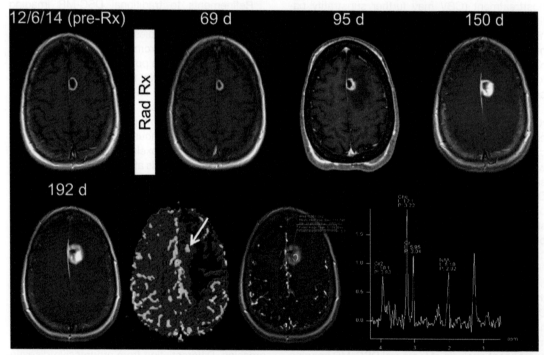

Fig. 9. A 60-year-old woman with stage 3A non–small cell lung carcinoma (NSCLC), following stereotactic radiosurgery for a rim-enhancing left frontal juxta-falcine brain metastasis at rostral cingulate gyrus with recurrent progressively enlarging enhancement and increasing vasogenic edema. DSC-MR imaging 192 days after treatment showed elevated rCBV (*white arrow*; approximately 4 times normal-appearing white matter) at the thickest enlarging region of enhancement, and MRS demonstrated an elevated choline/creatine ratio, consistent with recurrent metastasis rather than radiation necrosis.

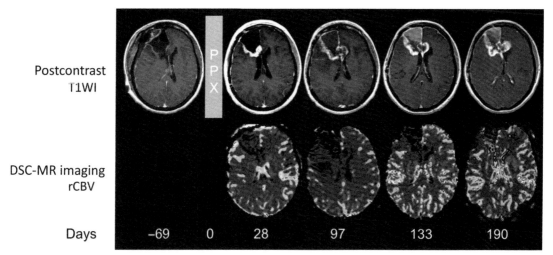

Fig. 10. A 38-year-old woman with right frontal and transcallosal GBM following resection and treatment with the radiation sensitizer paclitaxel poliglumex (PPX) plus temozolomide. Progressive enlargement of marginal enhancement at the resection cavity began 28 days after PPX treatment, but there was no corresponding elevation of rCBV on any subsequent imaging time points. Biopsy 205 days after PPX was consistent with pseudoprogression. T1WI, T1-weighted image.

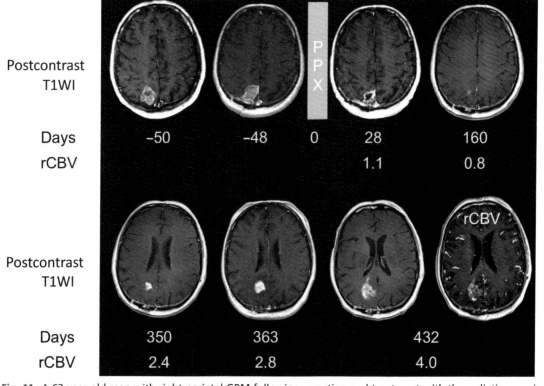

Fig. 11. A 63-year-old man with right parietal GBM following resection and treatment with the radiation sensitizer paclitaxel poliglumex (PPX) plus temozolomide. By 160 days after PPX, marginal enhancement at resection cavity has regressed but recurred 350 days after treatment with progressive enlargement and corresponding increase in mean enhancing lesion rCBV over subsequent imaging time points. Biopsy-proven recurrent GBM. T1WI, T1-weighted image.

kurtosis have predicted lesion destiny in GBMs with progressive postchemoradiation enhancement.[86] Similarly, fractional tumor volume using a single-voxel rCBV threshold with a cutoff of 1.0 depicted histologic tumor fraction in a study of 25 GBMs and correlated with OS better than mean rCBV after progressive enhancement.[87] Also patterns of change in rCBV and apparent diffusion coefficient (ADC) on subtracted combined rCBV-ADC histograms have been shown to distinguish PsP from PD.[88] Therefore, there is emerging evidence that rCBV analysis schemes capturing temporal (trends) and spatial (histogram) heterogeneity may outperform static measures of mean rCBV for distinguishing PsP and PD.

Although DSC-MR imaging seems to aid diagnosis of PsP following standard chemoradiotherapy, its applicability to PsP from immunotherapies is less certain. Pilot data demonstrated higher rCBV in recurrent GBMs treated with dendritic cell immunotherapy that progressed compared with stable disease (**Figs. 12** and **13**),[89] and recurrent tumor in GBMs treated with immunogene therapy also showed elevated rCBV.[90] These data, although preliminary, suggest that rCBV may be useful in identifying PD in patients treated with immunotherapeutics (**Fig. 14**), similar to the current paradigm for standard therapy. Immunotherapeutic approaches may each require independent validation of perfusion-derived metrics that most accurately depict disease burden. Because mounting an effective immune response may take several weeks or longer, perfusion changes may also demonstrate time courses distinct from those typically observed following standard therapy. Now that immunotherapeutics are in more widespread development, further studies will be required to specifically test these potential biomarkers following treatment regimens that quite clearly are distinct in their mechanism from conventional chemoradiation.

Predicting low-grade to high-grade transformation

Although LGGs are generally slow growing, malignant transformation to HGG (World Health Organization [WHO] III and IV) frequently occurs.[91] Predicting malignant transformation is difficult[92,93]; the risks, benefits, and timing of aggressive therapy remain controversial.[94,95] Because the survival benefit of early aggressive surgical or radiation therapy is debated,[96,97] some centers proceed with imaging surveillance of patients with LGGs, with the appearance of contrast-enhancement frequently viewed as a hallmark of malignant transformation despite lack of high specificity for tumor grade.[41,43,98]

Currently, there are no validated imaging biomarkers for predicting malignant transformation in LGGs that aid the decision on when to pursue aggressive therapy. There is evidence that initial

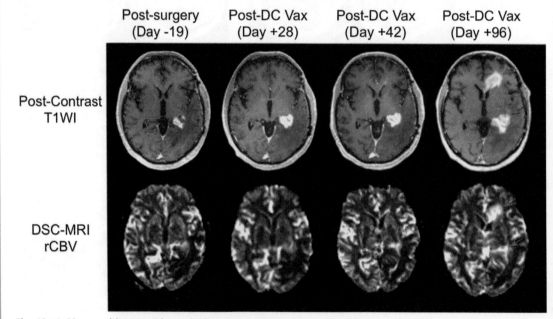

Fig. 12. A 68-year-old man with newly diagnosed GBM treated with dendritic cell vaccine therapy (DC Vax) plus placebo adjuvant therapy. Postcontrast T1-weighted images (T1WI) show progressive lesion enhancement over time and emergence of a new lesion near the frontal horn of the left lateral ventricle (*red arrows*). rCBV maps demonstrate increasing mean rCBV within the enhancing lesions, consistent with progression.

| | Pre-RT
(Day -108) | Post-RT/Pre-DC Vax
(Day -19) | Post-DC Vax
(Day +46) | Post-DC Vax
(Day +87) |

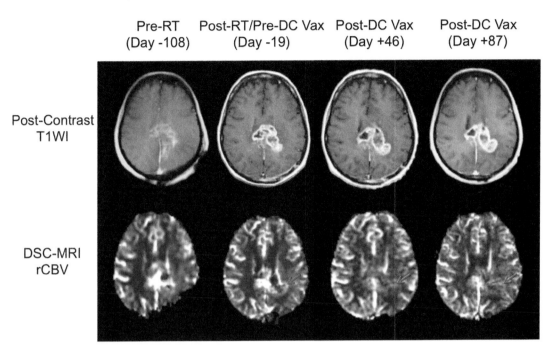

Post-Contrast T1WI

DSC-MRI rCBV

Fig. 13. A 60-year-old man with newly diagnosed GBM treated with dendritic cell vaccine therapy (DC Vax). Post-contrast T1-weighted images (T1WI) show emergence of a contrast-enhancing lesion crossing the corpus callosum. Serial rCBV maps demonstrate decreasing rCBV within the enhancing lesion over time (*red arrows*) consistent with treatment-related tissue changes. RT, radiotherapy.

tumor volume and growth rate and 6-month tumor growth of LGGs are significant predictors of time to transformation.[92,99,100] Conventional contrast-enhanced MR imaging is insensitive to early changes of transformation,[91] but DSC-MR imaging may be helpful (**Fig. 15**). rCBV has been associated with time to progression in LGGs and may identify LGGs that are actually HGGs, either misdiagnosed because of sampling error at pathologic examination or that have undergone angiogenesis with progression toward malignant transformation.[101] The longitudinal increase in rCBV, detected as early as 12 months before the appearance of contrast enhancement, has been

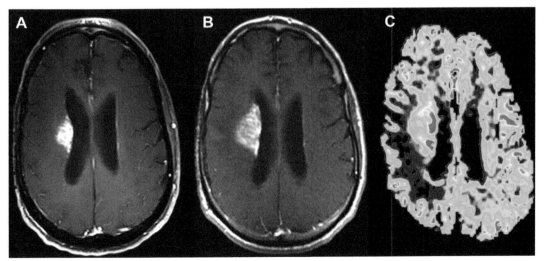

Fig. 14. A 66-year-old man with GBM treated with TMZ and rindopepimut vaccine for EGFRvIII-positive disease. Pretreatment (*A*) and posttreatment (*B*) postcontrast T1-weighted images demonstrate interval increased size of a right periventricular enhancing mass. Increased rCBV (*C*) is consistent with PD rather than treatment-related enhancement. EGFRvIII, epidermal growth factor receptor variant III.

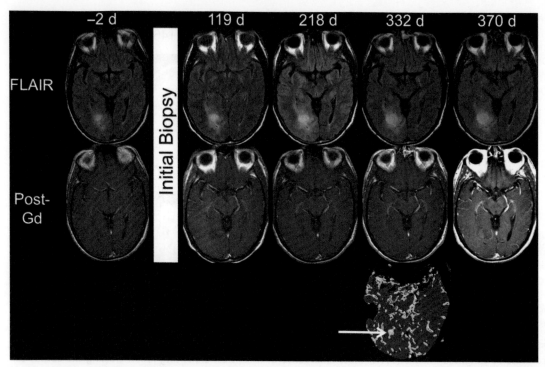

Fig. 15. A 65-year-old man with visual field loss and a nonenhancing FLAIR hyperintense right temporo-occipital lesion. Biopsy was consistent with a low-grade astrocytoma (WHO II). Subsequently, there was gradual increased FLAIR hyperintensity without enhancement. Three hundred thirty-two days after biopsy, lesion rCBV was notably elevated (*white arrow*) and the lesion was regraded as an oligoastrocytoma (WHO III) on second biopsy 370 days after initial biopsy. Elevated rCBV was consistent with either low-grade to high-grade transformation or undergrading of the initial lesion (DSC-MR imaging had not been performed previously).

shown to correlate with malignant transformation in LGGs, whereas relatively stable rCBV values indicate a lack of transformation.[102] Compared with nontransformers, LGGs undergoing anaplastic transformation have been shown to have significantly higher mean rCBV on initial, follow-up, and final magnetic resonance examinations.[103]

IMAGING PROTOCOLS

DSC-MR imaging protocols vary widely in the literature. Despite promising results from single-center studies and preliminary results from several multicenter trials, there remains a significant need to validate DSC-MR imaging techniques and standardize methods that provide clinically reliable measurements across multiple institutions. Compared with anatomic and diffusion MR imaging, intrasite and intersite reproducibility of DSC-MR imaging results are substantially more difficult to achieve[104,105] because of multiple factors impacting DSC-MR imaging signal, including arterial dispersion of contrast bolus,[106] the concentration-dependent

difference of T2* relaxivity between tissue and large vessels,[107] pulse sequence parameters including acquisition flip angle,[108] GRE versus SE preparation,[10] and TE.[109] Evidence suggests that for single-echo acquisitions, preload improves the clinical utility[7,110] and accuracy[11] of rCBV measures.[11] However, variations in preload dose and incubation time before dynamic acquisition may impact DSC-MR imaging signal and rCBV measurement.[110] Various DSC-MR imaging postprocessing techniques are available, the choice of which can also influence rCBV estimates.[108] Postprocessing software has recently been shown to significantly impact rCBV calculations.[111,112] Standardization of rCBV to a consistent scale helps eliminate the subjective selection of normal-appearing white matter, thereby reducing interpatient variability and facilitating quantitative comparison across studies.[113]

However, greater technical standardization is required, particularly in the setting of multicenter clinical brain tumor trials.[114] Efforts are currently being made by organizations, such as the Quantitative Imaging Biomarker Alliance, subgroups within the American Society of Neuroradiology,[13] and International Society of Magnetic Resonance in Medicine, to produce standardization documents that help guide the clinical practice of DSC-MR imaging and improve its reliability in multicenter trials, similar to what has been done for conventional MR imaging.[115]

SUMMARY

rCBV is a measure of microvascular density that augments conventional contrast-enhanced MR imaging in the initial evaluation and posttreatment monitoring of brain tumors. High lesion rCBV tends to distinguish tumor from nontumor, correspond with higher rather than lower tumor grade with worse prognosis, and designate biopsy sites with an increased likelihood of capturing the highest-grade portion of tumor. rCBV values at or compared with baseline may help with response assessment for cytotoxic (progression vs pseudoprogression) and antiangiogenic (response vs pseudoresponse) therapies. DSC-MR imaging protocols and postprocessing techniques vary widely in the literature, and validation with standardization of methods providing clinically reliable measurements is needed, particularly in the setting of multicenter clinical brain tumor trials.

REFERENCES

1. Shiroishi MS, Castellazzi G, Boxerman JL, et al. Principles of T *-weighted dynamic susceptibility contrast MRI technique in brain tumor imaging. J Magn Reson Imaging 2015;41(2):296–313.
2. Essig M, Nguyen TB, Shiroishi MS, et al. Perfusion MRI: the five most frequently asked clinical questions. AJR Am J Roentgenol 2013;201(3): W495–510.
3. Villringer A, Rosen BR, Belliveau JW, et al. Dynamic imaging with lanthanide chelates in normal brain: contrast due to magnetic susceptibility effects. Magn Reson Med 1988;6(2):164–74.
4. Rosen BR, Belliveau JW, Buchbinder BR, et al. Contrast agents and cerebral hemodynamics. Magn Reson Med 1991;19:285–92.
5. Weisskoff RM, Chesler D, Boxerman JL, et al. Pitfalls in MR measurement of tissue blood flow with intravascular tracers: which mean transit time? Magn Reson Med 1993;29(4):553–8.
6. Cha S, Knopp EA, Johnson G, et al. Intracranial mass lesions: dynamic contrast-enhanced susceptibility-weighted echo-planar perfusion MR imaging. Radiology 2002;223(1):11–29.
7. Boxerman JL, Schmainda KM, Weisskoff RM. Relative cerebral blood volume maps corrected for contrast agent extravasation significantly correlate with glioma tumor grade, whereas uncorrected

maps do not. AJNR Am J Neuroradiol 2006;27(4): 859–67.
8. Quarles CC, Gochberg DF, Gore JC, et al. A theoretical framework to model DSC-MRI data acquired in the presence of contrast agent extravasation. Phys Med Biol 2009;54(19):5749–66.
9. Boxerman JL, Rosen BR, Weisskoff RM. Signal-to-noise analysis of cerebral blood volume maps from dynamic NMR imaging studies. J Magn Reson Imaging 1997;7(3):528–37.
10. Schmainda KM, Rand SD, Joseph AM, et al. Characterization of a first-pass gradient-echo spin-echo method to predict brain tumor grade and angiogenesis. AJNR Am J Neuroradiol 2004;25(9): 1524–32.
11. Boxerman JL, Prah DE, Paulson ES, et al. The role of preload and leakage correction in gadolinium-based cerebral blood volume estimation determined by comparison with MION as a criterion standard. AJNR Am J Neuroradiol 2012;33(6): 1081–7.
12. Hu LS, Eschbacher JM, Dueck AC, et al. Correlations between perfusion MR imaging cerebral blood volume, microvessel quantification, and clinical outcome using stereotactic analysis in recurrent high-grade glioma. AJNR Am J Neuroradiol 2012;33(1):69–76.
13. Welker K, Boxerman J, Kalnin A, et al. ASFNR recommendations for clinical performance of MR dynamic susceptibility contrast perfusion imaging of the brain. AJNR Am J Neuroradiol 2015;36(6):E41–51.
14. Schmiedeskamp H, Straka M, Newbould RD, et al. Combined spin- and gradient-echo perfusion-weighted imaging. Magn Reson Med 2012;68(1): 30–40.
15. Vonken EJ, van Osch MJ, Bakker CJ, et al. Measurement of cerebral perfusion with dual-echo multi-slice quantitative dynamic susceptibility contrast MRI. J Magn Reson Imaging 1999;10(2): 109–17.
16. Hakyemez B, Erdogan C, Bolca N, et al. Evaluation of different cerebral mass lesions by perfusion-weighted MR imaging. J Magn Reson Imaging 2006;24(4):817–24.
17. Floriano VH, Torres US, Spotti AR, et al. The role of dynamic susceptibility contrast-enhanced perfusion MR imaging in differentiating between infectious and neoplastic focal brain lesions: results from a cohort of 100 consecutive patients. PLoS One 2013;8(12):e81509.
18. Toh CH, Wei KC, Chang CN, et al. Differentiation of brain abscesses from glioblastomas and metastatic brain tumors: comparisons of diagnostic performance of dynamic susceptibility contrast-enhanced perfusion MR imaging before and after mathematic contrast leakage correction. PLoS One 2014;9(10):e109172.

19. Ernst TM, Chang L, Witt MD, et al. Cerebral toxoplasmosis and lymphoma in AIDS: perfusion MR imaging experience in 13 patients. Radiology 1998;208(3):663–9.

20. Cha S, Pierce S, Knopp EA, et al. Dynamic contrast-enhanced T2*-weighted MR imaging of tumefactive demyelinating lesions. AJNR Am J Neuroradiol 2001;22(6):1109–16.

21. Cha S. Update on brain tumor imaging: from anatomy to physiology. AJNR Am J Neuroradiol 2006; 27(3):475–87.

22. Blasel S, Pfeilschifter W, Jansen V, et al. Metabolism and regional cerebral blood volume in autoimmune inflammatory demyelinating lesions mimicking malignant gliomas. J Neurol 2011; 258(1):113–22.

23. Hourani R, Brant LJ, Rizk T, et al. Can proton MR spectroscopic and perfusion imaging differentiate between neoplastic and nonneoplastic brain lesions in adults? AJNR Am J Neuroradiol 2008; 29(2):366–72.

24. Al-Okaili RN, Krejza J, Woo JH, et al. Intraaxial brain masses: MR imaging-based diagnostic strategy–initial experience. Radiology 2007;243(2): 539–50.

25. Law M, Yang S, Babb JS, et al. Comparison of cerebral blood volume and vascular permeability from dynamic susceptibility contrast-enhanced perfusion MR imaging with glioma grade. AJNR Am J Neuroradiol 2004;25(5):746–55.

26. Cha S, Tihan T, Crawford F, et al. Differentiation of low-grade oligodendrogliomas from low-grade astrocytomas by using quantitative blood-volume measurements derived from dynamic susceptibility contrast-enhanced MR imaging. AJNR Am J Neuroradiol 2005;26(2):266–73.

27. Lev MH, Ozsunar Y, Henson JW, et al. Glial tumor grading and outcome prediction using dynamic spin-echo MR susceptibility mapping compared with conventional contrast-enhanced MR: confounding effect of elevated rCBV of oligodendrogliomas [corrected]. AJNR Am J Neuroradiol 2004;25(2):214–21.

28. Sunwoo L, Choi SH, Yoo RE, et al. Paradoxical perfusion metrics of high-grade gliomas with an oligodendroglioma component: quantitative analysis of dynamic susceptibility contrast perfusion MR imaging. Neuroradiology 2015;57(11):1111–20.

29. Law M, Yang S, Wang H, et al. Glioma grading: sensitivity, specificity, and predictive values of perfusion MR imaging and proton MR spectroscopic imaging compared with conventional MR imaging. AJNR Am J Neuroradiol 2003;24(10): 1989–98.

30. Zonari P, Baraldi P, Crisi G. Multimodal MRI in the characterization of glial neoplasms: the combined role of single-voxel MR spectroscopy, diffusion imaging and echo-planar perfusion imaging. Neuroradiology 2007;49(10):795–803.

31. Pope WB, Sayre J, Perlina A, et al. MR imaging correlates of survival in patients with high-grade gliomas. AJNR Am J Neuroradiol 2005;26(10): 2466–74.

32. Schafer ML, Maurer MH, Synowitz M, et al. Low-grade (WHO II) and anaplastic (WHO III) gliomas: differences in morphology and MRI signal intensities. Eur Radiol 2013;23(10):2846–53.

33. Chaichana KL, McGirt MJ, Niranjan A, et al. Prognostic significance of contrast-enhancing low-grade gliomas in adults and a review of the literature. Neurol Res 2009;31(9):931–9.

34. Bonekamp D, Deike K, Wiestler B, et al. Association of overall survival in patients with newly diagnosed glioblastoma with contrast-enhanced perfusion MRI: Comparison of intraindividually matched T1- and T2(*)-based bolus techniques. J Magn Reson Imaging 2015;42(1):87–96.

35. Hirai T, Murakami R, Nakamura H, et al. Prognostic value of perfusion MR imaging of high-grade astrocytomas: long-term follow-up study. AJNR Am J Neuroradiol 2008;29(8):1505–10.

36. Jain R, Poisson L, Narang J, et al. Genomic mapping and survival prediction in glioblastoma: molecular subclassification strengthened by hemodynamic imaging biomarkers. Radiology 2013; 267(1):212–20.

37. Law M, Young RJ, Babb JS, et al. Gliomas: predicting time to progression or survival with cerebral blood volume measurements at dynamic susceptibility-weighted contrast-enhanced perfusion MR imaging. Radiology 2008;247(2):490–8.

38. Achrol AS, Liu T, Mitchell LA, et al. Quantitative volumetric magnetic resonance perfusion identifies a distinct vasculogenic molecular subtype of human glioblastoma associated with worse clinical outcomes. Neurosurgery 2015;62(Suppl 1):204–5.

39. Macyszyn L, Akbari H, Pisapia JM, et al. Imaging patterns predict patient survival and molecular subtype in glioblastoma via machine learning techniques. Neuro Oncol 2016;18(3):417–25.

40. Barajas RF Jr, Phillips JJ, Vandenberg SR, et al. Pro-angiogenic cellular and genomic expression patterns within glioblastoma influences dynamic susceptibility weighted perfusion MRI. Clin Radiol 2015;70(10):1087–95.

41. Maia AC, Malheiros SM, da Rocha AJ, et al. Stereotactic biopsy guidance in adults with supratentorial nonenhancing gliomas: role of perfusion-weighted magnetic resonance imaging. J Neurosurg 2004; 101(6):970–6.

42. Lefranc M, Monet P, Desenclos C, et al. Perfusion MRI as a neurosurgical tool for improved targeting in stereotactic tumor biopsies. Stereotact Funct Neurosurg 2012;90(4):240–7.

43. Macdonald DR. Low-grade gliomas, mixed gliomas, and oligodendrogliomas. Semin Oncol 1994;21(2):236–48.

44. Barker FG 2nd, Chang SM, Huhn SL, et al. Age and the risk of anaplasia in magnetic resonance-nonenhancing supratentorial cerebral tumors. Cancer 1997;80(5):936–41.

45. Ohgaki H, Kleihues P. Population-based studies on incidence, survival rates, and genetic alterations in astrocytic and oligodendroglial gliomas. J Neuropathol Exp Neurol 2005;64(6):479–89.

46. Chen CC, White NS, Farid N, et al. Pre-operative cellularity mapping and intra-MRI surgery: potential for improving neurosurgical biopsies. Expert Rev Med Devices 2015;12(1):1–5.

47. Friedman HS, Prados MD, Wen PY, et al. Bevacizumab alone and in combination with irinotecan in recurrent glioblastoma. J Clin Oncol 2009;27(28): 4733–40.

48. Chinot OL, Wick W, Cloughesy T. Bevacizumab for newly diagnosed glioblastoma. N Engl J Med 2014;370(21):2049.

49. Verhoeff JJ, Lavini C, van Linde ME, et al. Bevacizumab and dose-intense temozolomide in recurrent high-grade glioma. Ann Oncol 2010;21(8): 1723–7.

50. Schmainda KM, Prah M, Connelly J, et al. Dynamic-susceptibility contrast agent MRI measures of relative cerebral blood volume predict response to bevacizumab in recurrent high-grade glioma. Neuro Oncol 2014;16(6):880–8.

51. Kickingereder P, Wiestler B, Burth S, et al. Relative cerebral blood volume is a potential predictive imaging biomarker of bevacizumab efficacy in recurrent glioblastoma. Neuro Oncol 2015;17(8):1139–47.

52. Cao Y, Tsien CI, Nagesh V, et al. Survival prediction in high-grade gliomas by MRI perfusion before and during early stage of RT [corrected]. Int J Radiat Oncol Biol Phys 2006;64(3):876–85.

53. Bag AK, Cezayirli PC, Davenport JJ, et al. Survival analysis in patients with newly diagnosed primary glioblastoma multiforme using pre- and post-treatment peritumoral perfusion imaging parameters. J Neurooncol 2014;120(2):361–70.

54. Mangla R, Singh G, Ziegelitz D, et al. Changes in relative cerebral blood volume 1 month after radiation-temozolomide therapy can help predict overall survival in patients with glioblastoma. Radiology 2010;256(2):575–84.

55. Galban CJ, Chenevert TL, Meyer CR, et al. The parametric response map is an imaging biomarker for early cancer treatment outcome. Nat Med 2009; 15(5):572–6.

56. Lemasson B, Chenevert TL, Lawrence TS, et al. Impact of perfusion map analysis on early survival prediction accuracy in glioma patients. Transl Oncol 2013;6(6):766–74.

57. Leu K, Enzmann DR, Woodworth DC, et al. Hypervascular tumor volume estimated by comparison to a large-scale cerebral blood volume radiographic atlas predicts survival in recurrent glioblastoma treated with bevacizumab. Cancer Imaging 2014;14:31.

58. Harris RJ, Cloughesy TF, Hardy AJ, et al. MRI perfusion measurements calculated using advanced deconvolution techniques predict survival in recurrent glioblastoma treated with bevacizumab. J Neurooncol 2015;122(3):497–505.

59. Schmainda KM, Zhang Z, Prah M, et al. Dynamic susceptibility contrast MRI measures of relative cerebral blood volume as a prognostic marker for overall survival in recurrent glioblastoma: results from the ACRIN 6677/RTOG 0625 multicenter trial. Neuro Oncol 2015;17(8):1148–56.

60. Gilbert MR, Dignam JJ, Armstrong TS, et al. A randomized trial of bevacizumab for newly diagnosed glioblastoma. N Engl J Med 2014;370(8): 699–708.

61. Boxerman JL, Zhang Z, Safriel Y, et al. Early post-bevacizumab progression on contrast-enhanced MRI as a prognostic marker for overall survival in recurrent glioblastoma: results from the ACRIN 6677/RTOG 0625 Central Reader Study. Neuro Oncol 2013;15(7):945–54.

62. Norden AD, Drappatz J, Muzikansky A, et al. An exploratory survival analysis of anti-angiogenic therapy for recurrent malignant glioma. J Neurooncol 2009;92(2):149–55.

63. Ellingson BM, Cloughesy TF, Lai A, et al. Quantitative volumetric analysis of conventional MRI response in recurrent glioblastoma treated with bevacizumab. Neuro Oncol 2011;13(4):401–9.

64. Wen PY, Macdonald DR, Reardon DA, et al. Updated response assessment criteria for high-grade gliomas: response assessment in neuro-oncology working group. J Clin Oncol 2010; 28(11):1963–72.

65. Huang RY, Rahman R, Ballman KV, et al. The impact of T2/FLAIR evaluation per RANO criteria on response assessment of recurrent glioblastoma patients treated with bevacizumab. Clin Cancer Res 2016;22(3):575–81.

66. Boxerman JL, Zhang Z, Schmainda KM, et al. Early post-bevacizumab change in rCBV from DSC-MRI predicts overall survival in recurrent glioblastoma whereas 2D-T1 response status does not: results from the ACRIN 6677/RTOG 0625 multi-center study. Paper presented at: Radiological Society of North America 100th Scientific Assembly. Chicago, December 4, 2014.

67. Artzi M, Bokstein F, Blumenthal DT, et al. Differentiation between vasogenic-edema versus tumor-infiltrative area in patients with glioblastoma during bevacizumab therapy: a longitudinal MRI study. Eur J Radiol 2014;83(7):1250–6.

68. Akbari H, Macyszyn L, Da X, et al. Pattern analysis of dynamic susceptibility contrast-enhanced MR imaging demonstrates peritumoral tissue heterogeneity. Radiology 2014;273(2):502–10.

69. Jain R, Poisson LM, Gutman D, et al. Outcome prediction in patients with glioblastoma by using imaging, clinical, and genomic biomarkers: focus on the nonenhancing component of the tumor. Radiology 2014;272(2):484–93.

70. Batchelor TT, Sorensen AG, di Tomaso E, et al. AZD2171, a pan-VEGF receptor tyrosine kinase inhibitor, normalizes tumor vasculature and alleviates edema in glioblastoma patients. Cancer Cell 2007; 11(1):83–95.

71. LaViolette PS, Cohen AD, Prah MA, et al. Vascular change measured with independent component analysis of dynamic susceptibility contrast MRI predicts bevacizumab response in high-grade glioma. Neuro Oncol 2013;15(4):442–50.

72. Sorensen AG, Emblem KE, Polaskova P, et al. Increased survival of glioblastoma patients who respond to antiangiogenic therapy with elevated blood perfusion. Cancer Res 2012;72(2):402–7.

73. Batchelor TT, Gerstner ER, Emblem KE, et al. Improved tumor oxygenation and survival in glioblastoma patients who show increased blood perfusion after cediranib and chemoradiation. Proc Natl Acad Sci U S A 2013;110(47):19059–64.

74. Gerstner ER, McNamara MB, Norden AD, et al. Effect of adding temozolomide to radiation therapy on the incidence of pseudo-progression. J Neurooncol 2009;94(1):97–101.

75. Brandes AA, Franceschi E, Tosoni A, et al. MGMT promoter methylation status can predict the incidence and outcome of pseudoprogression after concomitant radiochemotherapy in newly diagnosed glioblastoma patients. J Clin Oncol 2008; 26(13):2192–7.

76. Brandsma D, Stalpers L, Taal W, et al. Clinical features, mechanisms, and management of pseudoprogression in malignant gliomas. Lancet Oncol 2008;9(5):453–61.

77. Fatterpekar GM, Galheigo D, Narayana A, et al. Treatment-related change versus tumor recurrence in high-grade gliomas: a diagnostic conundrum–use of dynamic susceptibility contrast-enhanced (DSC) perfusion MRI. AJR Am J Roentgenol 2012;198(1):19–26.

78. Barajas RF Jr, Chang JS, Segal MR, et al. Differentiation of recurrent glioblastoma multiforme from radiation necrosis after external beam radiation therapy with dynamic susceptibility-weighted contrast-enhanced perfusion MR imaging. Radiology 2009;253(2):486–96.

79. Hu LS, Baxter LC, Smith KA, et al. Relative cerebral blood volume values to differentiate high-grade glioma recurrence from posttreatment radiation effect: direct correlation between image-guided tissue histopathology and localized dynamic susceptibility-weighted contrast-enhanced perfusion MR imaging measurements. AJNR Am J Neuroradiol 2009;30(3):552–8.

80. Prager AJ, Martinez N, Beal K, et al. Diffusion and perfusion MRI to differentiate treatment-related changes including pseudoprogression from recurrent tumors in high-grade gliomas with histopathologic evidence. AJNR Am J Neuroradiol 2015; 36(5):877–85.

81. Young RJ, Gupta A, Shah AD, et al. MRI perfusion in determining pseudoprogression in patients with glioblastoma. Clin Imaging 2013;37(1):41–9.

82. Kong DS, Kim ST, Kim EH, et al. Diagnostic dilemma of pseudoprogression in the treatment of newly diagnosed glioblastomas: the role of assessing relative cerebral blood flow volume and oxygen-6-methylguanine-DNA methyltransferase promoter methylation status. AJNR Am J Neuroradiol 2011;32(2):382–7.

83. Gahramanov S, Muldoon LL, Varallyay CG, et al. Pseudoprogression of glioblastoma after chemo- and radiation therapy: diagnosis by using dynamic susceptibility-weighted contrast-enhanced perfusion MR imaging with ferumoxytol versus gadoteridol and correlation with survival. Radiology 2013; 266(3):842–52.

84. Boxerman JL, Ellingson BM, Jeyapalan S, et al. Longitudinal DSC-MRI for distinguishing tumor recurrence from pseudoprogression in patients with a high-grade glioma. Am J Clin Oncol 2014. [Epub ahead of print].

85. Di Chiro G, Oldfield E, Wright DC, et al. Cerebral necrosis after radiotherapy and/or intra-arterial chemotherapy for brain tumors: PET and neuropathologic studies. AJR Am J Roentgenol 1988; 150(1):189–97.

86. Baek HJ, Kim HS, Kim N, et al. Percent change of perfusion skewness and kurtosis: a potential imaging biomarker for early treatment response in patients with newly diagnosed glioblastomas. Radiology 2012;264(3):834–43.

87. Hu LS, Eschbacher JM, Heiserman JE, et al. Reevaluating the imaging definition of tumor progression: perfusion MRI quantifies recurrent glioblastoma tumor fraction, pseudoprogression, and radiation necrosis to predict survival. Neuro Oncol 2012;14(7):919–30.

88. Cha J, Kim ST, Kim HJ, et al. Differentiation of tumor progression from pseudoprogression in patients with posttreatment glioblastoma using multiparametric histogram analysis. AJNR Am J Neuroradiol 2014;35(7):1309–17.

89. Vrabec M, Van Cauter S, Himmelreich U, et al. MR perfusion and diffusion imaging in the follow-up of recurrent glioblastoma treated with dendritic cell

immunotherapy: a pilot study. Neuroradiology 2011;53(10):721–31.

90. Stenberg L, Englund E, Wirestam R, et al. Dynamic susceptibility contrast-enhanced perfusion magnetic resonance (MR) imaging combined with contrast-enhanced MR imaging in the follow-up of immunogene-treated glioblastoma multiforme. Acta Radiol 2006;47(8):852–61.

91. van den Bent MJ, Wefel JS, Schiff D, et al. Response assessment in neuro-oncology (a report of the RANO group): assessment of outcome in trials of diffuse low-grade gliomas. Lancet Oncol 2011;12(6):583–93.

92. Brasil Caseiras G, Ciccarelli O, Altmann DR, et al. Low-grade gliomas: six-month tumor growth predicts patient outcome better than admission tumor volume, relative cerebral blood volume, and apparent diffusion coefficient. Radiology 2009; 253(2):505–12.

93. Hathout L, Pope WB, Lai A, et al. Radial expansion rates and tumor growth kinetics predict malignant transformation in contrast-enhancing low-grade diffuse astrocytoma. CNS Oncol 2015;4(4):247–56.

94. Veeravagu A, Jiang B, Ludwig C, et al. Biopsy versus resection for the management of low-grade gliomas. Cochrane Database Syst Rev 2013;(4):CD009319.

95. van den Bent MJ. Chemotherapy for low-grade glioma: when, for whom, which regimen? Curr Opin Neurol 2015;28(6):633–938.

96. Johannesen TB, Langmark F, Lote K. Progress in long-term survival in adult patients with supratentorial low-grade gliomas: a population-based study of 993 patients in whom tumors were diagnosed between 1970 and 1993. J Neurosurg 2003;99(5): 854–62.

97. van den Bent MJ, Afra D, de Witte O, et al. Long-term efficacy of early versus delayed radiotherapy for low-grade astrocytoma and oligodendroglioma in adults: the EORTC 22845 randomised trial. Lancet 2005;366(9490):985–90.

98. Ginsberg LE, Fuller GN, Hashmi M, et al. The significance of lack of MR contrast enhancement of supratentorial brain tumors in adults: histopathological evaluation of a series. Surg Neurol 1998; 49(4):436–40.

99. Pallud J, Mandonnet E, Duffau H, et al. Prognostic value of initial magnetic resonance imaging growth rates for World Health Organization grade II gliomas. Ann Neurol 2006;60(3):380–3.

100. Rees J, Watt H, Jager HR, et al. Volumes and growth rates of untreated adult low-grade gliomas indicate risk of early malignant transformation. Eur J Radiol 2009;72(1):54–64.

101. Law M, Oh S, Babb JS, et al. Low-grade gliomas: dynamic susceptibility-weighted contrast-enhanced

perfusion MR imaging–prediction of patient clinical response. Radiology 2006;238(2):658–67.

102. Danchaivijitr N, Waldman AD, Tozer DJ, et al. Low-grade gliomas: do changes in rCBV measurements at longitudinal perfusion-weighted MR imaging predict malignant transformation? Radiology 2008;247(1):170–8.

103. Bobek-Billewicz B, Stasik-Pres G, Hebda A, et al. Anaplastic transformation of low-grade gliomas (WHO II) on magnetic resonance imaging. Folia Neuropathol 2014;52(2):128–40.

104. Prah MA, Stufflebeam SM, Paulson ES, et al. Repeatability of standardized and normalized relative CBV in patients with newly diagnosed glioblastoma. AJNR Am J Neuroradiol 2015; 36(9):1654–61.

105. Jafari-Khouzani K, Emblem KE, Kalpathy-Cramer J, et al. Repeatability of cerebral perfusion using dynamic susceptibility contrast MRI in glioblastoma patients. Transl Oncol 2015;8(3): 137–46.

106. Calamante F. Bolus dispersion issues related to the quantification of perfusion MRI data. J Magn Reson Imaging 2005;22(6):718–22.

107. Kjolby BF, Ostergaard L, Kiselev VG. Theoretical model of intravascular paramagnetic tracers effect on tissue relaxation. Magn Reson Med 2006;56(1): 187–97.

108. Paulson ES, Schmainda KM. Comparison of dynamic susceptibility-weighted contrast-enhanced MR methods: recommendations for measuring relative cerebral blood volume in brain tumors. Radiology 2008;249(2):601–13.

109. Thilmann O, Larsson EM, Bjorkman-Burtscher IM, et al. Effects of echo time variation on perfusion assessment using dynamic susceptibility contrast MR imaging at 3 tesla. Magn Reson Imaging 2004;22(7):929–35.

110. Hu LS, Baxter LC, Pinnaduwage DS, et al. Optimized preload leakage-correction methods to improve the diagnostic accuracy of dynamic susceptibility-weighted contrast-enhanced perfusion MR imaging in posttreatment gliomas. AJNR Am J Neuroradiol 2010;31(1):40–8.

111. Kelm ZS, Korfiatis PD, Lingineni RK, et al. Variability and accuracy of different software packages for dynamic susceptibility contrast magnetic resonance imaging for distinguishing glioblastoma progression from pseudoprogression. J Med Imaging (Bellingham) 2015;2(2): 026001.

112. Hu LS, Kelm Z, Korfiatis P, et al. Impact of software modeling on the accuracy of perfusion MRI in glioma. AJNR Am J Neuroradiol 2015; 36(12):2242–9.

113. Ellingson BM, Malkin MG, Rand SD, et al. Validation of functional diffusion maps (fDMs) as a

biomarker for human glioma cellularity. J Magn Reson Imaging 2010;31(3):538–48.

114. Wen PY, Cloughesy TF, Ellingson BM, et al. Report of the Jumpstarting Brain Tumor Drug Development Coalition and FDA clinical trials neuroimaging endpoint workshop (January 30, 2014, Bethesda MD). Neuro Oncol 2014; 16(Suppl 7):vii36–47.

115. Ellingson BM, Bendszus M, Boxerman J, et al. Consensus recommendations for a standardized brain tumor imaging protocol in clinical trials. Neuro Oncol 2015;17(9):1188–98.

Multiparametric Imaging Analysis
Magnetic Resonance Spectroscopy

O. Rapalino, MD[a], E.M. Ratai, PhD[a,b],*

KEYWORDS

- Magnetic resonance spectroscopy • N-acetyl aspartate • Choline • Glioma • Cerebral metastasis
- Lactate • 2-Hydroxyglutarate • Brain tumor

KEY POINTS

- Magnetic resonance spectroscopy (MRS) is a noninvasive technique that allows the study of metabolic processes and chemical environment in the brain parenchyma.
- MRS is one of the few diagnostic techniques that can be used for evaluation of low-grade neoplastic processes and for their differentiation from non-neoplastic entities.
- Despite many technical and reimbursement challenges to its use in routine clinical practice, MRS will continue to develop as an important and sensitive imaging tool for assessment of intracranial pathologies.

DISCUSSION OF PROBLEM/CLINICAL PRESENTATION

MRS allows the qualitative and quantitative assessment of specific metabolites in the brain parenchyma or intracranial extra-axial spaces. MRS analysis of brain tumors can be performed using ^{1}H (proton) MRS or, less frequently, with [31]P (phosphorus) or ^{13}C (carbon) MRS techniques. For ^{1}H MRS, the most common metabolites evaluated in routine clinical practice include N-acetyl aspartate (NAA), choline-containing compounds (Cho), creatine (Cr), myo-inositol (mI), lipid (Lip), and lactate (Lac) (Table 1). NAA is considered a neuronal metabolite and is decreased in processes with neuronal destruction or dysfunction.[1] Cr is a metabolite related to the cellular energy metabolism and is considered relatively stable in different pathologic processes affecting the central nervous system and useful as a reference metabolite. Cho are related to membrane turnover and their elevation is indicative of a process that results in increased glial proliferation and membrane synthesis (as seen with cellular proliferative disorders).[2,3] Lip peaks are often indicative of areas of necrosis and Lac peaks are directly originated from processes resulting in anaerobic metabolism. mI can be a marker of astrocytic metabolism and can be seen elevated in certain pathologic processes (see Table 1).

Common diagnostic problems encountered in routine clinical brain tumor imaging can be summarized as follows.

Is It Neoplastic or Not?

Non-neoplastic processes, including malformations of cortical development (such as focal

Disclosures: The authors have nothing to disclose.
[a] Neuroradiology Division, Department of Radiology, Massachusetts General Hospital, Boston, MA 02114, USA;
[b] MGH/HST Athinoula A. Martinos Center for Biomedical Imaging, Building 149, 13th Street, Room 2301, Charlestown, MA 02129, USA
* Corresponding author. Neuroradiology Division, Department of Radiology, Massachusetts General Hospital, Harvard Medical School, and A. A. Martinos Center for Biomedical Imaging, Building 149, 13th Street, Room 2301, Charlestown, MA 02129.
E-mail address: eratai@mgh.harvard.edu

mri.theclinics.com

Table 1
Metabolites evaluated with magnetic resonance spectroscopy in brain tumor imaging

Metabolite	Peak Configuration	Resonance (ppm)	Best Echo Time for Detection	Clinical Associations
NAA	Singlet	2.0	Short or long TE	Neuronal marker (not seen in non-neural brain tumors)
Cho	Singlet	3.22	Short or long TE	Membrane turnover marker and cellular proliferation
Cr	Singlets	3.03 and 3.9	Short or long TE	Cellular energy byproduct. Lower in necrosis[63]
mI	Multiplets	3.56	Short TE	Low-grade gliomas, gliomatosis[4]
Lip	Broad peaks	0.9, 1.3	Short TE	Tuberculomas, PCNSL, radiation necrosis
Lac	Doublet	1.33	1.5T = inverted at 135–144 ms 3T = 288 ms	Anaerobic metabolism marker Prominent if necrosis or hypoxia
Glx	Multiplets	2.1–2.4 ppm; 3.7 ppm	Short TE	Detected in GBM, astrocytomas and oligodendrogliomas
Taurine	Triplets	3.4	Short TE	Medulloblastomas
Alanine	Doublet	1.47	1.5 T = 144 ms	Meningiomas
Citrate[30,64]	Multiplets	2.6	3T = 35 ms and inverts at 97 ms	Gliomas, particularly aggressive pediatric types
Gly[65–67]	Singlet	3.55	3T = 160 ms[67]	Low-grade gliomas, central neurocytomas
2HG[31,68]	Multiplets	1.85, 2.01, 2.28, and 4.05	Best seen with spectral editing techniques 3T = 97 ms[68]	IDH mutations

Adapted from Chronaiou I, Stensjoen AL, Sjobakk TE, et al. Impacts of MR spectroscopic imaging on glioma patient management. Acta Oncol 2014;53(5):583.

cortical dysplasia) (**Fig. 1**), hamartomas, cerebral infarcts, infectious pathologies, inflammatory diseases (including demyelinating and vasculitic processes), and vascular pathologies (including capillary telangiectasias and cavernous malformations), can be difficult to differentiate from intra-axial or extra-axial intracranial neoplastic processes in conventional magnetic resonance (MR) studies (**Table 2**). MRS is a useful imaging tool to help in the differentiation and characterization of these pathologies. Neoplastic processes have metabolic byproducts related to their mitotic activity (Cho) and neuronal dysfunction (NAA) that can be detected by MRS and improve the accuracy of the clinical diagnosis (**Fig. 2**). The closer the MR spectrum is to a normal spectrum the more likely that the intracranial lesion is a benign process or developmental anomaly (see **Fig. 1**).

There is significant overlap in the Cho/NAA ratios, however, between non-neoplastic processes, such as tumefactive demyelinating lesions, infarcts, and infectious processes with neoplastic pathologies. Specific metabolic markers have been identified that may make this distinction more reliable (eg, glutamate/glutamine [Glx] for demyelination or 2-hydroxyglutarate [2HG] for isocitrate dehydrogenase [IDH] 1–mutant gliomas).

Is the Lesion a Primary or a Secondary Brain Tumor?

Several studies have shown the utility of MRS, particularly using the multivoxel technique for differentiation of glioblastoma from an intracerebral metastasis.[4] The assessment of normal-appearing brain parenchyma in the immediate

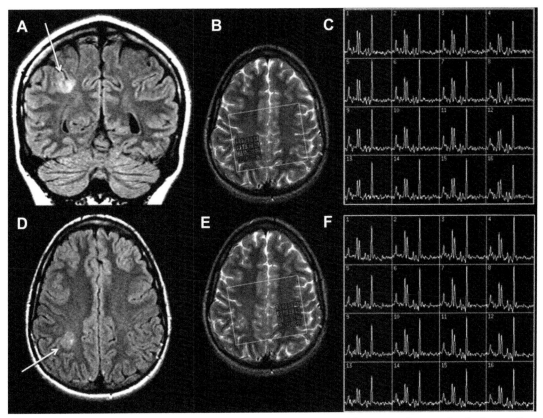

Fig. 1. Focal cortical dysplasia. A 13-year-old male patient presenting with nocturnal generalized seizures. Coronal (*A*) and axial (*D*) FLAIR images, axial T2-weighted images with corresponding intermediate (TE = 144 ms) TE spectra of a right parietal cortical dysplasia (*B*, *C*) and contralateral normal brain parenchyma (*E*, *F*). There is no significant difference in the metabolite ratios between the lesion compared with the ipsilateral surrounding and contralateral brain parenchyma. The yellow arrows point to the lesion.

vicinity of the tumor has been shown reliable, with glioblastoma cases showing higher Cho/NAA ratios compared with metastatic lesions[4] (**Figs. 3** and **4**).

Is It a High-Grade or Low-Grade Tumor?

Multiple studies have shown the value of MRS for predicting the histologic grade of glial tumors.[5] Higher Cho/NAA ratios have been associated with higher World Health Organization (WHO) grades among glial tumors[6–8] (see **Figs. 2** and **3**). The Cho/Cr ratio seems more accurate for the differentiation of high-grade versus low-grade gliomas (with sensitivity and specificity values of 80% and 76%, respectively).[9]

Where Is the Best Target for Surgery or Treatment?

MRS can provide a general overview of the metabolic profile of a brain tumor and indicate areas of higher clinical aggressiveness or histologic grade (with higher Cho/Cr ratios).[10,11] Multivoxel MRS

can guide the neurosurgeon for sampling the anatomic sites with the highest histologic grade in low-grade tumors[12] and increases the diagnostic accuracy of stereotactic and excisional biopsies[13,14] (see **Fig. 3**). There is also growing evidence of the potential use of 3-D volumetric MRS imaging (MRSI) to guide radiation treatment.[15,16] MRS can potentially identify areas with abnormal Cho/NAA ratios that can extend beyond the tumoral margins defined by conventional MR sequences[11,15,16] (see **Fig. 3**).

Radiation-Induced Changes or Recurrent High-Grade Tumor?

MRS, particularly when using multivoxel techniques, has been shown useful for the differentiation of radiation necrosis and recurrent high-grade glioma and recommended as an evidence level II diagnostic modality for this differentiation.[17] In general, areas with recurrent glioma have higher Cho/NAA ratios with variable Lip peaks. Pure radiation necrosis shows prominent Lip with relative decrease of the remaining metabolites compared

Table 2
Magnetic resonance spectroscopy features of intracranial neoplastic and non-neoplastic pathologies

Pathology	N-Acetyl Aspartate	Choline	Myo-inositol	Glutamate/ Glutamine	Glycine	Lactate	Lipid	Taurine	Alanine	Amino Acids	Succinate	2-Hydroxyglutarate	Comments
Glioblastoma and anaplastic gliomas[69]	--/---	++/+++				++	++					+	Necrotic areas with high Lac and Lip
Diffuse astrocytoma	-	+	++										
Pilocytic astrocytoma[36]	-	+				+	+	+				+	Decreased Cr
Medulloblastoma[22,41,42]	-	++/+++	+	+/++		+	+	+/++					Groups 3 and 4 show high taurine, lower Lip, and high Cr. SHH tumors show high Cho and Lip, with minimal taurine.[40] Also phosphocholine
Ependymoma[42]			++/+++	+/++				+					Also glycerophosphocholine in vitro[42]
Intracranial metastases	--					++	++						Relatively normal metabolites in the parenchyma surrounding the lesion. Absent NAA within the lesion
PCNSL[70]							+++						MRS obtained from non-necrotic lesions
Epidermoid cysts[71]						++			+	+			Aminoacids: valine, isoleucine and glycine
Meningioma	--/---	++							+				Alanine (up to 90% of cases)[45]
Piogenic abscess	-/--	+/++				++				++	++		Aminoacids, Lac, alanine, and acetate[72]
Tuberculoma[73]	-	+		++		+	++						Higher Cho/Cr and mI/Cr in tumors. Also peak at 3.8 ppm, possibly guanidinoacetate
Tumefactive demyelinating lesion (TDL)[74-76]	-/--	+/++			+								
Radiation necrosis	-	+		++			++						Higher Cho/Cr and mI/Cr in tumors

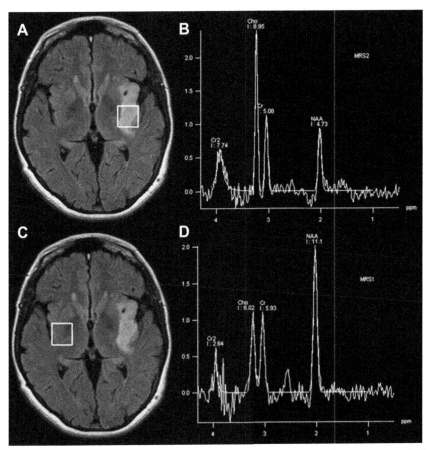

Fig. 2. Low-grade glioma. A 40-year-old woman presenting with partial complex seizures and with a biopsy-proved WHO grade II left insular oligoastrocytoma. Axial FLAIR images with MRS voxels and corresponding intermediate TE spectra from the lesional side (A, B) and contralateral side (C, D). The white boxes indicate the volume of interest of the obtained spectra, respectively. There is a clear increase of Cho/NAA values within the lesion compared to the contralateral brain parenchyma compatible with the clinical diagnosis of a low-grade glioma.

with the contralateral normal appearing brain parenchyma (Fig. 5). Relative ratios of intralesional Cho to contralateral Cr have also been shown to be a good marker to distinguish between radiation necrosis and recurrent high-grade tumor.[18] This distinction is not always black and white, however, because many cases have concurrent areas of neoplastic involvement and postradiation changes. In addition, elevated Lip can also be seen in high-grade gliomas near areas of central necrosis.

How to Identify Infiltrative (Recurrent) Tumor in Patients with Glioblastoma Treated with Antiangiogenic Treatment

Patients receiving antiangiogenic medications, such as bevacizumab, show rapid decrease or resolution of the intratumoral abnormal enhancement and the conventional MR sequences are difficult to interpret during the follow-up imaging of these cases. MRS has the potential to identify abnormal metabolic patterns suggestive of tumoral infiltration in progressive areas of fluid-attenuated inversion recovery (FLAIR) hyperintensity in patients treated with bevacizumab, despite the lack of abnormal enhancement.[19] A multicenter trial by the American College of Radiology Imaging Network demonstrated increased NAA/Cho and decreased Cho/Cr levels 8 weeks into the treatment with bevacizumab in patients with recurrent glioblastoma correlated with increased progression free survival rates.[20]

Can Treatment Response or Outcomes Be Predicted with Magnetic Resonance Spectroscopy?

Multiple studies have highlighted the potential role of MRS to predict treatment responses and outcome after treatment. The identification of 2HG in glial tumors with IDH1 mutations and glutamate in pediatric medulloblastomas is associated with better overall survival rates.[21,22] The decrease

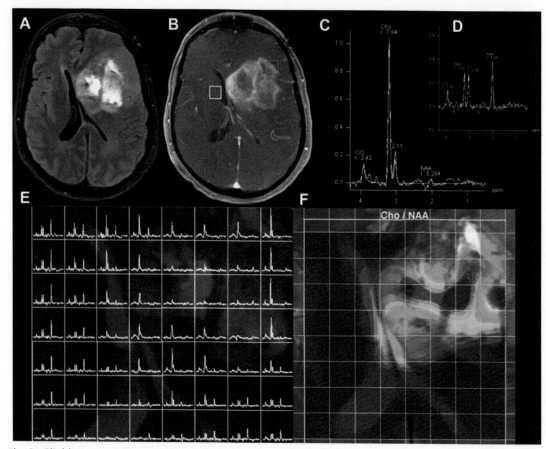

Fig. 3. Glioblastoma. A 65-year-old woman presenting with headache and right sided weakness. Pathology was consistent with glioblastoma. Axial FLAIR (*A*), postcontrast axial T1-weighted (*B*), individual spectra (TE = 144 ms) from the anterolateral margin of the enhancing mass (*blue* region of interest [*C*]) and contralateral brain (*yellow* region of interest [*D*]), spectral map (*E*), and metabolic (Cho/NAA) map (*F*). MR spectra are abnormal even in the adjacent brain parenchyma without conventional MR abnormalities in the left frontal and left parietal lobe. Spectral and metabolic maps clearly depict areas with the highest Cho/NAA ratios providing the best target for proper pathologic grading of the tumor.

of 2HG within glial tumors after treatment also correlate with functional status.[23] MRS, specifically the Lac-to-NAA ratio, may also be helpful in the prediction of potential sites of glioblastoma recurrence.[24] Increased Cho/NAA values 3 weeks after radiation treatment are associated with higher probability of early glioblastoma progression.[25]

PHYSICS

The MR spectra are derived from characteristic radiofrequency (RF) signals produced by certain nuclei when stimulated by an oscillating RF pulse in a static magnetic field. The nuclei that have been used for MRS include hydrogen (^{1}H) (high gyromagnetic ratio and abundance), phosphorus-31 (31P), and carbon-13 (13C), among others. These nuclei within different molecules produce different RF signatures depending on their electron densities, chemical structure, and magnetic properties of surrounding nuclei. The differences in the local magnetic field surrounding these individual nuclei during MRS are known as chemical shifts and are measured in parts per million (ppm) in relation to a reference compound (tetramethylsilane).[26] Tetramethylsilane has a chemical shift of 0 ppm. The chemical shift of different compounds is plotted along the X axis in the MR spectra. A large water peak is typically obtained at 4.7 ppm on ^{1}H-MRS that needs to be suppressed to appreciate smaller peaks related to other metabolites with a lower concentration in the brain parenchyma. MRS can be acquired using a single volume of interest using a single-voxel spectroscopy (SVS) or as 2-D or 3-D volumes of interest with multiple subdivisions known as multivoxel MRS, MRSI, or chemical

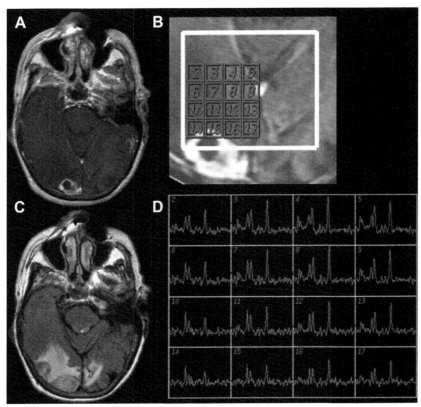

Fig. 4. Metastasis. A 90-year-old female patient with history of lung cancer presenting with new visual symptoms and headache. Pathology was consistent with metastatic adenocarcinoma. Axial T1 postcontrast (*A*), MRS grid superimposed on an axial T1 image (*B*), axial FLAIR (*C*), and multivoxel MRS (TE = 144 ms) (*D*). Metabolite ratios are relatively preserved within the areas of vasogenic edema (see voxels 7 and 11).

shift imaging (CSI). The CSI spectra can be displayed as an individual spectrum from a single subdivision, multiple spectra overlayed on conventional MR images (spectral maps), or concentration-dependent color-coded maps overlayed on conventional images (metabolic maps). Echo times (TEs) can have significant impact on the visualization of different metabolites in MRS, with short TE spectra displaying metabolites with short-echo and long-echo T2 relaxation times whereas long TE spectra only display metabolites with long T2 relaxation times (often with suppression of mI, Glx, and Lip peaks). Intermediate TEs (135–144 mms) are helpful for visualization of Lac that appears as an inverted doublet at 1.3 ppm.

The most common methods for spatial localization of MRS signals include the stimulated-echo acquisition mode (STEAM) and point-resolved spectroscopy (PRESS) techniques. Over the past decade, there has been increasing availability of faster MRS sequences using echo-planar techniques (echo-planar spectroscopic imaging) and spiral techniques.

IMAGING PROTOCOLS

MRS can be performed as a single-voxel acquisition or as a multivoxel acquisition. The choice of the best imaging protocol for a specific clinical case depends on the size of the lesion (large homogeneous lesions can be assessed with SVS but large heterogeneous lesions can be more accurately evaluated with 2-D or 3-D multivoxel MRS), anatomic location (pathologies located in the spinal cord, brainstem, and anterior temporal lobes near the skull are difficult to image with multivoxel MRS), and acquisition times (multivoxel MRS sequences usually take longer to acquire but recently developed spiral MRS sequences have markedly decreased the acquisition times). A reference spectrum is often acquired from the contralateral cerebral or cerebellar parenchyma when SVS techniques are used.

The choice of TEs depends on the specific clinical question and magnetic field strength. If MRS is needed as a metabolic screen for metabolic disorders or if short T2 relaxation metabolites are important for the clinical diagnosis (mI, Glx, Lip,

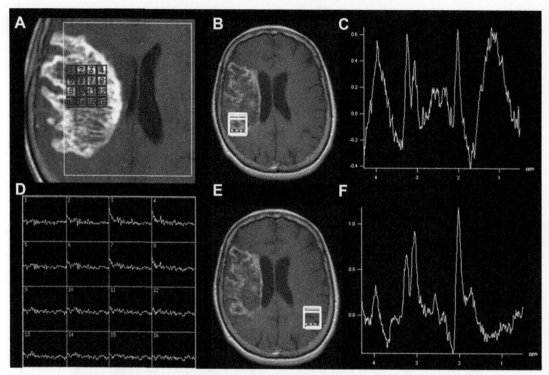

Fig. 5. Radiation necrosis. A 60-year-old male patient with an anaplastic astrocytoma treated with subtotal resection and chemoradiation. Reference axial postcontrast T1-weighted images showing the multivoxel grid (*A*), intralesional single voxel (*B*), and contralateral single voxel (*E*). The multivoxel spectra (*D*) were acquired approximately 6 months after radiation treatment. The single-voxel spectra from the lesion (*C*) and contralateral normal appearing brain parenchyma (*F*) were obtained approximately 1 year after radiation treatment. The lesion progressively decreased in size without treatment. There is diffuse decrease of metabolites within the evaluated areas on the multivoxel spectra and relatively decreased Cho/contralateral Cr ratios on the intralesional single-voxel spectrum compared with the contralateral normal spectrum, compatible with areas of necrosis related to prior radiation.

and so forth), a short TE spectrum should be acquired. If the MRS is performed for detection of Lac peaks, then an intermediate (at 1.5T) or long TE (at 3T) spectrum is ideal. Acquisition of MR spectra at 3T is usually preferred due to higher signal-to-noise ratios but susceptibility artifacts are more prominent at 3T making the acquisition of MRS near the skull base more challenging.

MRS has been shown valuable in the noninvasive diagnosis and follow-up imaging of brain tumors, with a sensitivity of approximately 80% and a sensitivity of 78.5%.[27] CSI seems more sensitive than SVS but the latter seems more specific.[27] The appropriate choices of the MRSI protocol and TE values are important to obtain the best possible imaging data.[27]

SPECIFIC PATHOLOGIES AND MAGNETIC RESONANCE SPECTROSCOPY FINDINGS
Glial Tumors

Multiple studies have documented a good correlation of WHO grade and metabolite ratios (Cho/ NAA, Cho/Cr, and Lip-Lac/Cr) (see **Table 2**).[7,28,29] A variety of gliomas may display high levels of citrate (not present in normal brain),[30] particularly in the pediatric population. A subgroup of glial tumors harboring IDH1 and carrying a better prognosis can now be identified using spectral-editing and 2-D correlation MRS techniques through the detection of an oncometabolite, called D-2HG (**Fig. 6**).[31–34] Pilocytic astrocytomas have been shown to have decreased Cr levels[35] and variable degrees of Cho/Cr ratios.[36]

Intracranial Metastases

There are significant differences in peritumoral metabolite ratios (lower Cho/Cr, lower Cho/NAA, and higher NAA/Cr) around intracerebral metastases compared with high-grade gliomas[29,37–39] (see **Figs. 3** and **4**).

Medulloblastomas

There are 4 major molecular subgroups of medulloblastoma based on their gene expression profile

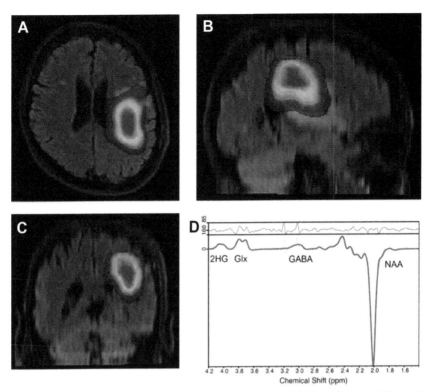

Fig. 6. IDH1 mutant glioma with 2HG metabolic imaging. Axial (A), coronal (B), and sagittal (C) metabolic maps of 2HG concentration in a low-grade glioma involving the left posterior frontal lobe. An individual spectral edited spectrum is also shown illustrating the position of the 2HG peak in relation to other metabolites (D). (*Courtesy of Dr O. Andronesi, Charlestown, MA.*)

and clinical characteristics: WNT, SHH, group 3, and group 4.[40] MRS is becoming a promising noninvasive tool for the differentiation and identification of these subgroups, with metabolic profiles markedly different between groups 3 and 4 (with high taurine, lower Lip, and high Cr) (**Fig. 7**) and

SHH tumors (high Cho and Lip and minimal taurine).[40,41] The presence of glutamate has been associated with increased survival rates.[22] A phosphocholine peak (3.208 ppm) has also been reported as another discriminatory marker for medulloblastomas.[42]

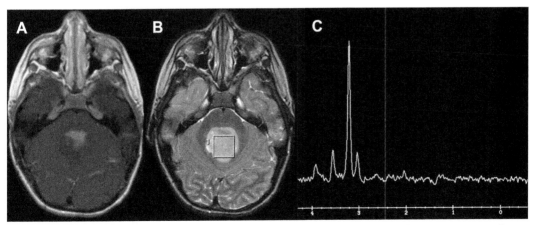

Fig. 7. Medulloblastoma. A 5-year-old boy presenting with nausea, vomiting, and diplopia. MR imaging demonstrates a large heterogeneously enhancing mass. Pathology was consistent with a medulloblastoma. Axial T1 postcontrast (A) and axial T2-weighted (B) (with MRS voxel) (1) and single-voxel MRS (C) (TE = 144 ms). MRS shows a prominent Cho peak and almost complete absence of NAA.

Atypical Teratoid Rhabdoid Tumors

Atypical teratoid rhabdoid tumors are characterized by prominent Lac/Lip, increased Cho, minimal NAA.[43]

Ependymomas

Relatively high mI and glycerophosphocholine (approximately 3.233 ppm in vitro) have been described within these tumors.[42,44]

Meningiomas

The extra-axial tumors, meningiomas, demonstrate high Cho peaks and often alanine peaks (**Fig. 8**). NAA is not seen or minimally detected. There are no reliable MRS findings that can be used to differentiate typical from atypical or malignant meningiomas.[45]

Intracranial Hemangiopericytomas

Intracranial hemangiopericytomas typically show increased Cho, prominent Lip/Lac peaks, decreased Cr, and marked decrease of NAA as well as increased mI and Glx peaks.[46]

Central Neurocytoma

Variable glycine, increased Glx, marked elevation of Cho, variable NAA, alanine/Lac.[47]

Primary Central Nervous System Lymphoma

Lip and Lac peaks from homogeneously enhancing components are useful for differentiation between primary central nervous system lymphoma (PCNSL) and glioblastoma or metastatic lesions[4,48] (**Fig. 9**).

PEARLS AND PITFALLS
Pearls

- Routine acquisition of multivoxel MRS using a short TE addresses most of the cases of brain tumors. Alternatively, single-voxel technique could be used if the multivoxel acquisitions are too long or not available. If single voxel is used, a contralateral spectrum should be obtained for comparison. An intermediate TE (eg, 144 ms) at 1.5T or long TE (eg, 288 ms) should be considered if the detection of Lac is important for the diagnosis. At 3 T, a TE of 288 ms is often used because at higher field

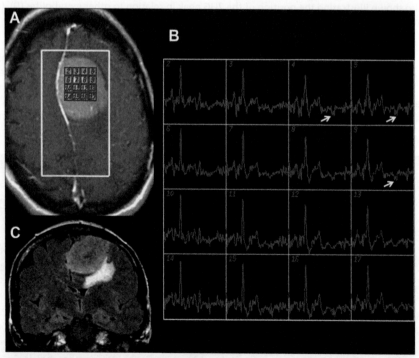

Fig. 8. Meningioma. A 60-year-old female patient with progressive headache and found to have a large left parafalcine meningioma. Axial postcontrast T1-weighted (*A*) with multivoxel MRS grid, multivoxel MR spectra (TE = 144 ms) (*B*), and coronal FLAIR (*C*) images. Small inverted doublets are seen at approximately 1.47 ppm suggestive of alanine peaks (*small yellow arrows*). The tumor also demonstrates increased Cho/Cr and markedly decreased NAA/Cr.

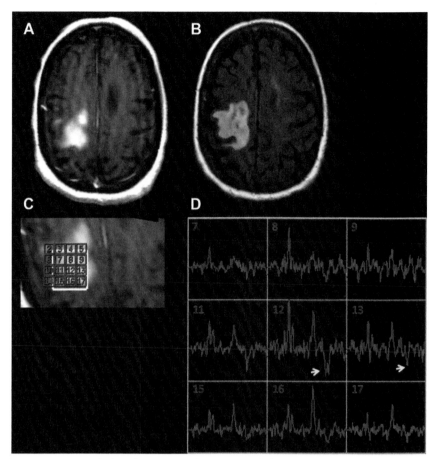

Fig. 9. Lymphoma. An 80-year-old female patient with progressive left sided weakness secondary to a large homogeneous enhancing mass in the right posterior frontal lobe. Pathology was consistent with diffuse large B-cell lymphoma. Axial postcontrast T1-weighted (*A*), axial FLAIR (*B*), MRS grid showing voxel placement overlaid on a T1-weighted image (*C*), and multivoxel MR spectra (TE = 144 ms) (*D*). There are prominent Lac (*yellow arrows*) and Lip peaks on the multivoxel MR spectra obtained from the regions of homogeneous enhancement, favoring the diagnosis of lymphoma.

strengths, Lac may show reduced or absent signal intensity at an intermediate TE.[49]
- The MRS should be planned in advance and previous imaging studies should be reviewed to determine the target of the study and the best way to approach it. Pathologies in difficult anatomic locations (eg, brainstem, spinal cord, or near the skull base) require manual shimming during the MRS acquisition.
- The presence of gadolinium does not significantly seem to affect the MRS, and the MRS acquisition can be performed after the postcontrast T1-weighted images to ensure that the enhancing lesions are properly included.[50]

Pitfalls

- The inclusion of bone or air-tissue interfaces in the voxel used for MRS significantly affect the technical quality of the spectra.

- MRS should always be interpreted in conjunction with the rest of the imaging findings and not as an isolated modality. Could the findings be related to artifact or suboptimal technique? Was the shimming adequate during the acquisition? Proper technique is of paramount importance for the appropriate interpretation of the clinical MRSI.

WHAT A REFERRING PHYSICIAN NEEDS TO KNOW

- MRS is an advanced MR technique that can be helpful in the differentiation of non-neoplastic versus neoplastic pathologies, noninvasive characterization of intracranial neoplasms, and evaluation of cases of radiation necrosis, among other clinical uses.
- MRS complements the information provided by the conventional MR imaging sequences

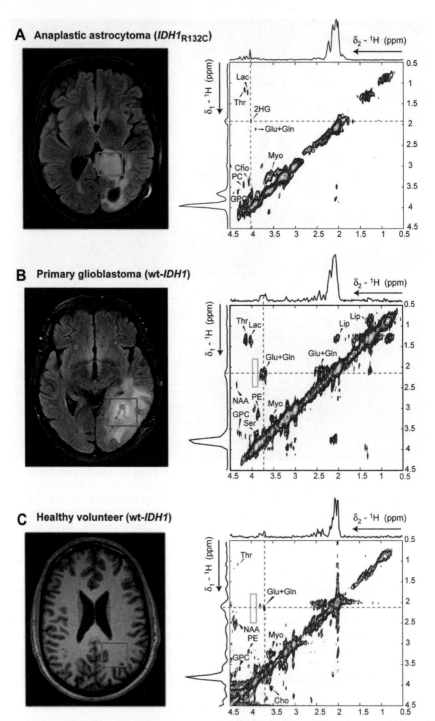

Fig. 10. 2-D COSY. Examples of in vivo 2-D LASER-COSY spectra at 3T from 2 patients, one with an IDH1-mutant anaplastic astrocytoma (*A*) and another with a primary glioblastoma (wild-type [wt]-IDH1) (*B*), compared with a spectrum obtained from a healthy volunteer (wt-IDH1) (*C*). There is a small peak at the 4.02/1.91 ppm intersection compatible with 2HG in the spectrum obtained from the anaplastic astrocytoma. This peak is absent in the primary glioblastoma and in the healthy control subject (*green rectangle*). (*From* Andronesi OC, Kim GS, Gerstner E, et al. Detection of 2-hydroxyglutarate in IDH-mutated glioma patients by in vivo spectral-editing and 2D correlation magnetic resonance spectroscopy. Sci Transl Med 2012;4(116):116ra4; with permission.)

and should always be interpreted in conjunction with the rest of the imaging studies.

FUTURE DIRECTIONS

Recent advances in MRSI have been focused toward shortening acquisition times. Fast MRSI has evolved from concepts related to spatial encoding using gradient switching during acquisition.[51] The proton echo-planar spectroscopic imaging (PEPSI) sequence uses standard-phase encoding in one direction, while phase encoding in the other direction is replaced by bipolar gradients, switching during data acquisition.[52] Spiral trajectories in k-space allow even faster encoding of spatial information due to faster gradient duty cycle.[53] Andronesi and colleagues[54] implemented a 3-D volumetric in vivo MRSI sequence using spiral trajectories at a spatial resolution of 1 cm³ with a total scan time of less than 2.5 min. These improvements in image quality and imaging time allow more routine acquisition of spectroscopic data in the clinical setting.

Other technical innovations include implementation of 3-D MRSI techniques with localization by adiabatic selective refocusing (LASER) pulses acquisition.[54] This sequence is designed to better compensate for chemical shift displacement errors, spatial nonuniformity of RF excitation, and contamination with subcutaneous Lip signal from tissues outside the region of interest using adiabatic pulses.[55,56]

Motion correction schemes applied in MR technology have brought many practical benefits. By using techniques, such as propeller MR imaging, it has become possible to oversample k-space and thereby compensate for motion.[57] As an alternative to these retrospective motion-correction techniques, it is also possible to prospectively correct motion using image-based navigators.[58–61]

Spectral editing techniques, such as 2-D J-resolved methods, allow for the detection of peaks that are otherwise hidden in the MR spectrum because many resonances of similar frequencies in the proton spectrum overlap. In spectral editing, selective and nonselective spin-echo spectra are acquired; the difference spectrum contains the target metabolite signal (eg, 2HG) while all other contributors are nulled. Another approach to visualize hidden MR resonances is 2-D correlation spectroscopy (COSY) and total correlation spectroscopy (TOCSY) imaging experiments. Compared with the 2-D J-resolved method, 2-D COSY and TOCSY provide increased spectral dispersion, which scales up with increasing main magnetic field strength and may have improved ability to unambiguously identify overlapping metabolites (**Fig. 10**).[32,62]

SUMMARY

MRS is a noninvasive technique that allows the study of metabolic processes and chemical environment in the brain parenchyma and has already demonstrated a tremendous diagnostic value in many clinical scenarios, particularly in the assessment of brain tumors and their differentiation from non-neoplastic pathologies and post-treatment changes. MRS is one of the few diagnostic techniques that can be used for evaluation of low-grade neoplastic processes and for their differentiation from non-neoplastic entities. Despite many technical and reimbursement challenges to its use in routine clinical practice, MRS will continue to develop as an important and sensitive imaging tool for assessment of intracranial pathologies.

REFERENCES

1. Urenjak J, Williams SR, Gadian DG, et al. Proton nuclear magnetic resonance spectroscopy unambiguously identifies different neural cell types. J Neurosci 1993;13(3):981–9.
2. Lin A, Ross BD, Harris K, et al. Efficacy of proton magnetic resonance spectroscopy in neurological diagnosis and neurotherapeutic decision making. NeuroRx 2005;2(2):197–214.
3. Gill SS, Thomas DG, Van Bruggen N, et al. Proton MR spectroscopy of intracranial tumours: in vivo and in vitro studies. J Comput Assist Tomogr 1990; 14(4):497–504.
4. Brandao LA, Castillo M. Adult brain tumors: clinical applications of magnetic resonance spectroscopy. Neuroimaging Clin N Am 2013;23(3):527–55.
5. Fudaba H, Shimomura T, Abe T, et al. Comparison of multiple parameters obtained on 3T pulsed arterial spin-labeling, diffusion tensor imaging, and MRS and the Ki-67 labeling index in evaluating glioma grading. AJNR Am J Neuroradiol 2014;35(11): 2091–8.
6. Devos A, Lukas L, Suykens JA, et al. Classification of brain tumours using short echo time 1H MR spectra. J Magn Reson 2004;170(1):164–75.
7. Dou W, Zhang M, Zhang X, et al. Convex-envelope based automated quantitative approach to multivoxel 1H-MRS applied to brain tumor analysis. PLoS One 2015;10(9):e0137850.
8. Sahin N, Melhem ER, Wang S, et al. Advanced MR imaging techniques in the evaluation of nonenhancing gliomas: perfusion-weighted imaging compared with proton magnetic resonance spectroscopy and tumor grade. Neuroradiol J 2013;26(5):531–41.

9. Wang Q, Zhang H, Zhang J, et al. The diagnostic performance of magnetic resonance spectroscopy in differentiating high-from low-grade gliomas: a systematic review and meta-analysis. Eur Radiol 2016; 26:2670–84.

10. Hall WA, Martin A, Liu H, et al. Improving diagnostic yield in brain biopsy: coupling spectroscopic targeting with real-time needle placement. J Magn Reson Imaging 2001;13(1):12–5.

11. Raschke F, Fellows GA, Wright AJ, et al. (1) H 2D MRSI tissue type analysis of gliomas. Magn Reson Med 2015;73(4):1381–9.

12. Bradac O, Vrana J, Jiru F, et al. Recognition of anaplastic foci within low-grade gliomas using MR spectroscopy. Br J Neurosurg 2014;28(5): 631–6.

13. Yao C, Lv S, Chen H, et al. The clinical utility of multimodal MR image-guided needle biopsy in cerebral gliomas. Int J Neurosci 2016;126:53–61.

14. Roder C, Skardelly M, Ramina KF, et al. Spectroscopy imaging in intraoperative MR suite: tissue characterization and optimization of tumor resection. Int J Comput Assist Radiol Surg 2014;9(4):551–9.

15. Parra NA, Maudsley AA, Gupta RK, et al. Volumetric spectroscopic imaging of glioblastoma multiforme radiation treatment volumes. Int J Radiat Oncol Biol Phys 2014;90(2):376–84.

16. Pirzkall A, Nelson SJ, McKnight TR, et al. Metabolic imaging of low-grade gliomas with three-dimensional magnetic resonance spectroscopy. Int J Radiat Oncol Biol Phys 2002;53(5):1254–64.

17. Ryken TC, Aygun N, Morris J, et al. The role of imaging in the management of progressive glioblastoma: a systematic review and evidence-based clinical practice guideline. J Neurooncol 2014; 118(3):435–60.

18. Rabinov JD, Lee PL, Barker FG, et al. In vivo 3-T MR spectroscopy in the distinction of recurrent glioma versus radiation effects: initial experience. Radiology 2002;225(3):871–9.

19. Artzi M, Bokstein F, Blumenthal DT, et al. Differentiation between vasogenic-edema versus tumor-infiltrative area in patients with glioblastoma during bevacizumab therapy: a longitudinal MRI study. Eur J Radiol 2014;83(7):1250–6.

20. Ratai EM, Zhang Z, Snyder BS, et al. Magnetic resonance spectroscopy as an early indicator of response to anti-angiogenic therapy in patients with recurrent glioblastoma: RTOG 0625/ACRIN 6677. Neuro Oncol 2013;15(7):936–44.

21. Natsumeda M, Igarashi H, Nomura T, et al. Accumulation of 2-hydroxyglutarate in gliomas correlates with survival: a study by 3.0-tesla magnetic resonance spectroscopy. Acta Neuropathol Commun 2014;2:158.

22. Wilson M, Gill SK, MacPherson L, et al. Noninvasive detection of glutamate predicts survival in pediatric medulloblastoma. Clin Cancer Res 2014;20(17): 4532–9.

23. Andronesi OC, Loebel F, Bogner W, et al. Treatment response assessment in IDH-mutant glioma patients by non-invasive 3D functional Spectroscopic Mapping of 2-Hydroxyglutarate. Clin Cancer Res 2016; 22:1632–41.

24. Deviers A, Ken S, Filleron T, et al. Evaluation of the lactate-to-N-acetyl-aspartate ratio defined with magnetic resonance spectroscopic imaging before radiation therapy as a new predictive marker of the site of relapse in patients with glioblastoma multiforme. Int J Radiat Oncol Biol Phys 2014;90(2):385–93.

25. Muruganandham M, Clerkin PP, Smith BJ, et al. 3-Dimensional magnetic resonance spectroscopic imaging at 3 Tesla for early response assessment of glioblastoma patients during external beam radiation therapy. Int J Radiat Oncol Biol Phys 2014; 90(1):181–9.

26. Barker PB. Clinical MR spectroscopy: techniques and applications. Cambridge (United Kingdom): Cambridge University Press; 2010.

27. Wang W, Hu Y, Lu P, et al. Evaluation of the diagnostic performance of magnetic resonance spectroscopy in brain tumors: a systematic review and meta-analysis. PLoS One 2014;9(11):e112577.

28. Bulik M, Jancalek R, Vanicek J, et al. Potential of MR spectroscopy for assessment of glioma grading. Clin Neurol Neurosurg 2013;115(2):146–53.

29. Caivano R, Lotumolo A, Rabasco P, et al. 3 Tesla magnetic resonance spectroscopy: cerebral gliomas vs. metastatic brain tumors. Our experience and review of the literature. Int J Neurosci 2013; 123(8):537–43.

30. Choi C, Ganji SK, Madan A, et al. In vivo detection of citrate in brain tumors by 1H magnetic resonance spectroscopy at 3T. Magn Reson Med 2014;72(2): 316–23.

31. Andronesi OC, Rapalino O, Gerstner E, et al. Detection of oncogenic IDH1 mutations using magnetic resonance spectroscopy of 2-hydroxyglutarate. J Clin Invest 2013;123(9):3659–63.

32. Andronesi OC, Kim GS, Gerstner E, et al. Detection of 2-hydroxyglutarate in IDH-mutated glioma patients by in vivo spectral-editing and 2D correlation magnetic resonance spectroscopy. Sci Transl Med 2012;4(116):116ra4.

33. Elkhaled A, Jalbert LE, Phillips JJ, et al. Magnetic resonance of 2-hydroxyglutarate in IDH1-mutated low-grade gliomas. Sci Transl Med 2012;4(116): 116ra5.

34. Choi C, Ganji SK, DeBerardinis RJ, et al. 2-hydroxyglutarate detection by magnetic resonance spectroscopy in IDH-mutated patients with gliomas. Nat Med 2012;18(4):624–9.

35. Panigrahy A, Krieger MD, Gonzalez-Gomez I, et al. Quantitative short echo time 1H-MR spectroscopy

of untreated pediatric brain tumors: preoperative diagnosis and characterization. AJNR Am J Neuroradiol 2006;27(3):560–72.

36. Porto L, Kieslich M, Franz K, et al. Spectroscopy of untreated pilocytic astrocytomas: do children and adults share some metabolic features in addition to their morphologic similarities? Childs Nerv Syst 2010;26(6):801–6.

37. Server A, Josefsen R, Kulle B, et al. Proton magnetic resonance spectroscopy in the distinction of high-grade cerebral gliomas from single metastatic brain tumors. Acta Radiol 2010;51(3):316–25.

38. Lee EJ, Ahn KJ, Lee EK, et al. Potential role of advanced MRI techniques for the peritumoural region in differentiating glioblastoma multiforme and solitary metastatic lesions. Clin Radiol 2013;68(12): e689–97.

39. Tsougos I, Svolos P, Kousi E, et al. Differentiation of glioblastoma multiforme from metastatic brain tumor using proton magnetic resonance spectroscopy, diffusion and perfusion metrics at 3 T. Cancer Imaging 2012;12:423–36.

40. Bluml S, Margol AS, Sposto R, et al. Molecular subgroups of medulloblastoma identification using noninvasive magnetic resonance spectroscopy. Neuro Oncol 2016;18:126–31.

41. Wu G, Pang H, Ghimire P, et al. (1)H magnetic resonance spectroscopy and diffusion weighted imaging findings of medulloblastoma in 3.0T MRI: a retrospective analysis of 17 cases. Neural Regen Res 2012;7(32):2554–9.

42. Davies NP, Wilson M, Harris LM, et al. Identification and characterisation of childhood cerebellar tumours by in vivo proton MRS. NMR Biomed 2008; 21(8):908–18.

43. Bruggers CS, Moore K. Magnetic resonance imaging spectroscopy in pediatric atypical teratoid rhabdoid tumors of the brain. J Pediatr Hematol Oncol 2014;36(6):e341–5.

44. Tugnoli V, Tosi MR, Barbarella G, et al. Magnetic resonance spectroscopy study of low grade extra and intracerebral human neoplasms. Oncol Rep 1998;5(5):1199–203.

45. Demir MK, Iplikcioglu AC, Dincer A, et al. Single voxel proton MR spectroscopy findings of typical and atypical intracranial meningiomas. Eur J Radiol 2006;60(1):48–55.

46. Mama N, Ben Abdallah A, Hasni I, et al. MR imaging of intracranial hemangiopericytomas. J Neuroradiol 2014;41(5):296–306.

47. Tlili-Graiess K, Mama N, Arifa N, et al. Diffusion weighted MR imaging and proton MR spectroscopy findings of central neurocytoma with pathological correlation. J Neuroradiol 2014;41(4): 243–50.

48. Mora P, Majos C, Castaner S, et al. (1)H-MRS is useful to reinforce the suspicion of primary central

nervous system lymphoma prior to surgery. Eur Radiol 2014;24(11):2895–905.

49. Lange T, Dydak U, Roberts TP, et al. Pitfalls in lactate measurements at 3T. AJNR Am J Neuroradiol 2006; 27(4):895–901.

50. Lima EC, Otaduy MC, Tsunemi M, et al. The effect of paramagnetic contrast in choline peak in patients with glioblastoma multiforme might not be significant. AJNR Am J Neuroradiol 2013;34(1):80–4.

51. Mansfield P. Spatial mapping of the chemical shift in NMR. Magn Reson Med 1984;1(3):370–86.

52. Posse S, Tedeschi G, Risinger R, et al. High speed 1H spectroscopic imaging in human brain by echo planar spatial-spectral encoding. Magn Reson Med 1995;33(1):34–40.

53. Adalsteinsson E, Spielman DM. Spatially resolved two-dimensional spectroscopy. Magn Reson Med 1999;41(1):8–12.

54. Andronesi OC, Gagoski BA, Sorensen AG. Neurologic 3D MR spectroscopic imaging with low-power adiabatic pulses and fast spiral acquisition. Radiology 2012;262(2):647–61.

55. Garwood M, Ugurbil K, Rath AR, et al. Magnetic resonance imaging with adiabatic pulses using a single surface coil for RF transmission and signal detection. Magn Reson Med 1989;9(1):25–34.

56. Andronesi OC, Ramadan S, Ratai EM, et al. Spectroscopic imaging with improved gradient modulated constant adiabaticity pulses on high-field clinical scanners. J Magn Reson 2010;203(2):283–93.

57. Tamhane AA, Arfanakis K. Motion correction in periodically-rotated overlapping parallel lines with enhanced reconstruction (PROPELLER) and turboprop MRI. Magn Reson Med 2009;62(1):174–82.

58. Hess AT, Andronesi OC, Tisdall MD, et al. Real-time motion and B0 correction for localized adiabatic selective refocusing (LASER) MRSI using echo planar imaging volumetric navigators. NMR Biomed 2012; 25(2):347–58.

59. Hess AT, Tisdall MD, Andronesi OC, et al. Real-time motion and B0 corrected single voxel spectroscopy using volumetric navigators. Magn Reson Med 2011;66(2):314–23.

60. Bogner W, Gagoski B, Hess AT, et al. 3D GABA imaging with real-time motion correction, shim update and reacquisition of adiabatic spiral MRSI. Neuroimage 2013;103:290–302.

61. Bogner W, Hess AT, Gagoski B, et al. Real-time motion- and B-correction for LASER-localized spiral-accelerated 3D-MRSI of the brain at 3T. Neuroimage 2013;88C:22–31.

62. Andronesi OC, Gagoski BA, Adalsteinsson E, et al. Correlation chemical shift imaging with low-power adiabatic pulses and constant-density spiral trajectories. NMR Biomed 2012;25(2):195–209.

63. Wyss M, Kaddurah-Daouk R. Creatine and creatinine metabolism. Physiol Rev 2000;80(3):1107–213.

64. Bluml S, Panigrahy A, Laskov M, et al. Elevated citrate in pediatric astrocytomas with malignant progression. Neuro Oncol 2011;13(10):1107–17.

65. Bobek-Billewicz B, Hebda A, Stasik-Pres G, et al. Measurement of glycine in a brain and brain tumors by means of 1H MRS. Folia Neuropathol 2010;48(3): 190–9.

66. Choi C, Ganji SK, DeBerardinis RJ, et al. Measurement of glycine in the human brain in vivo by 1H-MRS at 3 T: application in brain tumors. Magn Reson Med 2011;66(3):609–18.

67. Ganji SK, Maher EA, Choi C. In vivo H MRSI of glycine in brain tumors at 3T. Magn Reson Med 2016;75:52–62.

68. Choi C, Ganji S, Hulsey K, et al. A comparative study of short- and long-TE (1)H MRS at 3 T for in vivo detection of 2-hydroxyglutarate in brain tumors. NMR Biomed 2013;26(10):1242–50.

69. Guzman-De-Villoria JA, Mateos-Perez JM, Fernandez-Garcia P, et al. Added value of advanced over conventional magnetic resonance imaging in grading gliomas and other primary brain tumors. Cancer Imaging 2014;14:35.

70. Yamasaki F, Takayasu T, Nosaka R, et al. Magnetic resonance spectroscopy detection of high lipid levels in intraaxial tumors without central necrosis:

a characteristic of malignant lymphoma. J Neurosurg 2015;122(6):1370–9.

71. Bernabeu A, Lopez-Celada S, Alenda C, et al. Epidermoid cyst with a metabolite pattern mimicking a brain abscess. A magnetic resonance spectroscopy study. J Neuroimaging 2013;23(1):145–8.

72. Poptani H, Gupta RK, Jain VK, et al. Cystic intracranial mass lesions: possible role of in vivo MR spectroscopy in its differential diagnosis. Magn Reson Imaging 1995;13(7):1019–29.

73. Morales H, Alfaro D, Martinot C, et al. MR spectroscopy of intracranial tuberculomas: a singlet peak at 3.8 ppm as potential marker to differentiate them from malignant tumors. Neuroradiol J 2015;28(3):294–302.

74. Cianfoni A, Niku S, Imbesi SG. Metabolite findings in tumefactive demyelinating lesions utilizing short echo time proton magnetic resonance spectroscopy. AJNR Am J Neuroradiol 2007;28(2):272–7.

75. Lu SS, Kim SJ, Kim HS, et al. Utility of proton MR spectroscopy for differentiating typical and atypical primary central nervous system lymphomas from tumefactive demyelinating lesions. AJNR Am J Neuroradiol 2014;35(2):270–7.

76. Saindane AM, Cha S, Law M, et al. Proton MR spectroscopy of tumefactive demyelinating lesions. AJNR Am J Neuroradiol 2002;23(8):1378–86.

Interrogating Metabolism in Brain Cancer

Travis C. Salzillo, BS[a,b], Jingzhe Hu, BS[a,c], Linda Nguyen, BS[b],
Nicholas Whiting, PhD[a], Jaehyuk Lee, PhD[a], Joseph Weygand, BS[a,b],
Prasanta Dutta, PhD[a], Shivanand Pudakalakatti, PhD[a], Niki Zacharias Millward, PhD[a],
Seth T. Gammon, PhD[a], Frederick F. Lang, MD[d], Amy B. Heimberger, MD[d],
Pratip K. Bhattacharya, PhD[a,b,*]

KEYWORDS

- Metabolic imaging • Hyperpolarization • MRS • NMR • MRI • GC/MS • DNP • CEST

KEY POINTS

- Many existing and emerging techniques of interrogating metabolism in brain cancer are at an early stage of development.
- A few clinical trials that employ these techniques are in progress in patients with brain cancer to establish the clinical efficacy of these techniques.
- It is likely that in vivo metabolomics and metabolic imaging is the next frontier in brain cancer diagnosis and assessing therapeutic efficacy.

MR SPECTROSCOPY/NMR SPECTROSCOPY–BASED METABOLOMICS IN BRAIN TUMOR

Metabolomics is the "systematic study of the unique chemical fingerprints that specific cellular processes leave behind", the study of their small-molecule metabolite profiles.[1] Recently, metabolomics in cancer research is gaining considerable importance. The application of Nuclear Magnetic Resonance (NMR)-based and Magnetic Resonance Spectroscopy (MRS)-based metabolomics as applied to brain cancer is an evolving area of clinical use and investigation. In brain tumors, diagnosing tumor type and grade non-invasively has been a clinical challenge. ^{1}H MRS/NMR–based metabolomics has been explored to identify elevated metabolites in malignant tissue specifically in contrast with normal brain. Interestingly, most of the ^{1}H MRS in vivo studies to date have been done on the brain. This is primarily owing to the reduced effects of motion and lipid contamination in the brain. The global metabolic profile of live cells or cell extracts from established glioma models has been determined using standard NMR methods, and validated using tumor biopsies obtained from animal models or patients that have been imaged using high-resolution magic angle spinning spectroscopy.[2,3] Such approaches complement data to the in vivo findings.

Detected Metabolites Using ^{1}H MR Spectroscopy

^{1}H MRS is used extensively to monitor the steady-state levels of major endogenous cellular metabolites. For a full review of in vivo ^{1}H MRS-detectable

The authors have nothing to disclose.
[a] Department of Cancer Systems Imaging, MD Anderson Cancer Center, The University of Texas, Houston, TX, USA; [b] The University of Texas Health Science Center at Houston, Houston, TX, USA; [c] Department of Bioengineering, Rice University, Houston, TX, USA; [d] Department of Neurosurgery, MD Anderson Cancer Center, The University of Texas, Houston, TX, USA
* Corresponding author.
E-mail address: PKBhattacharya@mdanderson.org

mri.theclinics.com

metabolites, see De Graaf.[4] In the field of neurooncology, the most prevalent metabolites in the ^1H MR spectrum are N-acetylaspartate (NAA), total choline-containing metabolites (Cho), lactate (Lac), mobile lipids, creatine (Cre), glutamate (Glu), glutamine (Gln), Gln and Glu, glycine, glutathione, and 2-hydroxyglutarate (2-HG). The largest signal in normal healthy brain tissue is NAA and the NAA level typically decreases in gliomas.[5] The Cho signal is a composite of free choline, phosphocholine and glycerophosphocholine, which are the precursors and breakdown products of the main membrane phospholipid phosphatidylcholine. The intensity of this peak is associated with cell proliferation and cell signaling, and is typically increased in cancer.[6] Lactate is the end product of aerobic glycolysis and is enhanced in cancer as part of the Warburg effect.[7] Lipids (long chain fatty acids), especially lipid droplets known as mobile lipids or triglycerides, are rarely observed in the normal brain, but are often increased in glial tumors and are associated with cell death and increased necrosis.[8] The Cre signal is a composite of Cre and phosphocreatine, which are involved in energy metabolism via the creatine kinase reaction. Cre levels vary within normal brain regions and in some cases with tumorigenesis.[9] The amino acid Glu is the most abundant amino acid in the brain and an essential neurotransmitter. In gliomas, glutaminolysis is often required for tumor growth as an anaplerotic source of carbon complementary to glucose metabolism.[2] Finally, with the recent discovery of the isocitrate dehydrogenase (IDH) mutation, the most common mutation in oligodendroglioma and astrocytoma tumors,[10] increased levels of 2-HG, which is produced from α-ketoglutarate (α-KG) by mutant IDH, serve as a clear metabolic indicator for the presence of the mutation within a tumor and can also be detected by ^1H MRS when the mutation is present.

From a technical perspective, it is important to note that the length of the echo time (TE) used in ^1H MRS sequences defines which metabolites can be detected. Using a short TE (<50 ms), most metabolites can be observed, but overlappings between resonances often hampers proper quantification; on the other hand, when using a long TE (>120 ms), only a few metabolites remain visible, but their respective resonances can be readily identified and quantified.[9]

Detected Metabolites Using ^{13}C MR Spectroscopy

Early ^{13}C MRS/NMR investigations were used to monitor glucose metabolism and Lac turnover during steady-state hyperglycemia with stable isotopically labeled, [1-^{13}C] glucose in C6 glioma-bearing rats.[11] Labeling of glucose-derived [3-^{13}C] Lac, [4-^{13}C] Glu, [4-^{13}C] Gln, and [1-^{13}C] glycogen could all be detected. More important, increased labeled Lac with reduced labeling in Glu and Gln were observed when comparing tumor with normal contralateral brain, consistent with the Warburg effect and a reduction in flux into the tricarboxylic acid (TCA) cycle. ^{13}C MRS studies investigating glioblastoma (GBM) cells and a combination of ^{13}C-labeled glucose and ^{13}C-labeled Gln have also shed light on the possible role of Gln in high-grade brain tumors. Conversion of Gln to Lac via glutaminolysis was found to be sufficient to produce NADPH required for fatty acid synthesis. More recently, studies of primary human GBM models in mice infused with ^{13}C-labeled glucose further demonstrated not only increased glycolysis, but also active glucose metabolism via the TCA cycle to Glu and Gln, confirming that flux via pyruvate dehydrogenase was not suppressed in GBM. However, this study showed limited glutaminolysis.[12] Using ^{13}C MRS to probe the fate of ^{13}C-labeled acetate in orthotopic brain tumors, a recent investigation demonstrated that acetate is oxidized via the TCA cycle, together with glucose, to generate labeled Gln and Glu. This identifies an additional metabolite that could help to meet the high biosynthetic and bioenergetic demands of GBM tumor growth.[13] Future studies using additional ^{13}C-labeled substrates could be envisaged to shed further light on the metabolism of GBM and, as models are being developed, on the metabolism of lower grade brain tumors.

Clinical ^1H MR Spectroscopy

Numerous studies have highlighted the potential benefits of using ^1H MRS to estimate metabolite levels in brain tumors in the clinic.[14] When combined with similar spatial localization techniques that are used in generating anatomic MR images, this strategy can be used to produce maps of the variations in levels of choline containing compounds, Cre, NAA, Lac, and mobile lipids. With increased magnetic field strengths, improvements in scanner hardware and developments in software capabilities, the acquisition time for volumetric data is on the order of 5 to 10 minutes and the spatial resolution of the voxels obtained is typically 0.5 to 1 cm^3.[15] More recent advances in pulse sequence development and spectral editing schemes have facilitated the detection of metabolites with shorter T_2 relaxation times and lower signal-to-noise ratios such as Glu, Gln, Gln and Glu , and 2-HG, expanding the investigation of potential metabolic processes for both characterizing the spatial extent of gliomas and assessing therapeutic response.

For Tumor Characterization

The first studies to identify metabolic differences between gliomas and normal brain tissue date back to the mid-1990s and used a long TE (144 ms) ^{1}H MRS acquisition.[16,17] Since then, numerous studies have shown that elevated levels of Cho and reduced levels of NAA together can distinguish regions of tumor from normal brain,[18,19] define the spatial extent of abnormal metabolism owing to tumor beyond the contrast-enhancing lesion[20,21] guide the selection of the biopsy site to the most aggressive part of the tumor[22,23] and differentiate among tumor grades and types. The Cho-NAA index (CNI) is a metric that has been developed in the clinical setting to describe such changes and has been found to be more robust than ratios and absolute quantification.[24] These in vivo results have been confirmed by correlating with both ex vivo histologic characteristics from image-guided tissue samples and, more recently, ^{1}H high-resolution magic angle spinning spectroscopy of tumor biopsies to show that regions with increased Cho and reduced NAA relative to normal brain that have a high probability of corresponding to tumor.[22] However, despite the benefits of ^{1}H MRS imaging in improving sensitivity to metabolically active tumor and differentiating gliomas from metastatic disease,[25] other disease processes such as inflammation can also cause a reduction in neuronal function while increasing cellularity, so alone MRS is not specific enough to differentiate tumor from inflammation.[26]

For Predicting Outcome or Response to Therapy

In high-grade gliomas, higher Cho-to-Cre, higher Cho-to-NAA, higher Lac plus mobile lipids, and lower Cr-to-NAA abnormalities have been found to be associated with poor survival.[27] In low-grade gliomas, fewer data sets are available on the prognostic value of MRS in the clinic. In one study, increased Cre was found to be a significant predictor for tumor progression and for malignant tumor transformation in grade II gliomas. Gliomas with decreased Cre seemed to have longer progression-free times and later malignant transformation.[28] The information provided by MRS data is complementary to anatomic images and may often be more valuable than the contrast-enhancing lesion in assessing therapeutic response. The spatial extent of the metabolic lesion can also be used to plan focal therapy, such as external beam radiation therapy (RT) and gamma knife radiosurgery,[29] and to assess the response to therapy.[19] Alexander and colleagues[30] showed that the mean tumor Cho/NAA ratio and normalized Cho decreased from baseline to after completion of external beam RT. In this study, patients who exhibited more than a 40% decrease in normalized Cho between midradiotherapy and postradiotherapy studies were associated with shorter survival times and faster disease progression. The Lac/NAA ratio at the fourth week of RT and the change in normalized Cho/Cre between baseline and week 4 of RT were also predictive of the outcome, suggesting the possible benefit of adaptive, response-based radiation treatment.

Although a breadth of MR imaging methods can provide extensive anatomic and functional information about brain tumors, the current use of colocalized ^{1}H MRS/NMR metabolomics approaches provides valuable information that can help clinicians to determine tumor margins, distinguish between progression and pseudoprogression, characterize tumor grade and IDH status, and predict response to therapy. Additionally, preclinical studies of brain tumor models continue to shed light on the complexities of glioma metabolism, leading to an improved understanding of cellular events that could be targetable for new therapeutic approaches. Furthermore, methods currently optimized in the preclinical setting and most notably the use of hyperpolarized agents, are poised to enter the clinic and will enhance the steady-state metabolic data with dynamic flux information that could further improve the detection of tumors and the early monitoring of therapeutic response. Collectively, the breadth of existing and emerging MRS methodologies available for the metabolic imaging of brain tumors could improve current paradigms significantly on diagnosis, treatment, and response assessment, advancing personalized patient care and quality of life.

GAS CHROMATOGRAPHY/MASS SPECTROMETRY–BASED METABOLOMICS OF BRAIN CANCER

Besides NMR-based metabolomics, metabolomics based on gas chromatography/mass spectrometry are increasingly applied in brain cancer research but at this point are mostly restricted to ex vivo samples. However, mass spectrometry imaging is emerging as a powerful tool for directly determining the distribution of proteins, peptides, lipids, neurotransmitters, metabolites, and drugs in situ[31] and has enormous potential as a clinical tool for interrogating metabolism in brain cancer.

Gas Chromatography/Mass Spectrometry–Based Metabolomic Analysis of Cerebrospinal Fluid from Glioma Patients

Nakamizo and colleagues[32] analyzed cerebrospinal fluid from patients with glioma using gas chromatography/mass spectrometry to correlate metabolomic profiles based on World Health Organization tumor grades, tumor location, contrast in MR images, and IDH mutations. Samples were separated into 3 groups: grade I and II glioma, grade III glioma, and glioblastoma (GBM). Grades I and II and grade III samples did not differ in their metabolomic content. However, in GBM samples, citric and isocitric acid were increased compared with the other 2 groups, and lactic acid was higher relative to grades I and II samples. Succinic, fumaric, and malic acid were decreased in GBM samples relative to grades I and II and grade III gliomas. For samples that originated from tumors proximal to the ventricles, high-grade tumors possessed elevated levels of citric and isocitric acid, and low-grade tumors had elevated levels of lactic acid, compared with samples originating in tumors distal to the ventricles. In high-grade tumors that displayed gadolinium enhancement in MR images, citric and isocitric acid levels were higher than those tumors that did not display this enhancement. Levels of citric, isocitric, and lactic acid were higher in samples with mutated IDH than those with wild-type IDH, whereas the combined signal from pyruvate and oxaloacetic acid was decreased in the mutated IDH samples. The correlation between overall survival and concentrations of these metabolites was also investigated. It was found that in malignant glioma (grades III and IV), elevated levels of lactic acid were correlated to lower overall survival. Although not significant, there was a trend between elevated levels of citric and lactic acid and lower overall survival in all gliomas.

Metabolomic Patterns in Glioblastoma and Changes During Radiotherapy

Wibom and colleagues[33] examined the metabolic profile of GBM patients before and after radiotherapy. Extracellular fluid was extracted from the tumor and brain adjacent to tumor (BAT) via microdialysis before and during treatment, similar to the procedure performed by Tabatabaei and colleagues[34] and was analyzed with gas chromatography time-of-flight mass spectrometry. Reference samples were also collected subcutaneously from the abdomen. Tumor tissue was found to express lower levels of glucose than BAT and the subcutaneous tissue. Several amino acids were found in greater quantities in the tumor relative to the BAT, including the essential amino acids, L-threonine, allothreonine, L-tryptophan, L-arginine, L-lysine, and L-valine. Glycine and Glu levels were also increased in the tumor compared with the BAT. After radiotherapy was administered, Glu and Gln levels increased in both tumor and BAT regions. Ethanolamine and glycerol seemed to decrease in the tumor but increase in the BAT in addition to glycerol. Although the metabolic profile varied among the patients, it was suggested that the trends in the tumor metabolome could be monitored individually to help assess the efficacy of radiotherapy.

Metabolomic Screening of Glioma Patients Reveals Diagnostic and Prognostic Information

Moren and colleagues[35] conducted a study that compared the metabolic profiles of tumor samples and serum from different World Health Organization grades of GBM and oligodendroglioma via gas chromatography time-of-flight mass spectrometry. Correlations were determined between metabolite levels and survivability of the 2 diseases. Increased levels of 2-hydroxyglutaric acid, 4-aminobutyric acid (GABA), creatinine, glycerol-2-phosphate, glycerol-3-phosphate, ribitol, and myo-inositol were found in tumor samples, and lysine and 2-oxoisocaproic acid in serum from oligodendroglioma patients, relative to samples from GBM patients. Compared with oligodendroglioma samples, levels of mannitol and phenylalanine in GBM tumor samples and cysteine from serum were increased. Survival groups were split into short survival (4 months) and long survival (3 years), where the survival is measured as the time after diagnosis. In GBM, elevated levels of glycerol-3-phoshate, myo-inositol, ribitol, and fructose were associated with long survival. In oligodendroglioma levels of ribitol, myo-inositol and spermidine were higher for long survival patients, whereas short survival patients expressed elevated levels of glycine and aminomalonic acid.

Metabolomics of Human Cerebrospinal Fluid Identifies Signatures of Malignant Glioma

The first study to delineate the metabolic differences in cerebrospinal fluid samples between malignant and nonmalignant glioma patients was investigated by Locasale and colleagues[36] through the use of a liquid chromatography/tandem mass spectrometry. Several metabolites that were significantly altered between the malignant and nonmalignant samples were identified. A correlation between tumor size and metabolite levels was also determined. Acetylcarnitine, acetoacetate, phenylproplollc acid, and cholesteryl sulfate were correlated positively with tumor size whereas myo-inositol and cytidine were correlated negatively.

The Metabolomic Signature of Malignant Glioma Reflects Accelerated Anabolic Metabolism

The metabolic differences between various World Health Organization grades of glioma tumors were analyzed by Chinnaiyan and colleagues[37] via ultrahigh performance liquid chromatography/tandem mass spectrometry and gas chromatography/mass spectrometry platforms. There was a poor distinction of grade III tumors from either grade II or grade IV owing to overlap in their metabolomic profiles. Amino acid metabolism was altered in grade IV tumors, including increased levels of glutathione and tryptophan and a decrease in Cre levels. An analysis of lipid metabolism in grade IV tumors revealed higher levels of essential and medium chain fatty acids and metabolites associated with carnitine metabolism and lower levels of glycolipids, lysoplipids, and sterols. Although phosphoenolpyruvate and 3-phosphoglycerate levels were increased in grade IV tumors, there was an overall decrease in carbohydrate metabolism. Nucleotide metabolism, particularly pyrimidine catabolism, was found to increase in grade IV tumors. Random forest (RF) analysis was performed to determine which metabolites contributed the most to changes in global metabolism among the different grades of tumors. 2-HG was found to be the most significant biochemical that best delineates tumor grades. An investigation of glycolysis and the oxidative energy metabolism resulted in a more than 7-fold increase in the glycolytic intermediates 3-phosphoglycerate and phosphoenolpyruvate in grade IV tumors compared with grade II tumors. Furthermore, the metabolites 6-P-gluconate, ribose-5-phosphate, serine, and glycine, which contribute to the glycolytic pathway, are significantly increased in grade IV tumors. Interestingly, Gln, which is found to be a major component of tumorigenesis, was not found to be associated with tumor grade.

HYPERPOLARIZED MR IMAGING AND METABOLIC IMAGING IN BRAIN CANCER

MR imaging invaluably benefits many brain diseases patients due to its noninvasive investigation.

^{13}C MRS has been studied as another diagnostic modality in the brain tumor model of animals and in patients with brain tumor[38] because ^{13}C labeling compounds provide specific metabolic information with less background noise and can provide dynamic metabolic analysis with ^{13}C flux analysis.[39] However, the low inherent sensitivity compared with proton MRS must be compensated for in clinical applications. Recently, the novel rapid dissolution process of dynamic nuclear polarization technique was developed to retain strongly polarized nuclear spins in the liquid state.[40] This method can provide more than a 10,000-fold signal enhancement enough to investigate the metabolic changes at the cellular level. Many ^{13}C labeled compounds are used for detecting the abnormality of metabolic fluxes or the accumulation of metabolites in human cancer[41] such as succinate,[42] α-KG,[43,44] and pyruvate and ethyl pyruvate.[45–47] Hyperpolarized ^{13}C pyruvate and α-KG are now studied actively for brain cancer metabolism and the first clinical trial with hyperpolarized ^{13}C pyruvate in GBM patients is underway at the University of California, San Francisco (UCSF). This same group at UCSF conducted the first in human clinical study of metabolic imaging in prostate cancer using hyperpolarized ^{13}C pyruvate.[48]

[1-^{13}C] Pyruvate

A number of preclinical studies in brain tumors have shown that one can distinguish brain tumors from normal tissue by examining in vivo metabolism and assess early response to treatment of high-grade gliomas in animal models.[45,46] Recently, hyperpolarized ^{13}C pyruvate kinetic data were acquired from a healthy cynomolgus monkey brain using optimized ^{13}C coils and pulse sequences which demonstrated the feasibility of using hyperpolarized ^{13}C pyruvate for assessing in vivo metabolism for brain tumor patients in the near future,[47] like the first human clinical trial using ^{13}C metabolic imaging for prostate cancer.[48] All these findings suggest that hyperpolarization may be a promising tool for noninvasive cancer diagnosis and treatment assessment in the clinical setting.

[1-^{13}C] α-Ketoglutarate

Mutations in IDH 1 and 2 present in 70% of low-grade gliomas and 5-10% of glioblastoma in adults.[10] These mutations are associated with the production of the oncometabolite 2-HG instead of α-KG in the brain tumor, which contributes to the formation and malignant progression of gliomas.[49] This accumulated 2-HG can be detected using in vivo proton MRS acquisitions in patients on a 3T MR imaging scanner and this noninvasive 2-HG detection shows its feasibility as a diagnostic and prognostic biomarker.[50] Also, the injected hyperpolarized ^{13}C α-KG interrogated the accumulation of hyperpolarized 2HG[43] or the conversion to hyperpolarized ^{13}C Glu, a potential biomarker for glioma.[44]

Acetate Metabolism in the Brain

Many studies done 10 to 15 years ago show the high use of acetate directly in the brain and its specific use as a glial fuel.[51–53] Recently, this dependence on acetate as an energy source has been found not only in glial cells but also in GBM and brain metastases.[13] Most studies determine and compare the amount and rate of conversion of isotopically labeled acetate relative to labeled glucose using direct infusion techniques. In one such study, the kinetic parameters for 2-^{13}C acetate transport and conversion was determined by infusing the compound into rats at different rates.[54] The labeled compound was found to quickly accumulate in the brain, but its conversion to other metabolites is the rate-limiting step. With plasma concentrations around 2 to 3 mmol/L, the rate of acetate use was 0.5 μmol/g per minute and its transport into the brain was calculated to be 0.96 μmol/g per minute.[54] In addition, the ^{13}C label enrichment of the C4 position of Gln was 44% and the C4 position of Glu was 14% with 2-^{13}C acetate infusion.[54] Similar studies have been done in humans with plasma concentrations of 1 mmol/L and show similar incorporation of the ^{13}C label of acetate into Gln and Glu in the brain.[55–57]

The use of acetate in GBM and brain metastases was found using both ex vivo and in vivo NMR techniques after infusions of 1,2-^{13}C acetate in human orthotopic tumor mouse models. The acetate-to-glucose ratio in five GBM tumor models was around 5-fold higher than in normal control brain tissue. The rate of incorporation of acetate into the citric acid cycle was found to be directly correlated to the amount of acetyl-coenzyme A (CoA) synthetase enzyme 2 (ACSS2).[13] In humans, there are 3 acetyl-CoA synthetase enzymes— ACSS1, ACSS2, and ACSS3. Both ACSS1 and ACSS3 are found in the matrix of the mitochondria; however, ACSS2 is found mainly in the cytosol of the cell.[58,59] In GBM, the amount of ACSS2 was found to be directly correlated to the grade of the tumor with high staining in (100% positive) in grade IV tumors compared with normal brain tissue.[13]

These recent findings have initiated new metabolic research in acetate and cancer progression.[59]

Hyperpolarized 1-^{13}C Acetate

Acetate was one of the first compounds to be hyperpolarized using solid state dynamic nuclear polarization.[60,61] Since its initial polarization, several improvements in formulation and use of other techniques have significantly improved the percentage of polarization and increased the amount (final concentration) of hyperpolarized acetate that can be generated.[62–64] The compound has been polarized using both the preclinical dynamic nuclear polarization polarizer and the clinical polarizer.[65] Our laboratory recently reported a method of chemically converting hyperpolarized 1,2-^{13}C pyruvate to hyperpolarized 1-^{13}C acetate, ^{13}C-bicarbonate, and ^{13}C carbon dioxide using chemical reaction–induced multimolecular polarization.[66] Even with these improvements in 1-^{13}C acetate polarization, significant progress needs to be made for its rate of conversion to Gln, Glu, acetyl-CoA, and citrate to be useful in diagnostic imaging in the time scale of polarization (<5 minutes). A thorough discussion and execution of using hyperpolarized acetate to diagnosis metabolic changes in diabetic rats was published recently.[65] One of the main mechanisms acetyl-CoA gets shuttled into the mitochondria is through its conversion into acetylcarnitine through carnitineacetyltransferase-1 and then back to carnitine and acetyl-CoA in the mitochondria thorough carnitineacetyltransferase-2.[62] The Stodkilde–Jorgensen group could not detect a difference in the conversion rate of hyperpolarized acetate to acetylcarnitine in the time window of hyperpolarization and stated this is probably owing to low rate of conversion of the enzyme.[65] They observe similar results to the ^{13}C nonhyperpolarized infusion studies done in the brain; the transport of acetate into specific tissues is fast; however, the rate of conversion is the rate-limiting step and is significantly slower than hyperpolarized 1-^{13}C pyruvate. Another problem with 1-^{13}C acetate is that other metabolites that would incorporate the ^{13}C label such as citrate have similar chemical shifts to acetate. Using in vivo spectroscopy, it is thus difficult to separate the hyperpolarized resonance of hyperpolarized 1-^{13}C acetate from its metabolite 5-^{13}C citrate. Other compounds might be better suited to interrogate the citric acid cycle or fatty acid synthesis in the brain in the time scale of polarization.[42,67,68]

A recent paper by Rolf Gruetter's laboratory illustrates another method of using the hyperpolarization of 1-^{13}C acetate.[69] His group generated a pulse sequence that transferred the polarized signal in 1,2-^{13}C acetate from the carbonyl carbon (C1) to the methyl carbon (C2) in the brain of a rat and from the C1 position to a proton on the methyl group of acetate. This method allows for a whole new group of metabolites and chemical resonances to be observed. This transfer sequence could allow for hyperpolarized acetate to become clinical metabolic imaging agent.

Hyperpolarized Metabolic Spectroscopy in Brain Cancer Cell Lines

Hyperpolarized MRS has been applied in brain tumor cell line models in efforts to potentially inform medical decision making in novel and clinically useful ways. Various studies have used this technique, which could provide information on the diagnosis, treatment monitoring, and prognosis of brain tumors in a noninvasive manner.

With regard to diagnosing brain tumors, the differing signal levels provided by hyperpolarized ^{13}C-labeled pyruvate and ^{13}C-labeled Lac can be used to distinguish brain tumor and normal brain tissue. In one study, different GBM cell lines (U251 and U87) were used to generate orthotopic xenografts in the rat brain. Levels of ^{13}C-labeled pyruvate and ^{13}C-labeled Lac were elevated in the tumor tissue compared with the normal brain tissue.[45] Furthermore, the pattern of histopathology in the cell lines studied correlated with the amount of signal detected.[45] The U251 GBM cell line exhibits large areas of necrosis and hypoxia; in comparison, the U87 GBM cell line has very little necrosis and hypoxia. The signal to noise ratio of hyperpolarized ^{13}C-labeled Lac, pyruvate, and total carbon was significantly greater in U87 tumors than in U251 tumors; this was thought to be owing to the greater number of viable cells in the U87 line.

Compressed sensing has been used with hyperpolarized MRS to evaluate tumor tissues with heterogeneous metabolic profiles owing to varying levels of necrosis and hypoxia. Compressed sensing allows for the reduction of acquisition time and higher spatial resolution than conventional imaging; this permits the characterization of tumors with a heterogeneous nature like GBM.[46] Differentiation of tumor tissue that was hypoxic/necrotic, nonhypoxic/nonnecrotic, or normal brain tissue in an orthotopic human GBM xenograft model was possible using this technique. Specifically, highly necrotic and hypoxic tumor tissue had absent or low levels of ^{13}C-labeled pyruvate and ^{13}C-labeled Lac, whereas tumor tissue with minimal levels of necrosis and hypoxia had high levels of ^{13}C-labeled pyruvate and

^{13}C-labeled Lac.[46] If used in the clinic, hyperpolarized pyruvate with MRS and compressed sensing could be particularly useful in noninvasively determining tumor tissue types in GBM.

In addition to characteristic signal levels of hyperpolarized ^{13}C-labeled metabolites in tumor versus normal brain tissue, the apparent rate constant (k_{PL}) for the conversion of pyruvate to Lac can also be used to distinguish cancer and normal tissue. Orthotopic xenografts of C6 glioma had larger Lac/pyruvate ratios as well as a larger k_{PL} compared with normal tissue.[70] Furthermore, k_{PL} may even be a more robust marker than the Lac/pyruvate ratio in distinguishing cancerous brain tissue. The k_{PL} has significantly less variability than the Lac/pyruvate ratio when used to differentiate tumor tissue from normal brain tissue.[70]

Hyperpolarized techniques could also be applied to monitor treatment response in brain tumors; tumor response to RT and to different methods of chemotherapy, such as temozolomide (TMZ), everolimus, and LY294002, have been studied with hyperpolarized ^{13}C-labeled metabolites as a metric for response. TMZ is an alkylating agent used to treat brain tumors and is the first-line agent in treating GBM. Everolimus and LY294002 are drugs that target the PI3K/AKT/mammalian target of rapamycin pathway, which regulates the cell cycle. Using conversion of hyperpolarized pyruvate to Lac as a metric, tumor response to radiation treatment by a C6 glioma orthotopic tumor model was examined. By 72 hours after irradiation, the ratio of hyperpolarized Lac in tumor-to-maximum pyruvate in blood vessels was decreased by 34% compared with untreated tumors.[71]

Treatment with TMZ was found to decrease the hyperpolarized pyruvate/Lac ratio in an orthotopic rat model of human GBM.[72] This response could be detected just 1 day after TMZ treatment, whereas imaging-based evidence of tumor volume shrinkage owing to treatment did not occur until 5 to 7 days after treatment.[72] These results were supported by a second study that used a bioreactor to maintain GBM cells treated with TMZ during hyperpolarized imaging. TMZ-treated cells showed a decrease in conversion of hyperpolarized pyruvate to Lac compared with untreated cells.[73] Additionally, the authors of the study found that treatment with TMZ correlated with a decrease in pyruvate kinase, which is a glycolytic enzyme that indirectly controls pyruvate to Lac conversion.[73]

In hyperpolarized studies of everolimus treatment in an orthotopic rate model of GBM, a significant drop in hyperpolarized Lac/pyruvate ratio compared with control was observed 7 days after treatment.[74] At this same time point, conventional MR imaging was unable to detect a difference in tumor size between the treated and control group. It was not until 15 days after treatment that inhibition of tumor growth was appreciated on MR imaging.[74] Bioreactor studies of everolimus and LY294002 treated GBM cells support these results. Decreased hyperpolarized Lac levels were observed in cells treated with these drugs compared with untreated controls.[75,76] In addition to decreased hyperpolarized Lac levels, decreased phosphocholine levels were found to correlate with treatment using these agents.[75] This is expected because the PI3K/AKT/mammalian target of rapamycin pathway controls both the synthesis of phosphocholine and Lac via a common transcription factor hypoxia inducible factor-1-α.[75]

The balance between glycolysis and oxidative phosphorylation can provide important information regarding treatment response. Because many cancer cells derive most of their energy via glycolysis and normal cells via oxidative phosphorylation, the ability to detect if a tumor mainly uses one pathway over the other can indicate continued malignancy or positive response to treatment. One study was able to detect and quantify conversion of hyperpolarized ^{13}C-bicarbonate from ^{13}C-pyruvate in vivo for the first time.[77] Because CO_2 is a byproduct of the flux from pyruvate to acetyl-CoA, bicarbonate can be used as a surrogate marker for mitochondrial metabolism, which is predominant in normal cells. The study found that Lac levels were significantly greater in glioma, and bicarbonate levels were significantly greater in normal brain tissue.[77]

A bioreactor study of GBM cells with mutated IDH1 showed elevated levels of hyperpolarized 2-HG compared with GBM cells with wild-type IDH1.[75] IDH mutation was also found to correlate with decreased activity of branched chain amino acid transaminase.[44] Branched chain amino acid transaminase catalyzes the transamination of branched chain amino acids while converting α-KG to Glu. Thus, in cells with IDH1 mutation, a decrease in branched chain amino acid transaminase activity is expected to correlate with decreased Glu production. This was found to be the case in a bioreactor study of GBM cells with IDH1 mutation; hyperpolarized ^{13}C-Glu production was decreased in mutant cells compared with wild-type cells.[44] As biomarkers of metabolic imaging, hyperpolarized 2-HG and Glu may potentially provide useful information in regards to detecting IDH1 mutation and treatment monitoring of brain tumors with IDH1 mutation.

Currently, the main tool for cancer diagnosis and monitoring is ^{18}fluoro-2-deoxyglucose (FDG)-PET. In brain tumors, however, FDG-PET shows increased signal in surrounding brain tissue owing to the high uptake that masks the signal generated by the tumor itself.[71] Furthermore, pseudoprogression is a misleading phenomenon in which there is contrast enhancement of the tumor after treatment with radiotherapy or chemotherapy despite positive tumor response to the treatment. Diagnosis and treatment monitoring with hyperpolarized metabolic techniques could help mitigate this confounding clinical problem.

IMAGING INFLAMMATION IN THE BRAIN

Broadly, it is known that the heterogeneous microenvironment of brain tumors includes both the tumor and a variety of altered stromal components. These altered stromal components include a variety of cells such as the vascular epithelium and various infiltrative inflammatory cells. The genesis of the milieu has not yet been determined, but it is clear that the net effect of the local environment is mostly tumor supportive. Indeed, cells present at these sites do not behave as they would in their normal microenvironment. For example, tumor-associated macrophages and neutrophils exhibit a graded expression and functional pattern that is consistent with a tumor supportive role. When this tumor-supportive function is blocked, then glioma growth and progression is delayed.[78-80] In the case of the adaptive immune system there can be an abundance of regulatory T (Treg) cells[81,82] within the glioma that are immune suppressive and participate in blocking immune recognition and clearance of the glioma. Most recently, the immune checkpoints have been shown to be operational in a subset of glioma patients[83,84] and various inhibitors have shown promising results in preclinical models of glioma.[85,86] Such responses would have been unthinkable a decade ago. Currently, there are clinical trials underway at a host of institutions to study these immune checkpoint blockade inhibitors in the context of GBM and neuroblastomas.

There is a deep need to understand how and when the immune system begins to interact with the tumor environment and to understand how the status of the various types and states of the inflammatory cells might predict response to various classes of immune checkpoint inhibitors. There are starting points to dissect out these contributions, but each of the currently existing approaches has limitations. Broadly, people often interpret the flair phenomenon as inflammation, but this observation can also occur owing to increased vascular permeability in and around tumor sites. Indeed, when patients are treated with modern chemotherapy protocols, 20% to 30% of patients yield pseudoprogression, an increase in T2 bright areas owing to "inflammatory" processes. Effectively categorizing new tumor growth versus inflammation is critically important for managing patient care.[87] Similarly, phase-weighted MR imaging can also be used to find inflammatory lesions, but this again has been attributed primarily to an increase in the leaky blood vessels and an increase in accumulation of heme from hemoglobin at the site of inflammation. Similar to [111]indium oxine labeling of white blood cells for studying inflammation by SPECT imaging, macrophages have been loaded ex vivo with superparamagentic iron oxide nanoparticles and then their migration to otherwise T2 bright regions can be followed. Because these are T2* agents the tumor and surrounding brain tissue must be T2 bright a priori. The normal brain is well-suited for such an application, but as mentioned, an increase in vascular permeability can result in locally high concentrations of heme that also result in T2 darkening. In the context of spinal injury and traumatic brain injury, diffusion tensor imaging can be useful for detecting demyelination that is downstream of neuroinflammation.[88,89] However, particularly in the case of heterogeneous GBM assigning changes in diffusion to a specific cell type or biochemical pathway will be challenging. Classic targeting of surface receptors using contrast agents has been limited by the sensitivity of MR imaging relative to the abundance of surface receptors present on the cells and the requirement for breakdown of the blood–brain barrier.[90] Enzymatic amplification of the targeting signal might solve this problem. In preclinical models of inflammation, bis HT-DTPA-gadolinium uses a polymerization strategy for determining myeloperoxidase enzymatic activity in vivo.[91] This has shown to be selective in the context of myeloperoxidase $-/-$ mice.[92] However, this requires induction of free radical polymerization processes in vivo, this technique has not been adopted widely. Others have used MRS for studying changes in NAA, choline, and Cre levels, which correlate with changes in the neural tissue. However, it is not clear whether the subsequent increase NAA has been proven to be cell type specific through either cell depletion studies or knockout mice.[93] As such, there remains significant need for pathway, cell-type-specific molecular probes, or metabolic profiling for studying inflammation in the context of tumor initiation, growth, and treatment in vivo. Indeed, the need for enzymatic amplification and improvement in signal to noise ratio suggests that hyperpolarized MR imaging may be able to address several of the current limitations for imaging inflammation in the context of tumors in near future.

CHEMICAL EXCHANGE SATURATION TRANSFER IMAGING IN BRAIN CANCER

Chemical exchange saturation transfer (CEST) imaging offers enhanced indirect detection of exchangeable protons species, which can be endogenous such as hydroxyl, amide, and amine protons in peptides or exogenously introduced such as liposomes. There are several classification schemes of CEST techniques that are currently in use: (1) classification based on exchange type—protons, molecules, or compartments; (2) diamagnetic CEST or paramagnetic CEST (paraCEST).[94] The CEST mechanism relies on the selective RF saturation of exchangeable proton species that resonate at a different frequency relative to the bulk water (~ 4.75 ppm). The bulk water signal becomes attenuated to some extent after solute protons (micromolar to millimolar range) exchange with that of the bulk (~ 110 mol/L). Provided that the RF saturation is long enough (seconds range) and the solute exchange rates are sufficiently fast (millisecond residence time), significant saturation will eventually be visible on the bulk water signal (S_{sat}). Normalizing the original proton spectrum without saturation (S_0) with S_{sat} (S_{sat}/S_0) leads to the CEST spectrum or Z-spectrum. The inverted peaks in the Z-spectrum then correspond with the selectively saturated proton species and the bulk water peak is redefined to 0 ppm by convention. The asymmetric magnetization transfer ratio plot is subsequently obtained by subtracting the left half of the Z-spectrum (>0 ppm) from the right half to remove the bulk water signal for better visual representation.[94] For the diamagnetic CEST effect, the saturation frequency ranges from 0 to 7 ppm, whereas for paraCEST agents, the offset frequency range can be greater than 100 ppm, which offers a much cleaner saturation excitation profile.

The CEST signal is a function of CEST agent concentration, pH, temperature, magnetic parameters (relaxation rate, magnetic field strength), and imaging parameters (repetition time, RF irradiation amplitude, and power, as well as imaging sequence). For the CEST effect to be observed efficiently, a relatively slow to intermediate exchange rate on the MR time scale is required. If the exchange rate is too slow, the saturated protons could have relaxed back to equilibrium by the time it affects to the bulk water pool; if the exchange rate is too fast, not enough saturation on the solute proton pool will have been accumulated. The CEST effect also scales with B_0 owing to better spectrum separation, so more accurate selective saturation and a higher B_0 leads to longer $T_{1\ water}$, resulting in longer storage of saturation in the bulk water pool. However, the specific absorption rate increases quadratically with B_0, which places a constraint on sequence design and applications. Please refer to[94,95] for a comprehensive review of optimization and quantification techniques involved in CEST imaging. Herein, we focus on the potential applications of CEST to image brain cancer.

Glutamate Chemical Exchange Saturation Transfer

Glutamate is a major excitatory neurotransmitter in the brain that is restricted to the synaptic and perisynaptic space of glutamatergic synapses under normal physiologic conditions. Glu released by malignant gliomas has been shown to induce seizure and promote excitotoxicity, which help the invasion of tumor cells into normal tissues[96,97] CEST imaging of Glu (GluCEST) can provide noninvasive monitoring of Glu level in vivo, which can potentially be used to monitor disease progression and assess treatment efficacy.

GluCEST relies on the exchange of protons in the amine group with the bulk water. The resonance frequency of the amine protons is pH dependent and centered around 3 ppm relative to the bulk water resonance frequency.[98] In phantom studies at 7T and at a pH of 7, it has been demonstrated that under physiologic concentrations, the majority of the CEST effect with saturation at 3 ppm (Z-spectrum scale) came from Glu (~70%–75% of total CEST contrast), whereas other metabolites contribute relatively little (GABA ~12%, <6% from Cre, and minimal from other metabolites). In vivo experiment with middle cerebral artery occlusion–induced stroke models showed much higher GluCEST contrast compared with the normal contralateral side. GluCEST imaging offers a resolution of 0.27 × 0.27 × 2 mm for animal model and 1.9× 1.9 × 2 mm for human subjects with an imaging time of around 16 seconds per slice (1 average), which is much better compared with conventional chemical shift imaging techniques in terms of spatial and temporal resolution. The total scan time is around 12 minutes, including the acquisition of B0 and B1 maps needed for corrections.[98,99]

Glucose Chemical Exchange Saturation Transfer

Tumors tend to exhibit high glucose uptake, which forms the basis of FDG-PET. Noninvasive CEST imaging of unlabeled glucose (GlucoCEST) offers an alternative to assess glucose uptake in vivo without the use of ionizing radiation.[100] GlucoCEST rests on selective saturation of the hydroxyl protons of glucose at 1.2, 2.1, and 2.9 ppm. In two colorectal cancer models (LS174T and SW1222), GlucoCEST images taken 60 minutes after glucose infusion (1.1 mmol/kg, intraperitoneally) shows significant correlation with FDG-PET images (r^2 = 0.70; $P<.01$), offering a possible nonradioactive alternative and better spatial resolution (1 × 1 × 3 mm) to probe intratumoral heterogeneity that can readily be translated to GBM and other cancer systems.

Creatine Chemical Exchange Saturation Transfer

Creatine kinase reaction plays a vital role in energetics by regulating adenosine triphosphate reservoir (Cr + adenosine triphosphate + adenosine triphosphate + phosphocreatine + H^+). Reduced total Cre concentration has been shown to be a predictor for gliomas progression.[101–103] With traditional MRS techniques, it is possible to detect the total Cre (Cr + phosphocreatine), but not the individual components. CrEST imaging provides a way to assess the free Cre level in vivo with much improved spatial and temporal resolution.[104] However, quantification using only asymmetry analysis would be problematic owing to contributions from semisolid magnetization transfer and aliphatic nuclear Overhauser effect. So, the entire Z-spectrums for each pixel must be acquired for Lorentzian spectral fitting (5 components: free water, bound water, CrEST ~2 ppm, magnetization transfer, and CEST), which could lead to greatly increased scan time (~30 minutes for the brain). After fitting, the integral of Cre component in the brain tumor region was shown to decrease with disease progression in an intracranial cancer model, consistent with previous studies. And interestingly, the tumor margin as defined by the Cre map is sometimes larger than those obtained from traditional MR imaging contrast, such as proton density image, which may indicate that tumor could have negative impacts on the energetics of surrounding tissues.[105]

Amide Proton Transfer

CEST imaging of amide protons is based on saturation at 3.5 ppm from the water peak. Termed amide proton transfer, it is assumed to originate from the exchangeable amide protons of mobile tissue proteins and peptides. In tumors, amide proton transfer contrast increases as the tumor progresses, presumably owing to increased cellular amide proton content compared with normal tissues, whereas intracellular pH stays relatively constant.[94,105–108] In ischemic models, however, the amide proton transfer contrast is lower compared with the normal tissues, which could be attributed to lower amide proton exchange rate resulting from decreased intracellular pH.[109,110]

Paramagnetic Chemical Exchange Saturation Transfer

ParaCEST agents are mainly metal ion complexes, which offers protons exchanging slow enough for detection (eg, lanthanide groups, iron, and nickel). Aside from having a large chemical shift away from the bulk water pool, paraCEST agents can be designed to target specific biological processes and improve detection sensitivity by polymerization to increase the number of exchange sites per mole. They have been used to measure tissue pH, temperature, and enzymatic activity, as well as specific metabolite levels. But because paraCEST agents are administered exogenously, tissue perfusion and clearance tend to complicate the quantification of CEST contrast. One example of paraCEST agent for in vivo glioma detection is based on dendrimer labeled with Europium CEST agents and fluorescent labels for dual modality imaging ([DyLight 680]-Eu-G5PAMAM).[111] Ali and colleagues[111] have shown the paraCEST agent could be detected in the tumor region after around 10 minutes, primarily due to an impaired blood–brain barrier in the glioma models.

Superparamagnetic Iron Oxide Nanoparticles

Superparamagnetic iron oxide nanoparticles (SPION) act as T2-shortening agents, providing negative contrasts in MR imaging. They are available commercially and have been used extensively for cell labeling after modifications.[112,113] Recently, SPION has been conjugated with recombinant human epidermal growth factor for the in vivo detection of brain malignancies in C6 glioma models that overexpress epidermal growth factor receptor.[114] After 24 hours after intravenous injection (0.3 mg/kg), SPION–epidermal growth factor showed much better accumulation inside the tumor region compared with bare SPIONs; reflected laser scanning revealed internalization of SPION–epidermal growth factor inside the glioma cell cytoplasm.[114] It has also been shown that radiation sensitizes the glioma model for better uptake of SPIONs conjugated with antibodies targeting membrane heat shock protein 70.[115] These early preclinical studies were promising applications of SPIONs, but toxicity issues need to be further addressed before in vivo applications in human.

HYPERPOLARIZED XENON IMAGING IN THE BRAIN

Hyperpolarized xenon-129 (Xe)[116] has been developed for biomedical MR imaging over the last 25 years, with most emphasis on void-space and pulmonary imaging.[117,118] Because inhaled (or injected) xenon travels readily to the brain (and acts as an anesthetic),[119] it may also function as a novel contrast agent for brain imaging. Indeed, nonpolarized xenon gas has been used for enhancing computed tomography scans of the brain for decades.[120] In recent years, limited MR imaging studies have already successfully shown hyperpolarized ^{129}Xe gas dissolved in the brain tissue. Below is a brief overview of the current state of clinical and preclinical work applying hyperpolarized ^{129}Xe to brain MRS/MR imaging.

^{129}Xe has many physical and magnetic properties that make it well-suited for physiologic imaging. This inert gas (spin = 1/2) is nonradioactive, has no biological background signal, and dissolves readily into blood, tissue, and fat.[121] In fact, xenon's differential solubility (owing to a slight hydrophobicity) may be developed as a form of contrast to distinguish areas of the brain that are rich in water versus lipids.[116] Importantly, ^{129}Xe possesses an incredibly sensitive chemical shift range ($\delta > 7500$ ppm), which makes it well-suited to function as a spectroscopic chemical sensor.[122] Indeed, differences in chemical shift have been shown to distinguish ^{129}Xe inside cryptophane cages that are linked to different biological targets.[123] Furthermore, ^{129}Xe MR spectra are exceedingly simple to analyze, and typically only consist of a handful of sharp, well-resolved NMR peaks that correspond to different chemical and magnetic environments. The relaxation rate (T_1) of ^{129}Xe can also be used to differentiate contact with different tissue types,[124] as well as oxygenated versus deoxygenated blood.[125]

Because of its relatively low gyromagnetic ratio ($\gamma_{Xe}/\gamma_H \sim -0.28$) and natural abundance (~26%) compared with ^{1}H, the signal from ^{129}Xe at thermal equilibrium is insufficient for conventional MR imaging detection. ^{129}Xe gas can be hyperpolarized through spin-exchange optical pumping[126]—a two-step process where angular momentum from resonant, circularly polarized laser light is transferred to the electronic spins of an alkali metal vapor, then subsequently exchanged with the ^{129}Xe nuclei via gas phase collisions. This results in a buildup of ^{129}Xe nuclear spin polarization, which creates MR signal enhancement values of 4 to 5 orders of magnitude compared with thermal equilibrium—allowing ^{129}Xe MRS/MR imaging for biomedical studies. This enhanced signal decays over a time constant (T_1) that depends on the immediate environment of the gas, and can range from a few seconds to several hours. Spin-exchange optical pumping takes place in a dedicated 'hyperpolarizer'[127] that dispenses the polarized gas into a Tedlar bag for administration to the patient; owing to recent improvements in technology and methodology, ^{129}Xe nuclear spin polarization values of greater than 90% have been reported.[128]

Hyperpolarized ^{129}Xe can be administered to patients through either inhalation or intravenous injection, and it has been shown that both methods lead to comparable ^{129}Xe concentrations in the brain.[129] Owing to the decreased invasiveness of the procedure, gas inhalation is typically the method used for in vivo studies. In this case, the patient will inhale as much of the gas as possible (about 0.5 L) along with atmospheric air or O_2, followed by a breath hold (15–60 seconds). The xenon travels from the lungs to the brain relatively quickly (approximately 5 seconds).[130] For preclinical studies, the animal is usually intubated and an MR-compatible respirator controls the administration of the gas. For intravenous injections, the hyperpolarized ^{129}Xe is typically dissolved in saline or an emulsion (such as perflurbon or Intralipid) before injection. As with all hyperpolarized contrast agents, a major constraint is that the nonrenewable enhanced signal decays with time. When held in pristine laboratory conditions, hyperpolarized ^{129}Xe lasts for hours.[131] However, when administered in vivo, the enhanced signal is depleted over the course of about 1 minute owing to interactions with its environment. Indeed, the hyperpolarized T_1 of ^{129}Xe in the blood is only about 5 seconds, owing to the abundance of paramagnetic hemoglobin.[125] Additionally, the very act of acquiring a signal further depletes the magnetization of the contrast agent in a nonrenewable fashion. To combat this, many MR acquisitions take advantage of a 'fast low-angle shot' sequence to mitigate signal losses caused by RF pulsing. The silver lining to this time constraint is that the effective clearance rate of the ^{129}Xe MR signal can be quite fast to allow for multiple studies in a single patient session.

Since the initial demonstration of hyperpolarized ^{129}Xe MR imaging in a rat brain[132] and ^{129}Xe MRS in a human brain[130] in 1997, the field has grown steadily. ^{129}Xe brain MRS typically displays a handful of discernable peaks that can be attributed to ^{129}Xe in the gas phase, dissolved in blood, and dissolved in different brain tissues (ie, gray and white matter).[124,133] It has been shown that xenon has an increased proclivity for gray matter compared with white matter (with different T_1 rates), and perfusion between brain compartments can also be tracked.[124] A range of different administration methods, including inhalation and intravenous injection, have been compared and numerically modeled to show that inhalation is the preferred method of supplying the brain with hyperpolarized ^{129}Xe gas.[124] A differential distribution of ^{129}Xe signal in the cerebral cortex in rats was found after a pain stimulus (and corroborated with ^{1}H MR imaging), which is early work in the development of ^{129}Xe for functional MR imaging.[134] Indeed, ^{129}Xe may be developed further for functional MR imaging through an increase in concentration (owing to increased blood flow to regions of brain activity) and longer ^{129}Xe T_1 values in oxygenated blood (vs deoxygenated blood)[116]—acting as a proxy for blood oxygen level–dependent contrast imaging. It has also been shown that a perfusion deficit, such as one caused by a stroke, can be detected with changes in ^{129}Xe signal. Because ^{129}Xe is a safe, inert, and inhalable contrast agent, it may prove to be a safer MR contrast agent compared with injectable gadolinium-based tracers.[134]

Moving forward, several advances in hyperpolarized ^{129}Xe brain MRS/MR imaging are on the horizon. Most predominantly will be targeted imaging using functionalized biomarkers in the form of a cryptophane complex. As ^{129}Xe diffuses through the cage-shaped molecule, its chemical shift is changed—which allows it to be used as a sensitive chemical sensor that can differentiate whether the cage molecule is attached to a biomarker.[123] However, because the amount of ^{129}Xe associated with these targeted cryptophane cages at a given time is small, the resulting signal is often quite weak. One way around this is through a technique called hyperpolarized CEST, which saturates the "^{129}Xe in cryptophane" resonance while monitoring the increased depletion of the "^{129}Xe gas resonance" as the xenon transfers between the targeted cage complex and the spin reservoir.[135] This method can be used to indirectly detect the presence of low concentrations of transferrable species that are spectroscopically discernable, and has been recently demonstrated to show targeting of the human brain microvascular endothelial cells that comprise the blood–brain barrier.[136] Another potential improvement to detection sensitivity would be through the implementation of a remote detection protocol, where the step of RF encoding of nuclear spins is physically separated from the signal detection. This can be used to improve sensitivity through optimizing the detection filling factor; under this scenario, ^{129}Xe in the entire brain would be encoded at once, but then detected using a small surface coil placed over the jugular vein to monitor the ^{129}Xe as it exits the brain.[137]

Hyperpolarized xenon imaging applications in the brain are still at a nascent stage but this is a promising area that may provide some innovative applications to interrogate brain functions in real-time.

SUMMARY

This article reviews the existing and emerging techniques of interrogating metabolism in brain cancer from well-established proton MRS to the promising hyperpolarized metabolic imaging, GlucoCEST, hyperpolarized CEST, and imaging inflammation. Many of these techniques are at an early stage of development and clinical trials using these techniques are in progress in brain cancer patients to establish the clinical efficacy of these techniques. Nonetheless, it is likely that in vivo metabolomics and metabolic imaging is the next frontier in brain cancer diagnosis and assessing therapeutic efficacy; with the combined knowledge of genomics and proteomics a complete understanding of tumorigenesis in brain might be achieved.

REFERENCES

1. Bennett A. Growing pains for metabolomics. Scientist 2005;19:25-8.
2. DeBerardinis RJ, Mancuso A, Daikhin E, et al. Beyond aerobic glycolysis: transformed cells can engage in glutamine metabolism that exceeds the requirement for protein and nucleotide synthesis. Proc Natl Acad Sci U S A 2007;104:19345-50.
3. Elkhaled A, Jalbert LE, Phillips JJ, et al. Magnetic resonance of 2-hydroxyglutarate in IDH1-mutated low-grade gliomas. Sci Transl Med 2012;4: 116ra5.
4. De Graaf RA. In vivo NMR spectroscopy: principles and techniques. 2nd edition. Chichester, West Sussex (United Kingdom): John Wiley & Sons; 2007.
5. Zhu H, Barker PB. MR spectroscopy and spectroscopic imaging of the brain. Methods Mol Biol 2011;711:203-26.
6. Glunde K, Bhujwalla ZM, Ronen SM. Choline metabolism in malignant transformation. Nat Rev Cancer 2011;11:835-48.
7. Warburg O. On the origin of cancer cells. Science 1956;123:309-14.
8. Zoula S, Herigault G, Ziegler A, et al. Correlation between the occurrence of 1H-MRS lipid signal, necrosis and lipid droplets during C6 rat glioma development. NMR Biomed 2003;16:199-212.
9. Remy C, Arus C, Ziegler A, et al. In vivo, ex vivo, and in vitro one- and two-dimensional nuclear magnetic resonance spectroscopy of an intracerebral glioma in rat brain: assignment of resonances. J Neurochem 1994;62:166-79.
10. Dang L, White DW, Gross S, et al. Cancer-associated IDH1 mutations produce 2-hydroxyglutarate. Nature 2009;462:739-44.
11. Bouzier AK, Quesson B, Valeins H, et al. [1-(13)C] glucose metabolism in the tumoral and nontumoral cerebral tissue of a glioma-bearing rat. J Neurochem 1999;72:2445-55.
12. Marin-Valencia I, Yang C, Mashimo T, et al. Analysis of tumor metabolism reveals mitochondrial glucose oxidation in genetically diverse human glioblastomas in the mouse brain in vivo. Cell Metab 2012; 15:827-37.
13. Mashimo T, Pichumani K, Vemireddy V, et al. Acetate is a bioenergetic substrate for human glioblastoma and brain metastases. Cell 2014;159: 1603-14.
14. Nelson SJ. Assessment of therapeutic response and treatment planning for brain tumors using metabolic and physiological MRI. NMR Biomed 2011;24:734-49.
15. Nelson SJ, Ozhinsky E, Li Y, et al. Strategies for rapid in vivo 1H and hyperpolarized 13C MR spectroscopic imaging. J Magn Reson 2013;229:187-97.
16. Fulham MJ, Bizzi A, Dietz MJ, et al. Mapping of brain tumor metabolites with proton MR spectroscopic imaging: clinical relevance. Radiology 1992;185:675-86.
17. Negendank WG, Sauter R, Brown TR, et al. Proton magnetic resonance spectroscopy in patients with glial tumors: a multicenter study. J Neurosurg 1996; 84:449-58.
18. Dowling C, Bollen AW, Noworolski SM, et al. Preoperative proton MR spectroscopic imaging of brain tumors: correlation with histopathologic analysis of resection specimens. AJNR Am J Neuroradiol 2001;22:604-12.
19. Louis DN, Ohgaki H, Wiestler OD, et al. The 2007 WHO classification of tumours of the central nervous system. Acta Neuropathol 2007;114:97-109.
20. Di Costanzo A, Scarabino T, Trojsi F, et al. Multiparametric 3T MR approach to the assessment of cerebral gliomas: tumor extent and malignancy. Neuroradiology 2006;48:622-31.
21. Di Costanzo A, Trojsi F, Giannatempo GM, et al. Spectroscopic, diffusion and perfusion magnetic resonance imaging at 3.0 Tesla in the delineation of glioblastomas: preliminary results. J Exp Clin Cancer Res 2006;25:383-90.
22. Chang SM, Nelson S, Vandenberg S, et al. Integration of preoperative anatomic and metabolic physiologic imaging of newly diagnosed glioma. J Neurooncol 2009;92:401-15.
23. Croteau D, Scarpace L, Hearshen D, et al. Correlation between magnetic resonance

spectroscopy imaging and image-guided biopsies: semiquantitative and qualitative histopathological analyses of patients with untreated glioma. Neurosurgery 2001;49:823–9.

24. McKnight TR, Noworolski SM, Vigneron DB, et al. An automated technique for the quantitative assessment of 3D-MRSI data from patients with glioma. J Magn Reson Imaging 2001;13:167–77.

25. Caivano R, Lotumolo A, Rabasco P, et al. 3 Tesla magnetic resonance spectroscopy: cerebral gliomas vs. metastatic brain tumors. Our experience and review of the literature. Int J Neurosci 2013;123:537–43.

26. Venkatesh SK, Gupta RK, Pal L, et al. Spectroscopic increase in choline signal is a nonspecific marker for differentiation of infective/inflammatory from neoplastic lesions of the brain. J Magn Reson Imaging 2001;14:8–15.

27. Li X, Jin H, Lu Y, et al. Identification of MRI and 1H MRSI parameters that may predict survival for patients with malignant gliomas. NMR Biomed 2004; 17:10–20.

28. Hattingen E, Delic O, Franz K, et al. 1)H MRSI and progression-free survival in patients with WHO grades II and III gliomas. Neurol Res 2010;32:593–602.

29. Chan AA, Lau A, Pirzkall A, et al. Proton magnetic resonance spectroscopy imaging in the evaluation of patients undergoing gamma knife surgery for Grade IV glioma. J Neurosurg 2004;101:467–75.

30. Alexander A, Murtha A, Abdulkarim B, et al. Prognostic significance of serial magnetic resonance spectroscopies over the course of radiation therapy for patients with malignant glioma. Clin Invest Med 2006;29:301–11.

31. Shariatgorji M, Svenningsson P, Andrén PE. Mass spectrometry imaging, an emerging technology in neuropsychopharmacology. Neuropsychopharmacology 2014;39:34–49.

32. Nakamizo S, Sasayama T, Shinohara M, et al. GC/MS-based metabolomics analysis of cerebrospinal fluid (CSF) from glioma patients. J Neurooncol 2013;113:65–74.

33. Wibom C, Surowiec I, Moren L, et al. Metabolomic patterns in glioblastoma and changes during radiotherapy: a clinical microdialysis study. J Proteome Res 2010;9:2909–19.

34. Tabatabaei P, Bergstrom P, Henriksson R, et al. Glucose metabolites, glutamate and glycerol in malignant glioma tumors during radiotherapy. J Neurooncol 2008;90:35–9.

35. Moren L, Bergenheim AT, Ghasimi S, et al. Metabolomic screening of tumor tissue and serum in glioma patients reveals diagnostic and prognostic information. Metabolites 2015;5:502–20.

36. Locasale JW, Melman T, Song S, et al. Metabolomics of human cerebrospinal fluid identifies signatures of malignant glioma. Mol Cell Proteomics 2012;11. M111.014688.

37. Chinnaiyan P, Kensicki E, Bloom G, et al. The metabolomic signature of malignant glioma reflect accelerated anabolic metabolism. Cancer Res 2012;72:5878–88.

38. Ross B, Lin A, Harris K, et al. Clinical experience with 13C MRS in vivo. NMR Biomed 2003;16: 358–69.

39. Maher EA, Marin-Valencia I, Bachoo RM, et al. Metabolism of [U-13C] glucose in human brain tumors in vivo. NMR Biomed 2012;25:1234–44.

40. Ardenkjaer-Larsen JH, Fridlund B, Gram A, et al. Increase in signal-to-noise ratio of > 10,000 times in liquid-state NMR. Proc Natl Acad Sci U S A 2003;100:10158–63.

41. Kurhanewicz J, Vigneron DB, Brindle K, et al. Analysis of cancer metabolism by imaging hyperpolarized nuclei: prospects for translation to clinical research. Neoplasia 2011;13:81–97.

42. Bhattacharya P, Chekmenev EY, Perman WH, et al. Towards hyperpolarized 13C-succinate imaging of brain cancer. J Magn Reson 2007;186:150–5.

43. Chaumeil MM, Larson PE, Yoshihara HA, et al. Noninvasive in vivo assessment of IDH1 mutational status in glioma. Nat Commun 2013;4:2429.

44. Chaumeil MM, Larson PE, Woods SM, et al. Hyperpolarized [1-13C] glutamate: a metabolic imaging biomarker of IDH1 mutational status in glioma. Cancer Res 2014;74:4247–57.

45. Park I, Larson PEZ, Zierhut ML, et al. Hyperpolarized 13C magnetic resonance metabolic imaging: application to brain tumors. Neuro Oncol 2010;12: 133–44.

46. Park I, Hu S, Bok R, et al. Evaluation of heterogeneous metabolic profile in an orthotopic human glioblastoma xenograft model using compressed sensing hyperpolarized 3D 13C magnetic resonance spectroscopic imaging. Magn Reson Med 2013;70:33–9.

47. Park I, Larson PE, Tropp JL, et al. Dynamic hyperpolarized carbon-13 MR metabolic imaging of nonhuman primate brain. Magn Reson Med 2014; 71:19–25.

48. Nelson SJ, Kurhanewicz J, Vigneron DB, et al. Metabolic imaging of patients with prostate cancer using hyperpolarized [1-13C]pyruvate. Sci Transl Med 2014;5:198ra108.

49. Yan H, Parsons DW, Jin G, et al. IDH1 and IDH2 mutations in gliomas. N Engl J Med 2009;360: 765–73.

50. Choi C, Ganji SK, DeBerardinis RJ, et al. 2-hydroxyglutarate detection by magnetic resonance spectroscopy in IDH-mutated patients with gliomas. Nat Med 2012;18:624–9.

51. Zielke HR, Zielke CL, Baab PJ. Direct measurement of oxidative metabolism in the living brain by microdialysis: a review. J Neurochem 2009; 109(Suppl 1):24–9.

52. Waniewski RA, Martin DL. Preferential utilization of acetate by astrocytes is attributable to transport. J Neurosci 1998;18:5225–33.

53. Wyss MT, Magistretti PJ, Buck A, et al. Labeled acetate as a marker of astrocytic metabolism. J Cereb Blood Flow Metab 2011;31:1668–74.

54. Deelchand DK, Shestov AA, Koski DM, et al. Acetate transport and utilization in the rat brain. J Neurochem 2009;109:46–54.

55. Bluml S, Moreno-Torres A, Shic F, et al. Tricarboxylic acid cycle of glia in the in vivo human brain. NMR Biomed 2002;15:1–5.

56. Sailasuta N, Harris K, Tran T, et al. Minimally invasive biomarker confirms glial activation present in Alzheimer's disease: a preliminary study. Neuropsychiatr Dis Treat 2011;7:495–9.

57. Sailasuta N, Tran TT, Harris KC, et al. Swift Acetate Glial Assay (SAGA): an accelerated human 13C MRS brain exam for clinical diagnostic use. J Magn Reson 2010;207:352–5.

58. Comerford SA, Huang Z, Du X, et al. Acetate dependence of tumors. Cell 2014;159:1591–602.

59. Lyssiotis CA, Cantley LC. Acetate fuels the cancer engine. Cell 2014;159(7):1492–4.

60. Brindle K. Watching tumours gasp and die with MRI: the promise of hyperpolarised 13C MR spectroscopic imaging. Br J Radiol 2012;85:697–708.

61. Harada M, Kubo H, Abe T, et al. Selection of endogenous 13C substrates for observation of intracellular metabolism using the dynamic nuclear polarization technique. Jpn J Radiol 2010; 28:173–9.

62. Bastiaansen JA, Cheng T, Mishkovsky M, et al. In vivo enzymatic activity of acetylCoA synthetase in skeletal muscle revealed by (13)C turnover from hyperpolarized [1-(13)C]acetate to [1-(13)C] acetylcarnitine. Biochim Biophys Acta 2013;1830: 4171–8.

63. Flori A, Liserani M, Bowen S, et al. Dissolution dynamic nuclear polarization of non-self-glassing agents: spectroscopy and relaxation of hyperpolarized [1-(13)c]acetate. J Phys Chem A 2015;119: 1885–93.

64. Vuichoud B, Milani J, Bornet A, et al. Hyperpolarization of deuterated metabolites via remote cross-polarization and dissolution dynamic nuclear polarization. J Phys Chem B 2014;118:1411–5.

65. Koellisch U, Laustsen C, Norlinger TS, et al. Investigation of metabolic changes in STZ-induced diabetic rats with hyperpolarized [1-13C]acetate. Physiol Rep 2015;3:1–9.

66. Lee Y, Zacharias NM, Piwnica-Worms D, et al. Chemical Reaction-Induced Multi-molecular Polarization (CRIMP). Chem Commun (Camb) 2014; 50(86):13030–3.

67. Ball DR, Rowlands B, Dodd MS, et al. Hyperpolarized butyrate: a metabolic probe of short chain fatty acid metabolism in the heart. Magn Reson Med 2014;71:1663–9.

68. Ross BD, Bhattacharya P, Wagner S, et al. Hyperpolarized MR imaging: neurologic applications of hyperpolarized metabolism. AJNR Am J Neuroradiol 2010;31:24–33.

69. Mishkovsky M, Cheng T, Comment A, et al. Localized in vivo hyperpolarization transfer sequences. Magn Reson Med 2012;68:349–52.

70. Park J, Josan S, Jang T, et al. Metabolite kinetics in C6 rat glioma model using magnetic resonance spectroscopic imaging of hyperpolarized [1-13 C] pyruvate. Magn Reson Med 2012;68:1886–93.

71. Day SE, Kettunen MI, Cherukuri MK, et al. Detecting response of rat C6 glioma tumors to radiotherapy using hyperpolarized [1-13C]pyruvate and 13C magnetic resonance spectroscopic imaging. Magn Reson Med 2011;65:557–63.

72. Park I, Bok R, Ozawa T, et al. Detection of early response to temozolomide treatment in brain tumors using hyperpolarized 13C MR metabolic imaging. J Magn Reson Imaging 2011;33: 1284–90.

73. Park I, Mukherjee J, Ito M, et al. Changes in pyruvate metabolism detected by magnetic resonance imaging are linked to DNA damage and serve as a sensor of temozolomide response in glioblastoma cells. Cancer Res 2014;74:7115–24.

74. Chaumeil MM, Ozawa T, Park I, et al. Hyperpolarized 13C MR spectroscopic imaging can be used to monitor Everolimus treatment in vivo in an orthotopic rodent model of glioblastoma. Neuroimage 2012;59:193–201.

75. Ronen SM, Izquierdo-Garcia JL, Chaumeil MM, et al. Metabolic Imaging Biomarkers For Mutant Idh1 Gliomas. Neuro Oncol 2014;16(Suppl 3):Iii12.

76. Venkatesh HS, Chaumeil MM, Ward CS, et al. Reduced phosphocholine and hyperpolarized lactate provide magnetic resonance biomarkers of PI3K/Akt/mTOR inhibition in glioblastoma. Neuro Oncol 2012;14:315–25.

77. Park JM, Recht LD, Josan S, et al. Metabolic response of glioma to dichloroacetate measured in vivo by hyperpolarized 13C magnetic resonance spectroscopic imaging. Neuro Oncol 2013;15: 433–41.

78. Yan J, Kong LY, Gabrusiewicz K, et al. FGL2 as a multimodality regulator of tumor-mediated immune suppression and therapeutic target in gliomas. J Natl Cancer Inst 2015;107(8). pii: djv137.

79. Xu S, Wei J, Wang F, et al. Effect of miR-142-3p on the M2 macrophage and therapeutic efficacy against murine glioblastoma. J Natl Cancer Inst 2014;106(8). pii: dju162.

80. Wu A, Wei J, Kong LY, et al. Glioma cancer stem cells induce immunosupressive macrophages/microglia. Neuro Oncol 2010;12(11):1113–25.

81. Heimberger AB, Abou-Ghazal M, Reina-Ortiz C, et al. Incidence and prognostic impact of FoxP3+ regulatory T cells in human gliomas. Clin Cancer Res 2008;14(16):5166–72.

82. Fecci PE, Mitchell DA, Whitesides JF, et al. Increased regulatory T-cell fraction amidst a diminished CD4 compartment explains cellular immune defects in patients with malignant glioma. Cancer Res 2006;66(6):3294–302.

83. Garber ST, Hashimoto Y, Weathers SP, et al. Immune checkpoint blockade as a potential therapeutic target: surveying CNS malignancies. Neuro Oncol 2016. pii: now132.

84. Nduom EK, Wei J, Yaghi NK, et al. PD-L1 expression and prognostic impact in glioblastoma. Neuro Oncol 2016;18(2):195–205.

85. Reardon DA, Gokhale PC, Klein SR, et al. Glioblastoma eradication following immune checkpoint blockade in an orthotopic, immunocompetent model. Cancer Immunol Res 2016;4(2):124–35.

86. Wainwright DA, Chang AL, Dey M, et al. Durable therapeutic efficacy utilizing combinatorial blockade against IDO, CTLA-4, and PD-L1 in mice with brain tumors. Clin Cancer Res 2014; 20(20):5290–301.

87. Huang RY, Neagu MR, Reardon DA, et al. Pitfalls in the neuroimaging of glioblastoma in the era of anti-angiogenic and immuno/targeted therapy- detecting illusive disease, defining response. Front Neurol 2015;6:33.

88. Zakszewski E, Schmit B, Kurpad S, et al. Diffusion imaging in the rat cervical spinal cord. J Vis Exp 2015;98:52390.

89. Budde MD, Shah A, McCrea M, et al. Primary blast traumatic brain injury in the rat: relating diffusion tensor imaging and behavior. Front Neurol 2013; 4:154.

90. Serres S, O'Brien ER, Sibson NR. Imaging angiogenesis, inflammation, and metastasis in the tumor microenvironment with magnetic resonance imaging. Adv Exp Med Biol 2014;772:263–83.

91. Rodriguez E, Nilges M, Weissleder R, et al. Activatable magnetic Resonance imaging agents for myeloperoxidase sensing: mechanism of activation, stability, and toxicity. J Am Chem Soc 2010;132: 168–77.

92. Chen JW, Breckwoldt MO, Aikawa E, et al. Myeloperoxidase targeted imaging of active inflammatory lesions in murine experimental autoimmune encephalomyelitis. Brain 2014;131:1123–33.

93. Stadler KL, Ober CP, Feeney DA, et al. Multivoxel proton magnetic Resonance spectroscopy of inflammatory and neoplastic lesions of the canine brain at 3.0 T. Am J Vet Res 2014;75:982–9.

94. Van Zijl PC, Yadav NN. Chemical exchange saturation transfer (CEST): what is in a name and what isn't? Magn Reson Med 2011;65:927–48.

95. Kim J, Wu Y, Guo Y, et al. A review of optimization and quantification techniques for chemical exchange saturation transfer MRI toward sensitive in vivo imaging. Contrast Media Mol Imaging 2015;10:163–78.

96. Sontheimer H. A role for glutamate in growth and invasion of primary brain tumors. J Neurochem 2008;105:287–95.

97. de Groot J, Sontheimer H. Glutamate and the biology of gliomas. Glia 2011;59:1181–9.

98. Cai K, Haris M, Singh A, et al. Magnetic resonance imaging of glutamate. Nat Med 2012;18:302–6.

99. Crescenzi R, DeBrosse C, Nanga RP, et al. In vivo measurement of glutamate loss is associated with synapse loss in a mouse model of tauopathy. Neuroimage 2014;101:185–92.

100. Walker-Samuel S, Ramasawmy R, Torrealdea F, et al. In vivo imaging of glucose uptake and metabolism in tumors. Nat Med 2013;19:1067–72.

101. Hattingen E, Raab P, Franz K, et al. Prognostic value of choline and creatine in WHO grade II gliomas. Neuroradiology 2008;50:759–67.

102. Usenius JP, Vainio P, Hernesniemi J, et al. Choline-containing compounds in human astrocytomas studied by 1H NMR spectroscopy in vivo and in vitro. J Neurochem 1994;63:1538–43.

103. Chang L, McBride D, Miller BL, et al. Localized in vivo 1H magnetic resonance spectroscopy and in vitro analyses of heterogeneous brain tumors. J Neuroimaging 1995;5:157–63.

104. Haris M, Singh A, Cai K, et al. A technique for in vivo mapping of myocardial creatine kinase metabolism. Nat Med 2014;20:209–14.

105. Cai K, Singh A, Poptani H, et al. CEST signal at 2ppm (CEST@2ppm) from Z-spectral fitting correlates with creatine distribution in brain tumor. NMR Biomed 2015;28:1–8.

106. Zhou J, Lai B, Wilson DA, et al. Amide proton transfer (APT) contrast for imaging of brain tumors. Magn Reson Med 2003;50:1120–6.

107. Gillies R, Raghunand N, Garcia-Martin ML, et al. pH imaging. A review of pH measurement methods and applications in cancers. IEEE Eng Med Biol Mag 2004;23:57–64.

108. Sagiyama K, Mashimo T, Togao O, et al. In vivo chemical exchange saturation transfer imaging allows early detection of a therapeutic response in glioblastoma. Proc Natl Acad Sci U S A 2014;111:4542–7.

109. Ling W, Eliav U, Navon G, et al. Chemical exchange saturation transfer by intermolecular double-quantum coherence. J Magn Reson 2008; 194:29–32.

110. Yan G, Kléber AG. Changes in extracellular and intracellular pH in ischemic rabbit papillary-muscle. Circ Res 1992;71:460–70.

111. Ali MM, Bhuiyan MP, Janic B, et al. A nano-sized PARACEST-fluorescence imaging contrast agent

facilitates and validates in vivo CEST MRI detection of glioma. Nanomedicine (Lond) 2012;7:1827–37.

112. Li L, Jiang W, Luo K, et al. Superparamagnetic iron oxide nanoparticles as MRI contrast agents for non-invasive stem cell labeling and tracking. Theranostics 2013;3:595–615.

113. Chen CC, Ku MC, Jayaseema DM, et al. Simple SPION incubation as an efficient intracellular labeling method for tracking neural progenitor cells using MRI. PLoS One 2013;8:e56125.

114. Shevtsov MA, Nikolaev BP, Yakovleva LY, et al. Superparamagnetic iron oxide nanoparticles conjugated with epidermal growth factor (SPION-EGF) for targeting brain tumors. Int J Nanomedicine 2014;9: 273–87.

115. Shevtsov MA, Nikolaev BP, Ryzhov VA, et al. Ionizing radiation improves glioma-specific targeting of superparamagnetic iron oxide nanoparticles conjugated with cmHsp70.1 monoclonal antibodies (SPION–cmHsp70.1). Nanoscale 2015; 7(48):20652–64.

116. Goodson BM. Nuclear magnetic resonance of laser-polarized noble gases in molecules, materials, and organisms. J Magn Reson 2002;155: 157–216.

117. Albert MS, Gates GD, Driehuys B, et al. Biological magnetic resonance imaging using laser-polarized ^{129}Xe. Nature 1994;370:199–201.

118. Mugler JP III, Altes TA, Ruset IC, et al. Simultaneous magnetic resonance imaging of ventilation distribution and gas uptake in the human lung using hyperpolarized xenon-129. Proc Natl Acad Sci U S A 2010;107:21707–12.

119. Franks NP, Dickinson R, de Sousa SLM, et al. How does xenon produce anaesthesia? Nature 1998; 396:324.

120. Drayer BP, Wolfson SK, Reinmuth OM, et al. Xenon enhanced CT for analysis of cerebral integrity, perfusion, and blood flow. Stroke 1978;9.2:123–30.

121. Cherubini A, Bifone A. Hyperpolarized xenon in biology. Prog Nucl Magn Reson Spectrosc 2003; 42:1–30.

122. PeitraiB T, Gaede HC. Optically polarized ^{129}Xe in NMR spectroscopy. Adv Mater 1995;7:826–38.

123. Spence MM, Rubin SM, Dimitrov IE, et al. Functionalized xenon as a biosensor. Proc Natl Acad Sci U S A 2001;98:10654–7.

124. Kilian W, Seifert F, Rinneberg H. Dynamic NMR spectroscopy of hyperpolarized ^{129}Xe in human brain analyzed by an uptake model. Magn Reson Med 2004;51:843–7.

125. Wolber J, Cherubini A, Dzik-Jurasz ASK, et al. Spin-lattice relaxation of laser-polarized Xenon in human blood. Proc Natl Acad Sci U S A 1999;96: 3664–9.

126. Walker TG, Happer W. Spin-exchange optical pumping of Noble-Gas Nuclei. Rev Mod Phys 1997;69:629–42.

127. Ruset IC, Ketel S, Hersman FW. Optical pumping system design for large production of hyperpolarized ^{129}Xe. Phys Rev Lett 2006;96:053002.

128. Nikolaou P, Coffey AM, Walkup LL, et al. Near-unity nuclear polarization with an open-source ^{129}Xe hyperpolarizer for NMR and MRI. Proc Natl Acad Sci U S A 2013;110:14150–5.

129. Lavini C, Payne GS, Leach MO, et al. Intravenous delivery of hyperpolarized ^{129}Xe: a compartmental model. NMR Biomed 2000;13:238–44.

130. Mugler JP III, Driehuys B, Brookeman JR, et al. MR imaging and spectroscopy using hyperpolarized ^{129}Xe gas: preliminary human results. Magn Reson Med 1997;37:809–15.

131. Anger BC, Schrank G, Schoeck A, et al. Gas-phase spin relaxation of ^{129}Xe. Phys Rev A 2008;78: 043406.

132. Swanson SD, Rosen MS, Agranoff BW, et al. Brain MRI with laser-polarized ^{129}Xe. Magn Reson Med 1997;38:695–8.

133. Mazzanti M, Walvick RP, Zhou X, et al. Distribution of hyperpolarized xenon in the brain following sensory stimulation: preliminary MRI findings. PLoS One 2011;6:e21607.

134. Zhou X, Sun Y, Mazzanti M, et al. MRI of stroke using hyperpolarized ^{129}Xe. NMR Biomed 2010;24: 170–5.

135. Witte C, Martos V, Rose HM, et al. Live-cell MRI with xenon hyper-CEST biosensors targeted to metabolically-labeled cell-surface glycans. Angew Chem Int Ed Engl 2015;54:2806–10.

136. Schnurr M, Sydow K, Rose HM, et al. Brain endothelial cell targeting via a peptide-functionalized liposomal carrier for Xenon Hyper-CEST MRI. Adv Healthc Mater 2015;4:40–5.

137. Harel E, Schroder L, Xu S. Novel detection schemes of nuclear magnetic resonance and magnetic resonance imaging: applications from analytical chemistry to molecular sensors. Annu Rev Anal Chem (Palo Alto Calif) 2008;1: 133–63.

Response Assessment in Neuro-Oncology Criteria and Clinical Endpoints

Raymond Y. Huang, MD, PhD[a],*, Patrick Y. Wen, MD[b]

KEYWORDS

• RANO • Response assessment • Endpoints • Gliomas • Brain metastases

KEY POINTS

- The Response Assessment in Neuro-Oncology (RANO) Working Group is an international multidisciplinary group whose goal is to improve response criteria and define endpoints for neuro-oncology trials.
- The RANO criteria for high-grade gliomas attempt to address the issues of pseudoprogression, pseudoresponse, and nonenhancing tumor progression but remain a work in progress.
- RANO criteria have been developed for brain metastases and are in progress for meningiomas, leptomeningeal disease, spinal tumors, and pediatric tumors.
- The RANO group has also developed criteria for neurologic response (Neurologic Assessment in Neuro-Oncology [NANO]) and immunologic therapies (Immunotherapy RANO [iRANO]), and criteria for seizures and steroid use are in progress.

BACKGROUND AND SUMMARY OF CURRENT RESPONSE ASSESSMENT IN NEURO-ONCOLOGY CRITERIA

Progress in improving therapies for patients with brain tumors has been limited not only by the lack of effective treatments but also by the limitations and variability of the available response criteria used in clinical trials. The RANO Working Group was established in 2008 to address some of these limitations. The work of the RANO group has recently been summarized.[1]

After its introduction in 1990, the Macdonald criteria,[2] which used the product of the maximal cross-sectional enhancing diameters as the primary measure of tumor size, were widely adopted in neuro-oncology clinical trials. It gradually became clear, however, that the Macdonald criteria had several important limitations.[3,4] They included the failure account for pseudoprogression after chemoradiotherapy, a lack of definitions of measurable and nonmeasurable disease, and failure to assess nonenhancing tumor and pseudoresponse in patients who received antiangiogenic therapies, such as bevacizumab that reduced vascular permeability and contrast enhancement.[3,4] In 2010 the RANO criteria for

Disclosures: Dr R.Y. Huang is a consultant for Celldex Therapeutics and Agios Pharmaceuticas. Dr P.Y. Wen provides research support to Angiochem, Agios, AstraZeneca, Exelixis, Genentech/Roche, GlaxoSmithKline, Karyopharm, Merck, Novartis, Sanofi-Aventis, and Vascular Biogenics; he serves on the advisory board for Agios, Cavion, Cortice Bioscience, Genentech/Roche, Monteris, Novartis, Novocure, Regeneron, and Vascular Biogenic; he is a speaker at Merck and is on the data safety committee at Monteris and Tocagen.
[a] Division of Neuroradiology, Department of Radiology, Brigham and Women's Hospital, Harvard Medical School, 75 Francis Street, Boston, MA 02115, USA; [b] Division of Neuro-Oncology, Department of Neurology, Center for Neuro-Oncology, Dana-Farber/Brigham and Women's Cancer Center, Brigham and Women's Hospital, Harvard Medical School, Boston, MA 02215, USA
* Corresponding author.
E-mail address: ryhuang@partners.org

Magn Reson Imaging Clin N Am 24 (2016) 705–718
http://dx.doi.org/10.1016/j.mric.2016.06.003
1064-9689/16/© 2016 Elsevier Inc. All rights reserved.

high-grade gliomas were published to address some of the limitations of the Macdonald criteria[4] (**Box 1, Table 1**). As with the Macdonald criteria, the RANO criteria continued to use the product of the maximal cross-sectional enhancing diameters as the primary measure of tumor size and also took into account corticosteroid use and clinical status. The key features of the RANO criteria included

1. Definition of measurable disease as contrast-enhancing lesions with clearly defined margins by CT or MR imaging scan, with 2 perpendicular diameters of at least 10 mm, visible on 2 or more axial slices that are preferably, at most, 5 mm apart with 0-mm skip. Nonmeasurable disease was defined as either unidimensionally measurable lesions, masses with margins not clearly defined, or lesions with maximal perpendicular diameters less than 10 mm.
2. Allowing up to 5 measurable lesions
3. Introducing a minimum requirement for entry into clinical trials for recurrent gliomas by requiring a 25% increase in the sum of the products of perpendicular diameters of the contrast-enhancing lesions while on stable or increasing doses of corticosteroids
4. Addressing pseudoprogression by excluding patients within the first 12 weeks after completion of radiotherapy from clinical trials for recurrent disease unless the progression is clearly outside the radiation field (eg, beyond the high-dose region or 80% isodose line) or if there is pathologic confirmation of disease progression
5. Addressing "pseudoresponse" by requiring a repeat scan at 4 weeks or later to confirm the response
6. Introducing the concept of nonenhancing tumor progression. For patients to achieve a partial or complete response, in addition to 50% reduction or disappearance of the contrast-enhancing disease, respectively, there could not be an increase in the amount of nonenhancing tumor. For progression, in addition to a 25% increase in the sum of the products of perpendicular diameters of enhancing lesions compared with the smallest tumor measurement obtained either at baseline or best response, on stable or increasing doses of corticosteroids, a significant increase in T2/fluid-attenuated inversion recovery (FLAIR) nonenhancing lesion not caused by comorbid events (eg, radiation therapy, demyelination, ischemic injury, infection, seizures, postoperative changes, or other treatment effects) could

constitute progression. Given the difficulty in measuring nonenhancing disease, no specific criteria were recommended to determine progression of nonenhancing disease. This subjective assessment of nonenhancing disease remains an important limitation, allowing patients in cases of uncertainty regarding whether there is progression, to continue on treatment and remain under close observation (eg, evaluated at 4-week intervals). If subsequent evaluations suggest that the patient is in fact experiencing progression, then the date of progression is backdated to the time point at which this issue was first raised.

CURRENT ADOPTION OF RESPONSE ASSESSMENT IN NEURO-ONCOLOGY AND CHALLENGES

The RANO criteria have been increasingly adopted to assess response endpoints in recent high-grade glioma clinical trials.[5–12] To date it is not clear whether the new criteria have adequately addressed the challenges arising from pseudoprogression, pseudoresponse, and nonenhancing tumor progression. Although the 12-week cutoff in the RANO criteria seem to help reduce pseudoprogression, there is concern that pseudoprogression can occur beyond the 12-week cutoff. In a prospective series of 56 patients with glioblastoma who demonstrated conventional findings concerning for progression of disease post–radiation treatment, pseudoprogression occurred in 27 of 56 patients as determined by perfusion MR imaging technique, and 8 of these 27 patients (39%) developed pseudoprogression 3 months post–radiation therapy.[13] In this series, the overall survival (OS) was significantly longer in patients with pseudoprogression (35.2 months) compared with those who never experienced pseudoprogression (14.3 months, $P<.001$). These results highlight both the benefit and limitation of the RANO criteria in the assessment of pseudoprogression and modification of the current criteria to more accurately identify the patients with delayed pseudoprogression is necessary.

The impact of the inclusion of T2/FLAIR assessment in the RANO criteria has been examined in several retrospective studies. Radbruch and colleagues[14] evaluated serial MR imaging studies of 144 patients with glioblastoma and reported that 62% of the scans with progression on T2-weighted imaging alone were followed by progression of enhancing lesion during the next follow-up scan, in contrast to 32% of the those showing stable disease. In this study, a 15% threshold of tumor increment on T2-weighted

---

Box 1
Criteria for response assessment incorporating MR imaging and clinical factors

All measurable and nonmeasurable lesions must be assessed using the same techniques as baseline.

Complete response

Requires all of the following:

1. Complete disappearance of all enhancing measurable and nonmeasurable disease sustained for at least 4 weeks

2. No new lesions

3. Stable or improved nonenhancing (T2/FLAIR) lesions

   a. Patients must be off corticosteroids

   b. Stable or improved clinically

Note: Patients with nonmeasurable disease only cannot have a complete response. The best response possible is stable disease.

Partial response

Requires all of the following

1. Greater than or equal to 50% decrease compared with baseline in the sum of products of perpendicular diameters of all measurable enhancing lesions sustained for at least 4 weeks

2. No progression of nonmeasurable disease

3. No new lesions

4. Stable or improved nonenhancing (T2/FLAIR) lesions on same or lower dose of corticosteroids compared with baseline scan

   a. The corticosteroid dose at the time of the scan evaluation should be no greater than the dose at time of baseline scan.

   b. Stable or improved clinically

Note: Patients with nonmeasurable disease only cannot have a partial response. The best response possible is stable disease.

Stable disease

Requires all of the following

1. Does not qualify for complete response, partial response, or progression

2. Stable nonenhancing (T2/FLAIR) lesions on same or lower dose of corticosteroids compared with baseline scan. In the event that the corticosteroid dose has been increased, the last scan considered to show stable disease is the scan obtained when the corticosteroid dose was equivalent to the baseline dose.

   a. Stable clinically

Progression

Defined by any of the following

1. Greater than 25% increase in sum of the products of perpendicular diameters of enhancing lesions compared with the smallest tumor measurement obtained either at baseline (if no decrease) or best response, on stable or increasing doses of corticosteroid[a]

2. Significant increase in T2/FLAIR nonenhancing lesion on stable or increasing doses of corticosteroids compared with baseline scan or best response after initiation of therapy,[a] not due to comorbid events (eg, radiation therapy, demyelination, ischemic injury, infection, seizures, postoperative changes, or other treatment effects)

3. Any new lesion

4. Clear clinical deterioration not attributable to other causes apart from the tumor (eg, seizures, medication side effects, complications of therapy, cerebrovascular events, infection, etc.) or changes in corticosteroid dose

5. Failure to return for evaluation due to death or deteriorating condition

6. Clear progression of nonmeasurable disease

^a Stable doses of corticosteroids include patients not on corticosteroids.
From Wen PY, Macdonald DR, Reardon DA, et al. Updated response assessment criteria for high-grade gliomas: response assessment in neuro-oncology working group. J Clin Oncol 2010;28:1964 and 1969; with permission.

imaging was more superior in detecting relevant tumor progression compared with the 25% threshold, thus providing preliminary evidence that quantitative measurement of T2/FLAIR abnormalities may be an important response assessment endpoint.

In another retrospective study of 78 patients with recurrent glioblastoma treated by irinotecan-bevacizumab, Gállego Pérez-Larraya and colleagues[15] assessed progression by both RANO and Macdonald criteria and concluded that one-third of patients exhibited nonenhancing progression with stable or improved contrast enhancement. Although there was not a significant difference in progression-free survival (PFS) between the 2 criteria in this study, the use of RANO trended toward a shorter PFS. In contrast, a retrospective evaluation of randomized, phase II trial of bevacizumab with irinotecan or temozolomide in recurrent glioblastoma (Radiation Therapy Oncology Group [RTOG] 0625/American College of Radiation Imaging Network [ACRIN] 6677) revealed early progression based on 2-D measurement of enhancing disease after 8 and 16 weeks of therapy was highly associated with OS, whereas measurement based on FLAIR imaging or objective response based on reduction of enhancing disease during early post-treatment period did not correlate with survival outcome.[16]

The impact of T2/FLAIR assessment in the RANO criteria was recently retrospectively evaluated using imaging data of 163 patients from the randomized phase II BRAIN (AVF3708g) trial evaluating bevacizumab or bevacizumab and irinotecan in patients with recurrent glioblastoma.[17] Comparing to the Macdonald criteria, the RANO criteria resulted in 1.8 months shorter median PFS in this trial and captured at least 35% of patients who had nonenhancing tumor progression who would not have been captured in the next sequential imaging relying on Macdonald criteria.

The benefit of earlier detection of nonenhancing radiographic progression needs to be confirmed by determining residual survival benefit. Landmark analyses of progression determined by RANO criteria at 2, 4, and 6 months after bevacizumab treatment correlated with OS, although the exclusion of T2/FLAIR evaluation did not reduce such correlation.[17] With availability of effective post-progression therapies in the future, however, an earlier detection of nonenhancing tumor progression may become clinically important. Furthermore, moderate difference in PFS detected by inclusion of T2/FLAIR may account for the very different outcomes in patient-reported outcomes and neuropsychological testing data from the 2 phase III trials (AVAglio and RTOG 0825)

Table 1
Summary of the Response Assessment in Neuro-Oncology criteria for high-grade gliomas

	Complete Response	Partial Response	Stable Disease	Progressive Disease^a
T1-Gd+	None	≥50% ↓	<50% ↓– <25% ↑	≥25% ↑*
T2/FLAIR	Stable or ↓	Stable or ↓	Stable or ↓	↑*
New lesion	None	None	None	Present*
Corticosteroids	None	Stable or ↓	Stable or ↓	NA
Clinical status	Stable or ↑	Stable or ↑	Stable or ↑	↓*
Requirement for response	All	All	All	Any*

Abbreviations: ↓, decrease; ↑, increase; Gd+, gadolinium; NA, not applicable (increase in corticosteroids alone is not taken into account in determining progression in the absence of persistent clinical deterioration).
^a Progression occurs when any of the criteria with * is present.
From Wen PY, Macdonald DR, Reardon DA, et al. Updated response assessment criteria for high-grade gliomas: response assessment in neuro-oncology working group. J Clin Oncol 2010;28:1970; with permission.

evaluating the role of bevacizumab in newly diagnosed glioblastoma.[18,19] AVAglio used a RANO-like response criteria and found improvement in patient reported outcomes during the period of improved PFS.[18] RTOG 0825 used the Macdonald criteria and found that patients experienced decline in patient-reported outcomes at the end of the period of PFS. It is unclear whether the failure to detect nonenhancing disease progression using the Macdonald criteria may have accounted for this deterioration.[19]

2014 JUMPSTARTING BRAIN TUMOR DRUG DEVELOPMENT COALITION AND FOOD AND DRUG ADMINISTRATION WORKSHOP

In 2014, the Jumpstarting Brain Tumor Drug Development Coalition (JBTDDC), consisting of the National Brain Tumor Society, the Society for Neuro-Oncology, Accelerate Brain Cancer Cure, and the Musella Foundation, held an imaging endpoint workshop with the Food and Drug Administration (FDA).[20] This workshop provided support for the RANO criteria. It also clarified several issues and challenges related to the RANO criteria and imaging endpoints in neuro-oncology.[21] It was thought that single-arm studies using response as an endpoint might potentially be used for accelerated approval for agents that do not significantly affect vascular permeability, provided the response was of sufficient magnitude and durability. Issues that required clarification included the value of assessing T2/FLAIR progression; value of advanced imaging, such as T1 subtraction maps and volumetric imaging in defining contrast-enhancing disease; value of other advanced MR imaging and PET imaging; and the need to standardize imaging in neuro-oncology to reduce variability.

IMAGE STANDARDIZATION IN NEURO-ONCOLOGY

The JBTDDC and FDA workshop led to an international effort to standardize MR imaging in neuro-oncology to reduce variability and improve consistency in neuroimaging in clinical trials. The effort included many of the leaders in neuro-oncology and cooperative groups running brain tumor trials, neuroradiologists, and imaging physicists, with input from FDA, National Institutes of Health, and industry. Recently, a consensus MR imaging protocol was published that will be adopted for most neuro-oncology clinical trials in Europe and North America[21] and ideally adopted for routine imaging of all brain tumor patients.

NEXT ITERATION: ROLES OF ADVANCED IMAGING AND IMAGING STANDARDIZATION

Despite increasing adoption of the RANO criteria in recent clinical trials, there remain challenges in assessing pseudoprogression and nonenhancing tumor using conventional imaging methods. Advanced imaging techniques based on physiologic or metabolic properties of tissues, including perfusion-weighted imaging (PWI), diffusion-weighted imaging (DWI), and magnetic resonance spectroscopy (MRS), can potentially be more accurate objective endpoints correlating with the status of tumor and treatment efficacy. For these novel techniques to serve as standard clinical and research trial endpoints, it is important to validate their diagnostic accuracy and reproducibility. The ease and cost of clinical implementation of these imaging methods also need to be considered.

Magnetic Resonance–Perfusion-Weighted Imaging

Dynamic susceptibility contrast (DSC–MR imaging) is currently the most widely clinically used magnetic resonance–PWI (MR-PWI) technique that measures signal intensity change during passage of contrast bolus.[22,23] Due to its relative short imaging acquisition time and availability of post-processing software packages, this technique has been increasingly built into standard imaging protocol for imaging of brain tumors. The time-signal intensity curve derived from DSC–MR imaging can be quantified by several hemodynamic parameters, including relative cerebral blood volume (rCBV), relative peak height, and percentage of signal intensity recovery (PSR).[24] For patients with glioblastomas after chemoradiation therapy, relative peak height and rCBV were greater in progressive/recurrent tumor, whereas PSR was significantly lower.[25] DSC–MR imaging provides an accuracy of approximately 90% in distinguishing pseudoprogression from progression when combined with conventional imaging.[26] There is often coexistence of tumor and treatment-induced necrosis within regions of suspected tumor progression, and the fractional tumor burden measured by DSC–MR imaging correlates with the relative histologic fraction of viable tumor.[27] Whole-tumor evaluation using methods, such as histogram or voxel-based parametric response map, can account for spatial heterogeneity of post-treatment tumor and improve the accuracy of measuring tumor burden.[28,29]

DSC–MR imaging measures vascular permeability using pharmacokinetic parameters, allowing more accurate calculation of cerebral blood volume (CBV) compared with DSC–MR imaging.[30–32] This technique is however more challenging to implement clinically due to the need of pharmacokinetic modeling. Preliminary evidence with retrospective data have shown that dynamic contrast-enhanced (DCE)–MR imaging can distinguish pseudoprogression from progression after chemoradiation treatment[33,34] but there was no significant difference in the degree of improvement for diagnostic accuracy when directly compared with DCE–MR imaging.[26]

The diagnostic accuracy of MR-PWI can be highly dependent on imaging acquisition parameters and postprocessing methods. Notably, calculation of rCBV using DSC–MR imaging can be overestimated or underestimated due to presence of blood-brain barrier disruption, resulting in extravascular contrast leakage,[35] and additional correction to imaging acquisition and postprocessing to compensate for leakage is necessary.[36] Even with commercial software most commonly used, however, different implementations of perfusion MR imaging software modeling can affect the accuracy of leakage correction, rCBV calculation, and histologic correlations.[37] This highlights the importance of standardization of imaging methodology when applying advanced imaging techniques to imaging biomarker development.

Magnetic Resonance–Diffusion-Weighted Imaging

Magnetic resonance (MR)-DWI can noninvasively measure water diffusion properties within tissues. This imaging technique is installed on most clinical MR imaging scanners and can help differentiate brain tumor subtypes and tumor grades when combined with conventional MR imaging.[38–42] Apparent diffusion coefficient (ADC) is a parameter derived from MR-DWI that has been shown to correlate with tumor cellularity.[41,43,44] After chemoradiation treatment, progressive tumors demonstrate lower ADC values compared with necrosis and normal brain tissues.[45–47] Similar to MR-PWI, ADC values within regions of enhancement are often heterogeneous due to presence of tumor and necrotic tumor tissue, and histogram or voxel-based analysis of whole-tumor ADC can provide early prognostic information for PFS after treatment, with a sensitivity of 71% and a specificity of 69%.[48] Similar to MR-PWI, quantitative analysis of DWI parameters, including calculation of ADC values, can be affected by variations in MR imaging equipment and acquisition parameters.[49] Without standardization of acquisition techniques, such variability presents significant challenges during analysis of multicenter data.[50]

Magnetic Resonance Spectroscopy

MRS can measure concentrations of metabolites within tissues, and based on differences in N-acetyl aspartate (NAA), choline, creatine, and lactate levels, recurrent tumor can be distinguished from treatment-related necrosis.[51–54] After chemoradiation treatment, there is usually a transient increase in choline with progressive decreased NAA concentrations over time.[51,53,55–57] Choline-to-NAA ratio can differentiate recurrent glioma from radiation necrosis, with sensitivity and specificity of 0.88 and 0.86, respectively.[58] A combined model based on multiple MRS metabolic peaks has been applied to diagnosing gliomas,[59,60] and this approach may enhance the specificity of differentiating treatment response from tumor. Furthermore, multivoxel acquisition (chemical shift imaging) can acquire location-specific data within heterogeneous tissues and improve accuracy for diagnosing tumor progression.[55,61–65]

MRS has a lower spatial resolution limiting its ability to evaluate lesions that are less than 1.5 cm^3. This technique is also user dependent, requiring an experienced radiologist or technologist to specify regions of interest during imaging acquisition. Quantitative measurements of metabolic concentrations can also be affected by variations in MR equipment, pulse sequences, and data postprocessing methods.[66]

Advanced imaging in the setting of antiangiogenic treatment

T1 subtraction map Objective response rates from phase II clinical trials of patients with recurrent glioblastoma treated with bevacizumab using either the Macdonald or RANO criteria have been widely variable, ranging from 35% to 63%.[67–70] Due to the antipermeability effect of antiangiogenic treatment, the area of enhancement is typically faint and can be obscured by intrinsic T1 shortening near the enhancing area, thus resulting in significant interobserver variability in determining objective response based on T1-weighted imaging.[67] Analysis of the BRAIN trial imaging data using T1 subtraction maps derived from both pre– and post–contrast-enhanced T1-weighted imaging resulted in greater association between measured tumor volumes, OS, and PFS.[71] A clear trend was observed between the change in contrast-enhancing tumor volume and median PFS when the authors used contrast-enhanced T1-weighted subtraction maps (P = .0192) but not with conventional segmentation (P = .6234). In this study, receiver-operator curve analysis revealed T1-weighted subtraction maps after therapy were clearly superior at aiding identification of patients who had progression at 6 months (mean area under the curve 0.59 vs 0.67, P = .0294) and those who survived at 6 months (mean area under the curve 0.52 vs 0.61, P = .0202). This technique requires only simple postprocessing and can potentially improve both objective response and PFS as endpoints for OS.

T2 mapping In the current RANO criteria, assessment of T2/FLAIR abnormality for both objective response and progressive disease (PD) is qualitative based on investigator or independent reader's subjective interpretation of significant changes among serial MR studies. Attempts to construct objective criteria have been difficult because these apparent signal abnormalities on T2/FLAIR imaging can result from other pathologies besides nonenhancing tumor, including radiation effects, edema, ischemic injury, infection, seizures, and postoperative gliosis.[4] Quantitative measurements of T2/FLAIR abnormalities using the same method of measuring enhancing area resulted in a lower degree of interobserver agreement.[67] Qualitative evaluation based on tumor shape by identifying circumscribed T2/FLAIR lesions improves prediction of survival outcome of patients receiving antiangiogenic therapy,[72] although this approach remains subjective and likely requires substantial imaging expertise. Quantitative T2 mapping technique directly calculates T2 relaxation times of individual voxels based on fitting of T2-weighted imaging acquired at different echo times and has been explored to increase specificity for identifying tumor after antiangiogenic therapy.[73–75] Although this technique requires validation in prospective trials, it can be readily performed on clinical MR imaging by adding a dual-echo T2-weighted sequence and is promising both as an early post-treatment predictor and as a more accurate marker of tumor burden during antiangiogenic therapy.

Magnetic resonance–diffusion-weighted imaging Although ADC measurements within glioblastoma prior to initiation of bevacizumab have been shown to correlate with PFS and OS,[76–78] there has been a significant variability of reported changes in ADC after treatment.[79–81] Very low ADC lesions after treatment have been shown to represent chronic hypoxia, gelatinous necrotic tissue, or tumor.[82,83] The timing of imaging may be important for the association of ADC measurements and patient outcome. By measuring ADC changes between baseline and 6-week post-treatment MR imaging using voxel subtraction method, Ellingson and colleagues[84] generated a functional diffusion map for 77 patients with recurrent glioblastomas and demonstrated volume of tissue showing decreased ADC within both FLAIR and contrast-enhancing regions stratified OS (P = .0024; hazard ratio [HR] = 2.012). Tumor volumes with decreased ADC between 0.25 and 0.4 μm^2/ms within the functional diffusion map improved prediction of OS (HR = 2.679, P<.001). In another retrospective study of 52 patients with recurrent glioblastoma receiving bevacizumab who developed low ADC lesions during the first and second post-treatment MR imaging, the volume of the low-ADC lesion at the second post-treatment scan was inversely associated with OS, with larger volumes predicting shorter OS (HR = 1.01, P = .009).[85]

Magnetic resonance–perfusion-weighted imaging
Perfusion imaging techniques can measure the effect of antiangiogenic therapy on tumor vascularity and permeability; early post-treatment decrease in k-trans, a marker of vascular permeability as measured by DCE–MR imaging, is associated with improved PFS and OS.[86–88] Increased percent recovery, a marker of permeability on DSC–MR imaging 2 months after antiangiogenic treatment, predicted subsequent durable response at 6 month,[89] whereas increased peak height, a marker of microvascular density between baseline and 1 month, is associated with progression at 6 months.[90] Using normalized rCBV measurement on DSC–MR imaging, Schmainda and colleagues[91,92] demonstrated low CBV pretreatment and post-treatment as well as early decreased in rCBV are predictive of improved survival in patients with recurrent glioblastoma treated with bevacizumab.

Multimodality parametric approach to tissue classification
With improved speed of imaging acquisition and capability of image postprocessing and computation, the advantage of multimodality approach to imaging brain tumor is increasingly recognized. Recently, several groups have reported results from such approaches to classify newly diagnosed glioblastoma according to gene expression pattern and patient outcome.[59,93–96] Artzi and colleagues[97] applied unsupervised clustering analysis of DSC, DCE, DWI, and conventional MR imaging parameters to classify FLAIR abnormalities in patients with recurrent glioblastoma before and during antiangiogenic treatment. The classification model was then validated using

MRS as well as patient outcome, including PFS at week 8 after treatment. This type of complex, multifeature-based approach has the potential to be highly accurate and reproducible but its generalizability largely depends on standardization of imaging data acquisition.

ADDITIONAL RESPONSE ASSESSMENT IN NEURO-ONCOLOGY EFFORTS

In addition to improving the ability to define enhancing and nonenhancing tumor on neuroimaging studies, there have been extensive efforts to refine other aspects of the RANO criteria.

Neurologic Assessment in Neuro-Oncology

Currently both the Macdonald and RANO criteria take into account clinical status in determining tumor response. The evaluation of clinical status is subjective, however, although the RANO criteria do provide some guidance based on performance status.[4] The RANO group is developing a simple clinician reported outcome assessment tool to measure neurologic function and integrity across 9 neurologic domains routinely assessed

during an office physical examination.[98] This NANO scale is in the process of being evaluated for interobserver variability and may provide a much needed measure to quantify neurologic functions.

Immunotherapy Response Assessment in Neuro-Oncology

There is increasing interest in evaluating immunotherapies for a variety of brain tumors.[99,100] As with systemic tumors, such as melanoma, there is the potential for the immunotherapies to produce an inflammatory response that results in transient enlargement of the tumor or new lesions, complicating the assessment of tumor progression. The immune-related response criteria was proposed for systemic tumors to address this issue and recommended that patients with enlarging lesions have a repeat scan at least 4 weeks apart to confirm progression and that new lesions do not have to indicate progression but can be incorporated into the total tumor burden.[101] The RANO group recently published iRANO that incorporates some of the recommendations of immune-related response criteria, including the need to repeat the scans to confirm progression (**Fig. 1**). It suggests

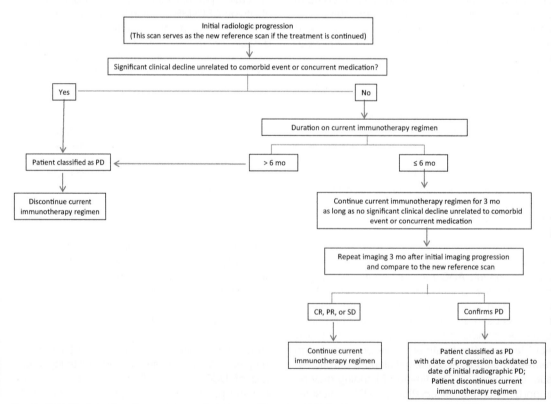

Fig. 1. iRANO algorithm for treatment decision making for radiologic progression. CR, complete response; PR, partial response; SD, stable disease. (*From* Okada H, Weller M, Huang R, et al. Immunotherapy response assessment in neuro-oncology: a report of the RANO working group. Lancet Oncol 2015;16:e538; with permission.)

Table 2
Summary of the proposed Response Assessment in Neuro-Oncology criteria for central nervous system metastases

Criterion	Complete Response	Partial Response	Stable Disease	Progressive Disease
Target lesions	None	≥30% Decrease in sum LD relative to baseline	<30% Decrease relative to baseline but <20% increase in sum LD relative to nadir	≥20% Increase in sum LD relative to nadir[a]
Nontarget lesions	None	Stable or improved	Stable or improved	Unequivocal PD[a]
New lesion(s)[b]	None	None	None	Present[a]
Corticosteroids	None	Stable or decreased	Stable or decreased	NA[c]
Clinical status	Stable or improved	Stable or improved	Stable or improved	Worse[a]
Requirement for response	All	All	All	Any[c]

Abbreviations: LD, longest dimension; NA, not applicable.

[a] Progression occurs when this criterion is met.

[b] New lesion = new lesion not present on prior scans and visible in at least 2 projections. If a new lesion is equivocal, for example, because of its small size, continued therapy may be considered, and follow-up evaluation clarifies if it represents truly new disease. If repeat scans confirm there is definitely a new lesion, then progression should be declared using the date of the initial scan showing the new lesion. For immunotherapy-based approaches, new lesions alone do not define progression (see "For immunotherapy-based approaches, new lesions alone do not define progression").

[c] Increase in corticosteroids alone is not taken into account in determining progression in the absence of persistent clinical deterioration.

From Lin NU, Lee EQ, Aoyama H, et al. Response assessment criteria for brain metastases: proposal from the RANO group. Lancet Oncol 2015;16:e274; with permission.

that within 6 months of initiating an immunotherapy, if a patient is clinically stable, the patient can remain on study for up to 3 months, even if the tumor has exceeded the 25% increase in area or if there is a new lesion.[102] If ultimately it is determined that the patients had PD, the date of progression is backdated to the initial time when this was considered.[102]

Response Assessment in Neuro-Oncology— Brain Metastases

There is increasing interest in developing novel therapies for brain metastases. The clinical trials to date, however, have used a variety of different response criteria and endpoints, compromising data interpretation and limiting the ability to do any cross-trial comparisons.[103,104] The RANO group recently proposed a criteria for response assessment for brain metastases.[105] To achieve consistency with Response Evaluation Criteria In Solid Tumors (RECIST) 1.1, 1-D measurements are used.[106] Measurable disease is defined as a contrast-enhancing lesion that can be accurately measured in at least 1-D with a minimum size of 10 mm. In a departure from RECIST 1.1, the brain is treated as a separate compartment and up to 5 target lesions can be chosen. Details of the

RANO brain metastases criteria are summarized in **Table 2**.

Other Response Assessment in Neuro-Oncology Efforts

In addition to the efforts discussed previously, the RANO group is developing response criteria for other tumors, including leptomeningeal disease,[107] meningiomas,[108,109] spinal tumors, and pediatric tumors[110] as well as refining recommendations for endpoints[111] and trial designs for high-grade gliomas.[112] In addition, there are ongoing efforts to develop criteria PET and use seizures and corticosteroid use as endpoints.[1]

SUMMARY

Although the RANO criteria for high-grade glioma aimed to address the limitations of Macdonald criteria by providing guidelines to reduce the impact of pseudoprogression and pseudoresponse, there remains room for further improvement. Advanced imaging techniques discussed in this article have the potential to supplement conventional imaging in diagnosing pseudoprogression and pseudoresponse, but there are several challenges related to validation and clinical implementation of these techniques for their use as clinical and clinical trial endpoints. In addition, there are extensive ongoing efforts by the RANO group to refine the RANO criteria for high-grade gliomas as well as developing response criteria for other tumors and other endpoints.

REFERENCES

1. Chang SM, Wen PY, Vogelbaum MA, et al. Response Assessment in Neuro-Oncology (RANO): more than imaging criteria for malignant glioma. Neuro Oncol Pract 2015;2(4):205–9.
2. Macdonald DR, Cascino TL, Schold SC, et al. Response criteria for phase II studies of supratentorial malignant glioma. J Clin Oncol 1990;8(7):1277–80.
3. van den Bent MJ, Vogelbaum MA, Wen PY, et al. End point assessment in gliomas: novel treatments limit usefulness of classical Macdonald's Criteria. J Clin Oncol 2009;27(18):2905–8.
4. Wen PY, Macdonald DR, Reardon DA, et al. Updated response assessment criteria for high-grade gliomas: response assessment in neuro-oncology working group. J Clin Oncol 2010;28(11):1963–72.
5. Taal W, Oosterkamp HM, Walenkamp AME, et al. Single-agent bevacizumab or lomustine versus a combination of bevacizumab plus lomustine in patients with recurrent glioblastoma (BELOB trial): a randomised controlled phase 2 trial. Lancet Oncol 2014;15(9):943–53.
6. Arakawa Y, Mizowaki T, Murata D, et al. Retrospective analysis of bevacizumab in combination with ifosfamide, carboplatin, and etoposide in patients with second recurrence of glioblastoma. Neurol Med Chir (Tokyo) 2013;53(11):779–85.
7. Nagpal S, Recht CK, Bertrand S, et al. Phase II pilot study of single-agent etirinotecan pegol (NKTR-102) in bevacizumab-resistant high grade glioma. J Neurooncol 2015;123(2):277–82.
8. Balaña C, Gil MJ, Perez P, et al. Sunitinib administered prior to radiotherapy in patients with non-resectable glioblastoma: results of a phase II study. Target Oncol 2014;9(4):321–9.
9. Soffietti R, Trevisan E, Bertero L, et al. Bevacizumab and fotemustine for recurrent glioblastoma: a phase II study of AINO (Italian Association of Neuro-Oncology). J Neurooncol 2014;116(3):533–41.
10. Muhic A, Poulsen HS, Sorensen M, et al. Phase II open-label study of nintedanib in patients with recurrent glioblastoma multiforme. J Neurooncol 2013;111(2):205–12.
11. Field KM, Simes J, Nowak AK, et al. Randomized phase 2 study of carboplatin and bevacizumab in recurrent glioblastoma. Neuro Oncol 2015;17(11):1504–13.
12. Lee EQ, Reardon DA, Schiff D, et al. Phase II study of panobinostat in combination with bevacizumab for recurrent glioblastoma and anaplastic glioma. Neuro Oncol 2015;17(6):862–7.
13. Nasseri M, Gahramanov S, Netto JP, et al. Evaluation of pseudoprogression in patients with glioblastoma multiforme using dynamic magnetic resonance imaging with ferumoxytol calls RANO criteria into question. Neuro Oncol 2014;16(8):1146–54.
14. Radbruch A, Lutz K, Wiestler B, et al. Relevance of T2 signal changes in the assessment of progression of glioblastoma according to the Response Assessment in Neurooncology criteria. Neuro Oncol 2012;14(2):222–9.
15. Gállego Pérez-Larraya J, Lahutte M, Petrirena G, et al. Response assessment in recurrent glioblastoma treated with irinotecan-bevacizumab: comparative analysis of the Macdonald, RECIST, RANO, and RECIST + F criteria. Neuro Oncol 2012;14(5):667–73.
16. Boxerman JL, Zhang Z, Safriel Y, et al. Early post-bevacizumab progression on contrast-enhanced MRI as a prognostic marker for overall survival in recurrent glioblastoma: results from the ACRIN 6677/RTOG 0625 Central Reader Study. Neuro Oncol 2013;15(7):945–54.
17. Huang RY, Rahman R, Ballman KV, et al. The impact of T2/FLAIR evaluation per RANO criteria on response assessment of recurrent glioblastoma patients treated with bevacizumab. Clin Cancer Res 2015;22(3):575–81.
18. Chinot OL, Wick W, Mason W, et al. Bevacizumab plus radiotherapy-temozolomide for newly diagnosed glioblastoma. N Engl J Med 2014;370(8):709–22.
19. Gilbert MR, Dignam JJ, Armstrong TS, et al. A randomized trial of bevacizumab for newly diagnosed glioblastoma. N Engl J Med 2014;370(8):699–708.
20. Wen PY, Cloughesy TF, Ellingson BM, et al. Report of the jumpstarting brain tumor drug development coalition and FDA clinical trials neuroimaging endpoint workshop (January 30, 2014, Bethesda MD). Neuro Oncol 2014;16(Suppl 7):vii36–47.
21. Ellingson BM, Bendszus M, Boxerman J, et al. Consensus recommendations for a standardized Brain Tumor Imaging Protocol in clinical trials. Neuro Oncol 2015;17(9):1188–98.
22. Rosen BR, Belliveau JW, Vevea JM, et al. Perfusion imaging with NMR contrast agents. Magn Reson Med 1990;14(2):249–65.
23. Villringer A, Rosen BR, Belliveau JW, et al. Dynamic imaging with lanthanide chelates in normal brain: contrast due to magnetic susceptibility effects. Magn Reson Med 1988;6(2):164–74.

24. Rosen BR, Belliveau JW, Buchbinder BR, et al. Contrast agents and cerebral hemodynamics. Magn Reson Med 1991;19(2):285–92.

25. Barajas RF, Chang JS, Segal MR, et al. Differentiation of recurrent glioblastoma multiforme from radiation necrosis after external beam radiation therapy with dynamic susceptibility-weighted contrast-enhanced perfusion MR imaging. Radiology 2009;253(2):486–96.

26. Kim HS, Ju Goh M, Kim N, et al. Which combination of MR imaging modalities is best for predicting recurrent glioblastoma? Study of diagnostic accuracy and reproducibility. Radiology 2014;273(3):831–43.

27. Hu LS, Eschbacher JM, Heiserman JE, et al. Reevaluating the imaging definition of tumor progression: perfusion MRI quantifies recurrent glioblastoma tumor fraction, pseudoprogression, and radiation necrosis to predict survival. Neuro Oncol 2012;14(7):919–30.

28. Baek HJ, Kim HS, Kim N, et al. Percent change of perfusion skewness and kurtosis: a potential imaging biomarker for early treatment response in patients with newly diagnosed glioblastomas. Radiology 2012;264(3):834–43.

29. Tsien C, Galbán CJ, Chenevert TL, et al. Parametric response map as an imaging biomarker to distinguish progression from pseudoprogression in high-grade glioma. J Clin Oncol 2010;28(13): 2293–9.

30. Tofts PS, Kermode AG. Measurement of the blood-brain barrier permeability and leakage space using dynamic MR imaging. 1. Fundamental concepts. Magn Reson Med 1991;17(2):357–67.

31. Tofts PS. Modeling tracer kinetics in dynamic Gd-DTPA MR imaging. J Magn Reson Imaging 1997; 7(1):91–101.

32. Tofts PS, Brix G, Buckley DL, et al. Estimating kinetic parameters from dynamic contrast-enhanced T(1)-weighted MRI of a diffusable tracer: standardized quantities and symbols. J Magn Reson Imaging 1999;10(3):223–32.

33. Larsen VA, Simonsen HJ, Law I, et al. Evaluation of dynamic contrast-enhanced T1-weighted perfusion MRI in the differentiation of tumor recurrence from radiation necrosis. Neuroradiology 2013; 55(3):361–9.

34. Bisdas S, Naegele T, Ritz R, et al. Distinguishing recurrent high-grade gliomas from radiation injury: a pilot study using dynamic contrast-enhanced MR imaging. Acad Radiol 2011;18(5):575–83.

35. Paulson ES, Schmainda KM. Comparison of dynamic susceptibility-weighted contrast-enhanced MR methods: recommendations for measuring relative cerebral blood volume in brain tumors. Radiology 2008;249(2):601–13.

36. Huang RY, Neagu MR, Reardon DA, et al. Pitfalls in the neuroimaging of glioblastoma in the era of antiangiogenic and immuno/targeted therapy - detecting illusive disease, defining response. Front Neurol 2015;6:33.

37. Hu LS, Kelm Z, Korfiatis P, et al. Impact of software modeling on the accuracy of perfusion MRI in glioma. AJNR Am J Neuroradiol 2015;36(12): 2242–9.

38. Yamasaki F, Kurisu K, Satoh K, et al. Apparent diffusion coefficient of human brain tumors at MR imaging1. Radiology 2005;235(3):985–91.

39. Guo AC, Cummings TJ, Dash RC, et al. Lymphomas and high-grade astrocytomas: comparison of water diffusibility and histologic characteristics. Radiology 2002;224(1):177–83.

40. Dorenbeck U, Grunwald IQ, Schlaier J, et al. Diffusion-weighted imaging with calculated apparent diffusion coefficient of enhancing extra-axial masses. J Neuroimaging 2005;15(4):341–7.

41. Sugahara T, Korogi Y, Kochi M, et al. Usefulness of diffusion-weighted MRI with echo-planar technique in the evaluation of cellularity in gliomas. J Magn Reson Imaging 1999;9(1):53–60.

42. Murakami R, Hirai T, Sugahara T, et al. Grading astrocytic tumors by using apparent diffusion coefficient parameters: superiority of a one- versus two-parameter pilot method1. Radiology 2009; 251(3):838–45.

43. Ellingson BM, Malkin MG, Rand SD, et al. Validation of functional diffusion maps (fDMs) as a biomarker for human glioma cellularity. J Magn Reson Imaging 2010;31(3):538–48.

44. Hayashida Y, Hirai T, Morishita S, et al. Diffusion-weighted imaging of metastatic brain tumors: comparison with histologic type and tumor cellularity. AJNR Am J Neuroradiol 2006;27(7):1419–25.

45. Hein PA, Eskey CJ, Dunn JF, et al. Diffusion-weighted imaging in the follow-up of treated high-grade gliomas: tumor recurrence versus radiation injury. AJNR Am J Neuroradiol 2004;25(2):201–9.

46. Asao C, Korogi Y, Kitajima M, et al. Diffusion-weighted imaging of radiation-induced brain injury for differentiation from tumor recurrence. AJNR Am J Neuroradiol 2005;26(6):1455–60.

47. Sundgren PC, Fan X, Weybright P, et al. Differentiation of recurrent brain tumor versus radiation injury using diffusion tensor imaging in patients with new contrast-enhancing lesions. Magn Reson Imaging 2006;24(9):1131–42.

48. Ellingson BM, Cloughesy TF, Lai A, et al. Quantitative probabilistic functional diffusion mapping in newly diagnosed glioblastoma treated with radiochemotherapy. Neuro Oncol 2013;15(3): 382–90.

49. Padhani AR, Liu G, Koh DM, et al. Diffusion-weighted magnetic resonance imaging as a cancer biomarker: consensus and recommendations. Neoplasia 2009;11(2):102–25.

50. Ellingson BM, Kim E, Woodworth DC, et al. Diffusion MRI quality control and functional diffusion map results in ACRIN 6677/RTOG 0625: a multicenter, randomized, phase II trial of bevacizumab and chemotherapy in recurrent glioblastoma. Int J Oncol 2015;46(5):1883–92.

51. Schlemmer HP, Bachert P, Herfarth KK, et al. Proton MR spectroscopic evaluation of suspicious brain lesions after stereotactic radiotherapy. AJNR Am J Neuroradiol 2001;22(7):1316–24.

52. Dowling C, Bollen AW, Noworolski SM, et al. Preoperative proton MR spectroscopic imaging of brain tumors: correlation with histopathologic analysis of resection specimens. AJNR Am J Neuroradiol 2001;22(4):604–12.

53. Rabinov JD, Lee PL, Barker FG, et al. In vivo 3-T MR spectroscopy in the distinction of recurrent glioma versus radiation effects: initial experience. Radiology 2002;225(3):871–9.

54. Prat R, Galeano I, Lucas A, et al. Relative value of magnetic resonance spectroscopy, magnetic resonance perfusion, and 2-(18F) fluoro-2-deoxy-D-glucose positron emission tomography for detection of recurrence or grade increase in gliomas. J Clin Neurosci 2010;17(1):50–3.

55. Rock JP, Scarpace L, Hearshen D, et al. Associations among magnetic resonance spectroscopy, apparent diffusion coefficients, and image-guided histopathology with special attention to radiation necrosis. Neurosurgery 2004;54(5):1111–7 [discussion: 1117–9].

56. Estève F, Rubin C, Grand S, et al. Transient metabolic changes observed with proton MR spectroscopy in normal human brain after radiation therapy. Int J Radiat Oncol Biol Phys 1998;40(2):279–86.

57. Kaminaga T, Shirai K. Radiation-induced brain metabolic changes in the acute and early delayed phase detected with quantitative proton magnetic resonance spectroscopy. J Comput Assist Tomogr 2005;29(3):293–7.

58. Zhang H, Ma L, Wang Q, et al. Role of magnetic resonance spectroscopy for the differentiation of recurrent glioma from radiation necrosis: A systematic review and meta-analysis. Eur J Radiol 2014; 83(12):2181–9.

59. Imani F, Boada FE, Lieberman FS, et al. Molecular and metabolic pattern classification for detection of brain glioma progression. Eur J Radiol 2014;83(2):e100–5.

60. Ranjith G, Parvathy R, Vikas V, et al. Machine learning methods for the classification of gliomas: Initial results using features extracted from MR spectroscopy. Neuroradiol J 2015; 28(2):106–11.

61. McKnight TR, von dem Bussche MH, Vigneron DB, et al. Histopathological validation of a three-dimensional magnetic resonance spectroscopy index as a predictor of tumor presence. J Neurosurg 2002;97(4):794–802.

62. Yang I, Huh NG, Smith ZA, et al. Distinguishing glioma recurrence from treatment effect after radiochemotherapy and immunotherapy. Neurosurg Clin N Am 2010;21(1):181–6.

63. Weybright P, Sundgren PC, Maly P, et al. Differentiation between brain tumor recurrence and radiation injury using MR spectroscopy. AJR Am J Roentgenol 2005;185(6):1471–6.

64. Zeng Q-S, Li C-F, Zhang K, et al. Multivoxel 3D proton MR spectroscopy in the distinction of recurrent glioma from radiation injury. J Neurooncol 2007; 84(1):63–9.

65. Smith EA, Carlos RC, Junck LR, et al. Developing a clinical decision model: MR spectroscopy to differentiate between recurrent tumor and radiation change in patients with new contrast-enhancing lesions. AJR Am J Roentgenol 2009;192(2):W45–52.

66. Oz G, Alger JR, Barker PB, et al. Clinical Proton MR Spectroscopy in Central Nervous System Disorders. Radiology 2014;270(3):658–79.

67. Friedman HS, Prados MD, Wen PY, et al. Bevacizumab alone and in combination with irinotecan in recurrent glioblastoma. J Clin Oncol 2009;27(28):4733–40.

68. Kreisl TN, Kim L, Moore K, et al. Phase II trial of single-agent bevacizumab followed by bevacizumab plus irinotecan at tumor progression in recurrent glioblastoma. J Clin Oncol 2009;27(5):740–5.

69. Vredenburgh JJ, Desjardins A, Herndon JE, et al. Phase II trial of bevacizumab and irinotecan in recurrent malignant glioma. Clin Cancer Res 2007;13(4):1253–9.

70. Vredenburgh JJ, Desjardins A, Herndon JE, et al. Bevacizumab plus irinotecan in recurrent glioblastoma multiforme. J Clin Oncol 2007;25(30):4722–9.

71. Ellingson BM, Kim HJ, Woodworth DC, et al. Recurrent glioblastoma treated with bevacizumab: contrast-enhanced T1-weighted subtraction maps improve tumor delineation and aid prediction of survival in a multicenter clinical trial. Radiology 2014;271(1):200–10.

72. Nowosielski M, Wiestler B, Goebel G, et al. Progression types after antiangiogenic therapy are related to outcome in recurrent glioblastoma. Neurology 2014;82(19):1684–92.

73. Ellingson BM, Cloughesy TF, Lai A, et al. Quantification of edema reduction using differential quantitative T2 (DQT2) relaxometry mapping in recurrent glioblastoma treated with bevacizumab. J Neurooncol 2011;106(1):111–9. Available at: http://www.ncbi.nlm.nih.gov/pubmed/21706273. Accessed November 8, 2011.

74. Hattingen E, Jurcoane A, Daneshvar K, et al. Quantitative T2 mapping of recurrent glioblastoma under bevacizumab improves monitoring for

non-enhancing tumor progression and predicts overall survival. Neuro Oncol 2013;15(10):1395–404.

75. Ellingson BM, Lai A, Nguyen HN, et al. Quantification of nonenhancing tumor burden in gliomas using effective T2 maps derived from dual-echo turbo spin-echo MRI. Clin Cancer Res 2015; 21(19):4373–83.

76. Pope WB, Kim HJ, Huo J, et al. Recurrent glioblastoma multiforme: ADC histogram analysis predicts response to bevacizumab treatment. Radiology 2009;252(1):182–9.

77. Pope WB, Qiao XJ, Kim HJ, et al. Apparent diffusion coefficient histogram analysis stratifies progression-free and overall survival in patients with recurrent GBM treated with bevacizumab: a multi-center study. J Neurooncol 2012;108(3): 491–8.

78. Rahman R, Hamdan A, Zweifler R, et al. Histogram analysis of apparent diffusion coefficient within enhancing and nonenhancing tumor volumes in recurrent glioblastoma patients treated with bevacizumab. J Neurooncol 2014;119(1):149–58.

79. Gerstner ER, Chen P-J, Wen PY, et al. Infiltrative patterns of glioblastoma spread detected via diffusion MRI after treatment with cediranib. Neuro Oncol 2010;12(5):466–72.

80. Jain R, Scarpace LM, Ellika S, et al. Imaging response criteria for recurrent gliomas treated with bevacizumab: role of diffusion weighted imaging as an imaging biomarker. J Neurooncol 2010; 96(3):423–31.

81. Nowosielski M, Recheis W, Goebel G, et al. ADC histograms predict response to anti-angiogenic therapy in patients with recurrent high-grade glioma. Neuroradiology 2011;53(4):291–302.

82. Rieger J, Bähr O, Müller K, et al. Bevacizumab-induced diffusion-restricted lesions in malignant glioma patients. J Neurooncol 2010;99(1):49–56.

83. Gerstner ER, Frosch MP, Batchelor TT. Diffusion magnetic resonance imaging detects pathologically confirmed, nonenhancing tumor progression in a patient with recurrent glioblastoma receiving bevacizumab. J Clin Oncol 2009; 28(6):e91–3.

84. Ellingson BM, Cloughesy TF, Lai A, et al. Graded functional diffusion map-defined characteristics of apparent diffusion coefficients predict overall survival in recurrent glioblastoma treated with bevacizumab. Neuro Oncol 2011;13(10): 1151–61.

85. Zhang M, Gulotta B, Thomas A, et al. Large-volume low apparent diffusion coefficient lesions predict poor survival in bevacizumab-treated glioblastoma patients. Neuro Oncol 2016;18(5):735–43.

86. Batchelor TT, Sorensen AG, di Tomaso E, et al. AZD2171, a pan-VEGF receptor tyrosine kinase inhibitor, normalizes tumor vasculature and alleviates edema in glioblastoma patients. Cancer Cell 2007;11(1):83–95.

87. Sorensen AG, Batchelor TT, Zhang W-T, et al. A "vascular normalization index" as potential mechanistic biomarker to predict survival after a single dose of cediranib in recurrent glioblastoma patients. Cancer Res 2009;69(13):5296–300.

88. Emblem KE, Bjornerud A, Mouridsen K, et al. T(1)- and T(2)(*)-dominant extravasation correction in DSC-MRI: part II-predicting patient outcome after a single dose of cediranib in recurrent glioblastoma patients. J Cereb Blood Flow Metab 2011;31(10): 2054–64.

89. Essock-Burns E, Lupo JM, Cha S, et al. Assessment of perfusion MRI-derived parameters in evaluating and predicting response to antiangiogenic therapy in patients with newly diagnosed glioblastoma. Neuro Oncol 2011;13(1):119–31.

90. Jain R, Gutierrez J, Narang J, et al. In vivo correlation of tumor blood volume and permeability with histologic and molecular angiogenic markers in gliomas. AJNR Am J Neuroradiol 2011;32(2): 388–94.

91. Schmainda KM, Prah M, Connelly J, et al. Dynamic-susceptibility contrast agent MRI measures of relative cerebral blood volume predict response to bevacizumab in recurrent high-grade glioma. Neuro Oncol 2014;16(6):880–8.

92. Schmainda KM, Zhang Z, Prah M, et al. Dynamic susceptibility contrast MRI measures of relative cerebral blood volume as a prognostic marker for overall survival in recurrent glioblastoma: results from the ACRIN 6677/RTOG 0625 multicenter trial. Neuro Oncol 2015;17(8):1148–56.

93. Gevaert O, Mitchell LA, Achrol AS, et al. Glioblastoma multiforme: exploratory radiogenomic analysis by using quantitative image features. Radiology 2014;273(1):168–74.

94. Gutman DA, Cooper LAD, Hwang SN, et al. MR imaging predictors of molecular profile and survival: multi-institutional study of the TCGA glioblastoma data set. Radiology 2013;267(2):560–9.

95. Jain R, Poisson L, Narang J, et al. Genomic mapping and survival prediction in glioblastoma: molecular subclassification strengthened by hemodynamic imaging biomarkers. Radiology 2013;267(1):212–20.

96. Macyszyn L, Akbari H, Pisapia JM, et al. Imaging patterns predict patient survival and molecular subtype in glioblastoma via machine learning techniques. Neuro Oncol 2015;18(3): 417–25.

97. Artzi M, Bokstein F, Blumenthal DT, et al. Differentiation between vasogenic-edema versus tumor-infiltrative area in patients with glioblastoma during

bevacizumab therapy: a longitudinal MRI study. Eur J Radiol 2014;83(7):1250–6.

98. Nayak L, DeAngelis L, Wen P, et al. The Neurologic Assessment in Neuro-Oncology (NANO) Scale: A Tool to Assess Neurologic Function for Integration in the Radiologic Assessment in Neuro-Oncology (RANO) Criteria (S22.005). Neurology 2014;82(10 Suppl):S22.005.

99. Preusser M, Lim M, Hafler DA, et al. Prospects of immune checkpoint modulators in the treatment of glioblastoma. Nat Rev Neurol 2015; 11(9):504–14.

100. Reardon DA, Freeman G, Wu C, et al. Immunotherapy advances for glioblastoma. Neuro Oncol 2014;16(11):1441–58.

101. Wolchok JD, Hoos A, O'Day S, et al. Guidelines for the evaluation of immune therapy activity in solid tumors: immune-related response criteria. Clin Cancer Res 2009;15(23):7412–20.

102. Okada H, Weller M, Huang R, et al. Immunotherapy response assessment in neuro-oncology: a report of the RANO working group. Lancet Oncol 2015; 16(15):e534–42.

103. Lin NU, Lee EQ, Aoyama H, et al. Challenges relating to solid tumour brain metastases in clinical trials, part 1: patient population, response, and progression. A report from the RANO group. Lancet Oncol 2013;14(10):e396–406.

104. Lin NU, Wefel JS, Lee EQ, et al. Challenges relating to solid tumour brain metastases in clinical trials, part 2: neurocognitive, neurological, and quality-of-life outcomes. A report from the RANO group. Lancet Oncol 2013;14(10):e407–16.

105. Lin NU, Lee EQ, Aoyama H, et al. Response assessment criteria for brain metastases: proposal from the RANO group. Lancet Oncol 2015;16(6): e270–8.

106. Eisenhauer EA, Therasse P, Bogaerts J, et al. New response evaluation criteria in solid tumours: revised RECIST guideline (version 1.1). Eur J Cancer 2009;45(2):228–47.

107. Chamberlain M, Soffietti R, Raizer J, et al. Leptomeningeal metastasis: a Response Assessment in Neuro-Oncology critical review of endpoints and response criteria of published randomized clinical trials. Neuro Oncol 2014;16(9):1176–85.

108. Rogers L, Barani I, Chamberlain M, et al. Meningiomas: knowledge base, treatment outcomes, and uncertainties. A RANO review. J Neurosurg 2015; 122(1):4–23.

109. Kaley T, Barani I, Chamberlain M, et al. Historical benchmarks for medical therapy trials in surgery- and radiation-refractory meningioma: a RANO review. Neuro Oncol 2014;16(6):829–40.

110. Warren KE, Poussaint TY, Vezina G, et al. Challenges with defining response to antitumor agents in pediatric neuro-oncology: a report from the response assessment in pediatric neuro-oncology (RAPNO) working group. Pediatr Blood Cancer 2013;60(9):1397–401.

111. Reardon DA, Galanis E, DeGroot JF, et al. Clinical trial end points for high-grade glioma: the evolving landscape. Neuro Oncol 2011; 13(3):353–61.

112. Galanis E, Wu W, Cloughesy T, et al. Phase 2 trial design in neuro-oncology revisited: a report from the RANO group. Lancet Oncol 2012;13(5): e196–204.

Radiomics in Brain Tumors
An Emerging Technique for Characterization of Tumor Environment

Aikaterini Kotrotsou, PhD[a], Pascal O. Zinn, MD, PhD[b],
Rivka R. Colen, MD[a,*]

KEYWORDS

- Radiomics • Radiogenomics • Big data • Brain tumors • Texture analysis

KEY POINTS

- Radiomics refers to the extraction of a large array of quantitative features from imaging that can be correlated with the demographic and genomic profile of the patient.
- Radiomic analysis has the potential to serve as a noninvasive technique for accurate characterization of tumor microenvironment.
- Incorporating simple imaging features, such as tumor location, involvement of eloquent cortex, and extent of the tumor, can improve understanding of tumor genomic profile and aid in therapy planning.

INTRODUCTION

Brain tumor is the growth of abnormal cells in the brain and ranges from noncancerous (benign) to malignant. Glioblastoma (GBM) is the most aggressive type of brain tumor, rising from glial cells, characterized by rapid growth and invasion into nearby brain tissue. GBM has an incidence of 3.19 cases per 100,000 adults per year and average age at diagnosis is 64 years.[1,2] The current line of treatment for patients with GBM involves maximal safe excision of the tumor followed by radiotherapy plus concomitant and adjuvant chemotherapy.[3,4] However, this paradigm of treatment has proven insufficient because most treatments cannot eradicate all tumor cells, explaining the high rate of progression; most patients with GBM survive approximately 12 to 15 months, and only 5% live for more than 5 years.[1,3,4] Another important factor that greatly reduces the efficacy of current therapy is the heterogeneity of gliomas.[5–7] In addition, analysis of histologic specimens highlights the intertumoral and intratumoral differences.[5,7,8] Against this background, research in the field is focused on identifying markers for patient stratification at the point of diagnosis and for follow-up.

MRI is a well-established technique for imaging evaluation of brain tumors because of its high soft tissue contrast.[9,10] Current standard of care involves acquisition of high-resolution MRI scans (<2 mm through plane resolution) that allow for tumor visualization, shape and size determination, and initial staging before surgery[10,11] (**Fig. 1**). Using more advanced imaging techniques, such

This research is partially funded by the John S. Dunn Sr. Distinguished Chair in Diagnostic Imaging Fund, MD Anderson Brain Tumor Center Program, and MD Anderson Cancer Center startup funding.
The authors have nothing to disclose.
[a] Department of Diagnostic Radiology, The University of Texas MD Anderson Cancer Center, 1400 Pressler Street, Houston, TX 77030, USA; [b] Department of Neurosurgery, Baylor College of Medicine, 1 Baylor Plaza, Houston, TX 77030, USA
* Corresponding author. Department of Diagnostic Radiology, The University of Texas MD Anderson Cancer Center, 1400 Pressler Street, Unit 1482, Room # FCT 16.5037, Houston, TX 77030.
E-mail address: rcolen@mdanderson.org

mri.theclinics.com

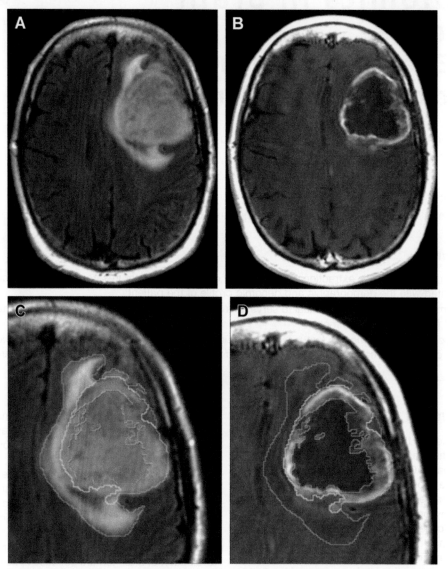

Fig. 1. Grade IV glioma on high-resolution anatomic MRI. A 60-year-old man with enhancing left frontal tumor. (*A*) Axial fluid attenuation inversion recovery MRI shows well-circumscribed intra-axial hyperintense with minimal surrounding vasogenic edema. (*B*) Axial gadolinium-enhanced T1-weighted MRI shows hypointense necrotic core with marginal enhancement. (*C, D*) Tumor along with the three-dimensional manual segmentation performed using 3D Slicer v. 4.3.1 (https://www.slicer.org). Edema/invasion is depicted in blue, contrast enhancement in yellow, and necrosis in red.

as diffusion weighted imaging, dynamic susceptibility contrast MRI, and magnetic resonance spectroscopy (MRS), it is now possible to probe the tumor cellularity and its vascular dynamics[12–16] (**Fig. 2**). Quantitative MRI allows for macroscopic, detailed, three-dimensional representation of the tumor and the surrounding environment without the need of invasive procedures, such as biopsy or surgery. Although, the information obtained from MRI is at the tissue/organ level and cannot substitute histologic findings, extracted quantitative parameters are believed to reflect various pathophysiologic aspects of the tissue under examination. Additionally, these parameters are suitable for statistical comparisons with clinical and genomic factors, and longitudinal analysis.

Recent findings have revealed that imaging contains complementary information with demographic and genomic data, giving rise to radiomics.[17,18] The combination of imaging features with demographic information, such as age, sex,

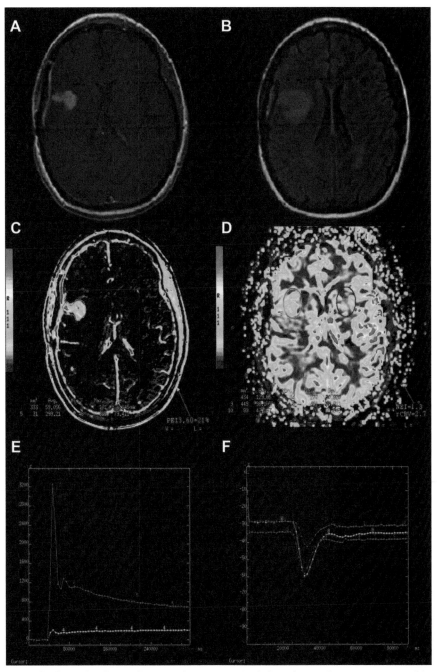

Fig. 2. Progressive high-grade glioma diagnosed postoperatively by advanced MRI. A 62-year-old woman with right frontal tumor. (*A*) Axial gadolinium-enhanced T1-weighted MRI shows an enhancing right frontal lesion, surrounded by vasogenic edema as shown in the axial fluid attenuation inversion recovery MRI (*B*). Dynamic contrast-enhanced map shows elevated leakage characteristics 21%, with elevation in the concentration time curve of the enhancing tumor region as shown (*C*, *E*). Dynamic susceptibility contrast map shows high relative cerebral blood volume values of 2.7 in the enhancing tumor, with high peak signal intensity curve (*green curve*) when compared with contralateral normal-appearing gray matter (*D*, *F*). Analysis for dynamic contrast-enhanced and dynamic susceptibility contrast was performed on General Electric workstation, Waukesha, WI, USA.

overall survival, and progression-free survival, presents a new opportunity to classify patients into survival groups and determine risk of recurrence based on a noninvasive assessment at the time of diagnosis or during therapy. Furthermore, correlating imaging features with genomic information (often referred as radiogenomics) highlights the important conclusion that information obtained at the tissue/organ level (macroscopic level) is directly linked to underlying physiologic, cellular processes (microscopic level).[19]

Consequently, radiomics has the potential to improve diagnosis and therapy planning of numerous cancers. In parallel, a by-product of radiomics is the generation of large-volume data that are currently accumulating in computers and servers, and are expected to increase daily. This article provides a summary of the current findings in radiomics of brain tumors with a focus on MRI, and also identifies future directions. In addition, an introduction to the concept of big data and its significance in medicine is presented.

RADIOMICS: EMERGING CLINICAL APPLICATIONS

Radiomics refers to the extraction of a large array of quantitative features from imaging that is correlated with the demographic and genomic profile of the patient. These imaging features comprise of descriptors of size, shape, volume, intensity distribution (extracted from the histogram), and texture patterns. Different imaging modalities (eg, MRI, computed tomography, ultrasound) and different sequences (T1-weighted, T2-weighted, fluid attenuation inversion recovery [FLAIR], diffusion weighted imaging) are used as the base for extracting these features. The complete set of imaging features obtained for a patient using the images available is called the "radiome."

One of the first attempts to correlate imaging findings with histology was published in 1988, highlighting that enhancing areas in MRIs and computed tomography scans overlapped with areas of neovascularity and cell proliferation as determined through biopsy.[20] Since then a plethora of studies have been published looking into the prognostic value of specific imaging features and correlations with genomic findings.[21–25] This section reviews the research findings on radiomics for GBM using MRI. The discussion is split into three separate sections, according to the level/complexity of the imaging features presented: (1) Visually AcceSAble Rembrandt Images (VASARI) features, (2) volumetric imaging features, and (3) texture analysis–derived features.

Visually AcceSAble Rembrandt Images Features

Incorporating simple imaging features, such as tumor location, involvement of eloquent cortex, and extent of the tumor, can improve understanding of tumor genomic profile and aid in therapy planning. Several groups have evaluated the use of such information in the context of predicting patient survival and making correlations with genomic signatures.[21–23,26,27] However, effectively combining imaging features with demographic or genomic information requires imaging features to be independent of the approach used, reviewer/radiologist evaluation, and data collection site. The aforementioned requirements allow for robust and reproducible results, and validation across data obtained from different sites. To address these issues, the cancer research community introduced the VASARI features,[28] a comprehensive list of standardized imaging features that can be obtained through typical clinical scans.

The first study using VASARI features was published by Gutman and colleagues[29] and investigated the association of VASARI features with genomic information and patient survival. Presurgical MRIs of 75 patients obtained from the Cancer Imaging Archive database (http://cancerimagingarchive.net/)[30] were evaluated by three neuroradiologists and results showed that increased length of the major axis obtained from the T2-weighted FLAIR image and the presence of contrast-enhanced tumor (>33%) are associated with poor survival.[29] Furthermore, results revealed associations between VASARI features and GBM mutation status; epidermal growth factor mutant GBMs were larger than wild-type epidermal growth factor GBMs, whereas TP53 mutant GBMs were smaller than wiled-type GBMs.[29]

Since then, more findings on the correlation of VASARI features and demographic/genomic information have been published.[19,31–36] In 2014, using a larger patient cohort (104 The Cancer Genome Atlas patients), Colen and colleagues[31] reported that deep white matter tract and ependymal involvement suggests poor survival. At the same study, mitochondrial pathway was identified at the top canonical pathway in GBMs with invasive phenotypes.[31] The most recent study on the subject was published on 2015 by Rao and colleagues[35]; the authors using a combination of three VASARI features (volume-class, hemorrhage, and T1/FLAIR ratio) partitioned patients into two distinct survival groups with survival difference of 12 months. It should be noted that in this study findings were validated on an independent set of 48 patients (training set, 43 patients).

Volumetric Imaging Features

The adoption of quantitative measurements is envisioned as a major advantage in the radiology field. VASARI features could be characterized as the first attempt in the transitioning from qualitative radiologic evaluation to accurate, reproducible, quantitative measurements. As highlighted in the previous section the size of the tumor (longer axis) is linked to genomic information and can predict survival; in addition over the past 5 years it became evident that three-dimensional segmentation (ie, volume) would allow one to grasp the whole tumor rather than information from a single slice.

Volumetric analysis provides a snapshot of the entire tumor, and partitions of the tumor that reflect specific imaging phenotypes; in the case of GBM, contrast-enhancing tumor (CE), nonenhancing edema/invasion, or necrotic portion. Typically, volumetric measurements are based on high-resolution precontrast/postcontrast T1-weighted images and FLAIR images. Different approaches ranging from manual delineation to fully automated segmentation have been adopted by researchers.[37] These methods are characterized by specific advantages and disadvantages; however, the investigation of those is not the subject of this article.

A large body of literature exists demonstrating that tumor volume (preoperatively or postoperatively) is associated with overall survival and progression-free survival.[25,27,38–42] Other well-known factors associated with good prognosis are younger age and higher preoperative Karnofsky Performance Status (KPS) score; thus, further studies assessed the additive benefit of combining volumetric information with demographic data in predicting overall survival.[23,43–47] Toward this goal, Park and colleagues[22] proposed a preoperative prognostic scale that evaluated tumor location, KPS, and tumor volume; results identified three distinct survival groups. A favorable prognosis was reported in patients with tumors away from the eloquent cortex (motor-speech/middle cerebral artery score $\leq$2), good performance status (KPS $\geq$80), and tumor volume less than 50 cm^3.[22] Further looking into the genomic associations of volumetric/demographic information and therefore moving toward the radiogenomics field, Zinn and colleagues[41] presented VAK, a three-point scoring system that evaluates volume, age, and KPS. Two classes with significant survival differences were

presented (VAK-A and VAK-B; P<.05), and VAK-specific molecular configuration was identified.

In the radiogenomics field, the first large-scale study using volumetric information obtain from MRIs along with the tumor's genomic profile was published by Zinn and colleagues.[25] Zinn and colleagues classified patients into two groups based on the volume of edema (obtained using the FLAIR sequence) and further identified main cancer genomic components associated with cell migration and invasion. Additionally, Iliadis and colleagues[39] reported that the volume of necrosis was a negative prognostic factor of progression-free survival and was inversely correlated with MGMT protein–positive tumor cells. Another MRI-based study by Naeini and colleagues[48] has shown that the volume of CE, central necrosis, and the ratio of FLAIR hyperintensity to the combined volume of CE and necrosis are significantly different between mesenchymal and nonmesenchymal GBM subtypes, suggesting that volumetric features may be linked to molecular subtypes. In a recent study by Colen and colleagues,[40] necrosis was associated with different molecular pathways in males (TP53) than females (MYC).

Texture Analysis–Derived Features

Texture analysis comprises of a wide range of techniques that evaluate gray level patterns, pixel interrelationships, and spectral patterns inside a region of interest (ROI). As an image postprocessing technique it can be applied to any type of imaging; the first publications on the subject were on images obtained from satellites.[49,50] Almost two decades later, the method was applied in radiographic images.[51,52] In the pipeline of texture analysis and feature extraction, the first and most important step is selection of an appropriate ROI. The selected ROI should be large enough to capture the tumor heterogeneity, reflect image appearances/phenotypes, and not involve dominant variations resulting from mixture of image phenotypes (ie, selecting an ROI that incorporates both CE and necrotic portions). For more methodologic considerations about texture analysis, see the study by Kotrotsou and colleagues.[53]

Texture analysis yields quantitative features that can be used for (1) classification, (2) correlation with demographic data (eg, survival), and (3) correlation with genomic data (**Fig. 3**). This section is organized based on the aforementioned applications of texture analysis in brain tumors.

Texture analysis features for discrimination of tissue/tumor type

One of the earliest applications of texture analysis was tissue characterization.[54,55] Schad and

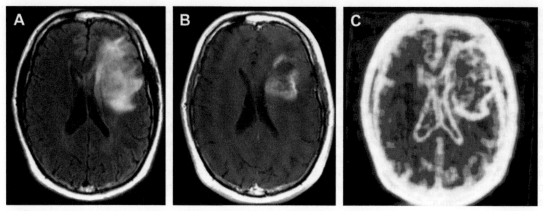

Fig. 3. Voxel-based texture analysis of high-grade gliomas. A 60-year-old man with enhancing left frontal tumor. Axial FLAIR and gadolinium-enhanced T1-weighted MRI (*A, B*) show a necrotic core with marginal enhancement and minimal edema. The voxel-based entropy map (*C*) calculated using the axial FLAIR image shows higher entropy compared with the contralateral normal-appearing white matter.

colleagues[55] reported the use of first- and second-order texture features for identifying tumor phenotypes (tumor, edema) and healthy tissue (gray matter, white matter, and cerebrospinal fluid). After extracting the features from T1- and T2-weighted images, a four-layer hierarchical decision tree was constructed for discrimination of the five aforementioned classes. Notably, this preliminary analysis yielded only one misclassification error. Using a larger dataset, 88 patients with various types of intracranial tumors and six healthy volunteers, Kjaer and colleagues[56] further explored the potential of texture analysis to differentiate among various tissue types (as described previously by Schad and colleagues[55]) and among different tumor types. Nachimuthu and Baladhandapani[57] suggested that combining information obtained through volumetric texture analysis from MRI and MRS improved the sensitivity of the classifier to distinguish among tumoral tissues and normal brain tissue. Combining volumetric texture features with features obtained from MRS yielded 99.15% accuracy in discriminating high-versus low-grade gliomas.[57]

Because conventional imaging has not been consistently able to differentiate among different tumor types, some studies have used texture features alone or in conjunction with other imaging-derived features for tumor type and grade classification. The first indication that texture analysis could differentiate among tumor types was published by Kjaer and colleagues.[56] One of the first comprehensive analyses on the subject was published by Sasikala and Kumaravel[58]; the authors looked into various classification techniques and computational effort for differentiating normal, benign, and malignant brain tumors.

Based on their findings, all classification techniques performed similarly (98% accuracy in leave-one-out cross-validation); however, the genetic algorithm achieved maximum performance using the least number of features.[58] A later study on 102 patients with a variety of histologically proven brain tumors found that texture features extracted from conventional MRI and perfusion MRI can be used to distinguish metastases from gliomas and high- from low-grade gliomas.[59] Similarly, Mouthuy and colleagues[60] obtained perfusion and texture parameters from 50 patients to discriminate GBM from metastasis. Applying three-dimensional texture analysis and using a separate cohort for validation, Georgiadis and colleagues[61] achieved 77.14% accuracy in discriminating metastatic, malignant, and benign brain tumors. In a cohort of 40 patients with different grades of gliomas (low grade [n = 8] and high grade [n = 32]), Ryu and colleagues[62] demonstrated a significant increase in apparent diffusion coefficient (ADC) entropy in high-grade gliomas compared with low-grade gliomas. In addition to assessing the performance of texture analysis in adult brain tumors, a study by Fetit and colleagues[63] reported that MRI texture analysis can also be used in the case of pediatric brain tumors. Furthermore, Rodriguez Gutierrez and colleagues[64] studied 40 children with posterior fossa tumors and evaluated the performance of texture features extracted from contrast-enhanced anatomic MRIs and ADC maps. They reported that ADC histogram features resulted in the best tumor type classification, whereas higher-order ADC features yielded the best subtype discrimination.[64] Similar research has been published by various authors.[65–67] Hu and colleagues[68] performed image-guided biopsy and texture analysis on the sites of biopsy to discriminate between high- and low-grade gliomas; the results (81.8% accuracy in validation set) suggest that texture features may provide a better picture of the tumor heterogeneity and therefore guide biopsy.

In addition to its capabilities in discriminating tumor type and grade, another exciting application of texture analysis is its potential to help neurosurgeons identify tumor boundaries, and invading cells beyond the borders of edema/invasion.[69] In a preliminary study published in 2003, authors reported significant textural differences among the peritumoral normal-appearing white matter and white matter regions away from the tumor.[70] The authors also reported improved results when using a three-dimensional approach for feature calculation.[70] Later, a study assessing the impact of gray levels when using the gray-level co-occurrence matrix highlighted that identifying the appropriate number of gray levels could further improve the sensitivity and specificity of the classification.[71]

Texture analysis features for assessing survival
Yang and colleagues[66] evaluated the predicted performance of various texture methods for predicting 12-month survival. Although the accuracy of their results was relatively low (area under the curve, 0.69; confidence interval 0.56–0.79), they suggest that texture features could be a method to predict survival at the time of imaging.[66] Brynolfsson and colleagues[72] identified texture features of ADC maps and assessed their performance in predicting survival; using 23 patients who were treated with radiotherapy and chemotherapy postsurgically, they performed texture analysis on the ADC maps for the residual enhancing tumor. By principal component analysis, authors identified ADC texture characteristics, which seem to hold pretreatment prognostic information, independent of known clinical prognostic factors.[72] A later investigation, driven by the potential of dynamic susceptibility contrast MRI to evaluate functional changes in cerebral blood volume (CBV), assessed the potential of texture features extracted by relative CBV (rCBV) maps to predict survival.[73] Preliminary results on a small cohort of 24 patients with GBM confirmed associations between radiomic features obtained from rCBV maps and overall survival.

Texture analysis features for predicting genomic profiling
It is also feasible to use texture features for the prediction of the presence of a gene. In GBM, methylation of the MGMT promoter has been identified as a strong predictive factor of favorable survival in patients undergoing chemotherapy.[74] Levner and colleagues[75] used texture features extracted from conventional MRIs (T2-weighted, FLAIR, and postcontrast T1-weighted) for prediction of MGMT methylation status. S-transform texture features obtained from the MRIs of 59 patients (53% methylation frequency) were used to train and validate a neural network to predict patients' methylation status. Neural network was able to achieve an average accuracy greater than 87% for the prediction of MGMT methylation status.[75] Similarly, Drabycz and colleagues[76] presented a preliminary study that evaluated visually assessed and computer-calculated texture features for prediction of MGMT methylation status. Results confirmed an earlier finding by Eoli and colleagues[77] that ring enhancement is associated with unmethylated status, and further showed that combining visually assessed with computer-calculated texture features improved the predictive power of the model.[76]

BIG DATA IN MEDICINE: IMPROVING 7 BILLION LIVES

In recent years, big data has rapidly developed into a strong focus that attracts overwhelming attention from academia, industry, and governments worldwide.[78–80] Although not strictly defined, the term "big data" first appeared in the mid-1990s, gradually becoming noted, and being ushered in as a new buzzword everywhere on the Internet, conferences, scientific publications, competitions, and start-up companies.[81–85] Researchers and policymakers are beginning to realize the potential benefit of appropriately "reading" these torrents of data and extracting useful information.

Life sciences and medicine have been highly affected by the generation of large-scale data, especially by omics information.[86] Data-driven medicine will allow the effective integration and accurate analysis of multisource information (demographics, clinical data, genomic data, imaging/radiomic data), which will lead to better predictions and individualized medicine. The management and consulting firm McKinsey alleged that if US health care were to properly use big data for patient planning, costs would be reduced by 8% and the sector would create more than $300 billion per year.[87] It may be argued that the double-helix structure of DNA that contains one's personal DNA fingerprint, as proposed by Watson and Crick[88] in 1953, launched the big data era in life sciences. Nowadays, one's personal genome, which is comprised of 100 gigabytes of data, can be mapped in just a few days for a few thousand dollars.[89] One can imagine that the size and complexity of data generated will only increase, as the cost of generating these data is continuously decreasing. Notably in 2010, Schadt and colleagues[90] referred to an expectation of exabyte of data being produced in 5 years' time just by sequencing DNA, RNA, and other omics.

In the radiogenomics field, this expectation is far higher because genomic and imaging/radiomic data are included. Approximately 8 GB of data are generated per patient as estimated by Bibault and colleagues[91]; however, this estimation is far from reality because it includes only raw data. Until recently radiology was primarily a qualitative field, but in recent years image postprocessing has been heavily integrated in the clinical setting; thus, if one accounts for the postprocessing data produced per patient the 8 GB estimation is far from being true. An additional 8 to 10 GB of data is produced per patient through radiomic analysis in the research setting, leading to an approximate 18 GB total volume per patient. Accounting for 1.6 million new patients in the United States alone, it is expected that zettabyte (10^{21}) of data will be created in clinic and research settings in the following years around the world.[92]

SUMMARY

Radiomic analysis has the potential to serve as a noninvasive technique for accurate characterization of tumor microenvironment, thus improving diagnosis and monitoring of treatment response.[93] One of the selling points of radiomic analysis is its ability to be integrated in any current study and in the clinic. This article summarizes several findings in MRI of GBM that indicate its ability to become a powerful biomarker that can be used for tumor grading, prognosis, and identification of genomic profile. It is expected that further studies will test and establish a robust methodology, which is required for subsequent validation and clinical use. Furthermore, the sensitivity and specificity of radiomics will be better defined by studies that include larger sample sizes from multiple centers. Additionally, clinical trials are needed to further validate the importance and additive role of radiomics in a clinical setting.

REFERENCES

1. Ostrom QT, Gittleman H, Farah P, et al. CBTRUS statistical report: primary brain and central nervous system tumors diagnosed in the United States in 2006-2010. Neuro Oncol 2013;15(Suppl 2):ii1–56.

2. DeAngelis LM. Brain tumors. N Engl J Med 2001; 344:114–23.

3. Stupp R, Mason WP, van den Bent MJ, et al. Radiotherapy plus concomitant and adjuvant temozolomide for glioblastoma. N Engl J Med 2005;352: 987–96.

4. Weller M, Cloughesy T, Perry JR, et al. Standards of care for treatment of recurrent glioblastoma: are we there yet? Neuro Oncol 2013;15(1):4–27.

5. Gatenby RA, Grove O, Gillies RJ. Quantitative imaging in cancer evolution and ecology. Radiology 2013;269(1):8–15.

6. Wen PY, Kesari S. Malignant gliomas in adults. N Engl J Med 2008;359(5):492–507.

7. Brennan CW, Verhaak RG, McKenna A, et al. The somatic genomic landscape of glioblastoma. Cell 2013;155(2):462–77.

8. Louis DN. Molecular pathology of malignant gliomas. Annu Rev Pathol 2006;1:97–117.

9. Jenkinson MD, Du Plessis DG, Walker C, et al. Advanced MRI in the management of adult gliomas. Br J Neurosurg 2007;21(6):550–61.

10. Kao HW, Chiang SW, Chung HW, et al. Advanced MR imaging of gliomas: an update. Biomed Res Int 2013;2013:970586.

11. Kondziolka D, Lunsford LD, Martinez AJ. Unreliability of contemporary neurodiagnostic imaging in evaluating suspected adult supratentorial (low-grade) astrocytoma. J Neurosurg 1993;79(4):533–6.

12. Rees J. Advances in magnetic resonance imaging of brain tumours. Curr Opin Neurol 2003;16(6): 643–50.

13. Rosen BR, Belliveau JW, Vevea JM, et al. Perfusion imaging with NMR contrast agents. Magn Reson Med 1990;14(2):249–65.

14. Stadnik TW, Chaskis C, Michotte A, et al. Diffusion-weighted MR imaging of intracerebral masses: comparison with conventional MR imaging and histologic findings. AJNR Am J Neuroradiol 2001; 22(5):969–76.

15. Prat R, Galeano I, Lucas A, et al. Relative value of magnetic resonance spectroscopy, magnetic resonance perfusion, and 2-(18F) fluoro-2-deoxy-D-glucose positron emission tomography for detection of recurrence or grade increase in gliomas. J Clin Neurosci 2010;17(1):50–3.

16. Schlemmer HP, Bachert P, Herfarth KK, et al. Proton MR spectroscopic evaluation of suspicious brain lesions after stereotactic radiotherapy. AJNR Am J Neuroradiol 2001;22(7):1316–24.

17. Lambin P, Petit SF, Aerts HJ, et al. The ESTRO Breur Lecture 2009. From population to voxel-based radiotherapy: exploiting intra-tumour and intra-organ heterogeneity for advanced treatment of non-small cell lung cancer. Radiother Oncol 2010;96:145–52.

18. Price SJ. The role of advanced MR imaging in understanding brain tumour pathology. Br J Neurosurg 2007;21(6):562–75.

19. Colen R, Foster I, Gatenby R, et al. NCI workshop report: clinical and computational requirements for correlating imaging phenotypes with genomics signatures. Transl Oncol 2014;7(5):556–69.

20. Earnest F, Kelly PJ, Scheithauer BW, et al. Cerebral astrocytomas: histopathologic correlation of MR and CT contrast enhancement with stereotactic biopsy. Radiology 1988;166(3):823–7.

21. Pope WB, Sayre J, Perlina A, et al. MR imaging correlates of survival in patients with high-grade gliomas. AJNR Am J Neuroradiol 2005;26(10): 2466–74.

22. Park JK, Hodges T, Arko L, et al. Scale to predict survival after surgery for recurrent glioblastoma multiforme. J Clin Oncol 2010;28(24):3838–43.

23. Lacroix M, Abi-Said D, Fourney DR, et al. A multivariate analysis of 416 patients with glioblastoma multiforme: prognosis, extent of resection, and survival. J Neurosurg 2001;95(2):190–8.

24. Hammoud MA, Sawaya R, Shi W, et al. Prognostic significance of preoperative MRI scans in glioblastoma multiforme. J Neurooncol 1996;27(1):65–73.

25. Zinn PO, Mahajan B, Sathyan P, et al. Radiogenomic mapping of edema/cellular invasion MRI-phenotypes in glioblastoma multiforme. PLoS One 2011;6:e25451.

26. Chaichana KL, Pendleton C, Chambless L, et al. Multi-institutional validation of a preoperative scoring system which predicts survival for patients with glioblastoma. J Clin Neurosci 2013;20(10): 1422–6.

27. Schoenegger K, Oberndorfer S, Wuschitz B, et al. Peritumoral edema on MRI at initial diagnosis: an independent prognostic factor for glioblastoma? Eur J Neurol 2009;16(7):874–8.

28. Wiki for the VASARI feature set The National Cancer Institute Web site. 2015. Available at: https://wiki.cancerimagingarchive.net/display/Public/VASARI+Research+Project. Accessed March 25, 2015.

29. Gutman DA, Cooper LA, Hwang SN, et al. MR imaging predictors of molecular profile and survival: multi-institutional study of the TCGA glioblastoma data set. Radiology 2013;267:560–9.

30. Prior FW, Clark K, Commean P, et al. TCIA: an information resource to enable open science. Conf Proc IEEE Eng Med Biol Soc 2013;2013:1282–5.

31. Colen RR, Vangel M, Wang J, et al. Imaging genomic mapping of an invasive MRI phenotype predicts patient outcome and metabolic dysfunction: a TCGA glioma phenotype research group project. BMC Med Genomics 2014;7:30.

32. Gevaert O, Mitchell LA, Achrol AS, et al. Glioblastoma multiforme: exploratory radiogenomic analysis by using quantitative image features. Radiology 2014;273(1):168–74.

33. Jain R, Poisson LM, Gutman D, et al. Outcome prediction in patients with glioblastoma by using imaging, clinical, and genomic biomarkers: focus on the nonenhancing component of the tumor. Radiology 2014;272(2):484–93.

34. Nicolasjilwan M, Hu Y, Yan C, et al. Addition of MR imaging features and genetic biomarkers strengthens glioblastoma survival prediction in TCGA patients. J Neuroradiol 2015;42(4):212–21.

35. Rao A, Rao G, Gutman DA, et al, TCGA Glioma Phenotype Research Group. A combinatorial radiographic phenotype may stratify patient survival and be associated with invasion and proliferation characteristics in glioblastoma. J Neurosurg 2016; 124:1008–17.

36. Mazurowski MA, Desjardins A, Malof JM. Imaging descriptors improve the predictive power of survival models for glioblastoma patients. Neuro Oncol 2013;15(10):1389–94.

37. Parmar C, Rios Velazquez E, Leijenaar R, et al. Robust radiomics feature quantification using semi-automatic volumetric segmentation. PLoS One 2014;9(7):e102107.

38. Grabowski MM, Recinos PF, Nowacki AS, et al. Residual tumor volume versus extent of resection: predictors of survival after surgery for glioblastoma. J Neurosurg 2014;121:1115–23.

39. Iliadis G, Kotoula V, Chatzisotiriou A, et al. Volumetric and MGMT parameters in glioblastoma patients: survival analysis. BMC Cancer 2012;12:3.

40. Colen RR, Wang J, Singh SK, et al. Glioblastoma: imaging genomic mapping reveals sex-specific oncogenic associations of cell death. Radiology 2015;275(1):215–27.

41. Zinn PO, Sathyan P, Mahajan B, et al. A novel volume-age-KPS (VAK) glioblastoma classification identifies a prognostic cognate microRNA-gene signature. PLoS One 2012;7:e41522.

42. Zhang Z, Jiang H, Chen X, et al. Identifying the survival subtypes of glioblastoma by quantitative volumetric analysis of MRI. J Neurooncol 2014;119(1): 207–14.

43. Buckner JC. Factors influencing survival in high-grade gliomas. Semin Oncol 2003;30:10–4.

44. Donato V, Papaleo A, Castrichino A, et al. Prognostic implication of clinical and pathologic features in patients with glioblastoma multiforme treated with concomitant radiation plus temozolomide. Tumori 2007;93(3):248–56.

45. Chaichana KL, Chaichana KK, Olivi A, et al. Surgical outcomes for older patients with glioblastoma multiforme: preoperative factors associated with decreased survival. Clinical article. J Neurosurg 2011;114:587–94.

46. Filippini G, Falcone C, Boiardi A, et al. Prognostic factors for survival in 676 consecutive patients with newly diagnosed primary glioblastoma. Neuro Oncol 2008;10:79–87.

47. Tait MJ, Petrik V, Loosemore A, et al. Survival of patients with glioblastoma multiforme has not improved between 1993 and 2004: analysis of 625 cases. Br J Neurosurg 2007;21:496–500.

48. Naeini KM, Pope WB, Cloughesy TF, et al. Identifying the mesenchymal molecular subtype of glioblastoma using quantitative volumetric analysis of anatomic magnetic resonance images. Neuro Oncol 2013;15(5):626–34.

49. Kaizer H. A quantification of textures on aerial photographs. Tech Note 1955;121.

50. Darling E, Joseph R. Pattern recognition from satellite altitudes. IEEE Trans Syst Sci Cybernetics 1968;1(4):38–47.

51. Hall E, Kruger R, Dwyer S, et al. A survey of preprocessing and feature extraction techniques for radiographic images. IEEE Trans Comput 1971;100(9):1032–44.

52. Lerski R, Barnett E, Morley P, et al. Computer analysis of ultrasonic signals in diffuse liver disease. Ultrasound Med Biol 1979;5(4):341–3.

53. Kotrotsou A, Zinn PO, Colen RR. MRI texture analysis for brain tumors: concept and clinical relevance. American Society of Neuroradiology. 53rd Annual Meeting. Chicago, IL, April 25–30, 2015.

54. Lerski RA, Straughan K, Schad LR, et al. MR image texture analysis: an approach to tissue characterization. Magn Reson Imaging 1993;11(6):873–87.

55. Schad LR, Blüml S, Zuna I. MR tissue characterization of intracranial tumors by means of texture analysis. Magn Reson Imaging 1993;11(6):889–96.

56. Kjaer L, Ring P, Thomsen C, et al. Texture analysis in quantitative MR imaging. tissue characterisation of normal brain and intracranial tumours at 1.5 T. Acta Radiol 1995;36(2):127–35.

57. Nachimuthu DS, Baladhandapani A. Multidimensional texture characterization: on analysis for brain tumor tissues using MRS and MRI. J Digit Imaging 2014;27(4):496–506.

58. Sasikala M, Kumaravel N. A wavelet-based optimal texture feature set for classification of brain tumours. J Med Eng Technol 2008;32(3):198–205.

59. Zacharaki EI, Wang S, Chawla S, et al. Classification of brain tumor type and grade using MRI texture and shape in a machine learning scheme. Magn Reson Med 2009;62(6):1609–18.

60. Mouthuy N, Cosnard G, Abarca-Quinones J, et al. Multiparametric magnetic resonance imaging to differentiate high-grade gliomas and brain metastases. J Neuroradiol 2012;39(5):301–7.

61. Georgiadis P, Cavouras D, Kalatzis I, et al. Enhancing the discrimination accuracy between metastases, gliomas and meningiomas on brain MRI by volumetric textural features and ensemble pattern recognition methods. Magn Reson Imaging 2009;27(1):120–30.

62. Ryu YJ, Choi SH, Park SJ, et al. Glioma: application of whole-tumor texture analysis of diffusion-weighted imaging for the evaluation of tumor heterogeneity. PLoS One 2014;9(9):e108335.

63. Fetit AE, Novak J, Rodriguez D, et al. MRI texture analysis in paediatric oncology: a preliminary study. Stud Health Technol Inform 2013;190:169–71.

64. Rodriguez Gutierrez D, Awwad A, Meijer L, et al. Metrics and textural features of MRI diffusion to improve classification of pediatric posterior fossa tumors. AJNR Am J Neuroradiol 2014;35(5):1009–15.

65. Fatima K, Arooj A, Majeed H. A new texture and shape based technique for improving meningioma classification. Microsc Res Tech 2014;77(11):862–73.

66. Yang D, Rao G, Martinez J, et al. Evaluation of tumor-derived MRI-texture features for discrimination of molecular subtypes and prediction of 12-month survival status in glioblastoma. Med Phys 2015;42(11):6725.

67. Eliat PA, Olivie D, Saikali S, et al. Can dynamic contrast-enhanced magnetic resonance imaging combined with texture analysis differentiate malignant glioneuronal tumors from other glioblastoma? Neurol Res Int 2012;2012:195176.

68. Hu LS, Ning S, Eschbacher JM, et al. Multi-parametric MRI and texture analysis to visualize spatial histologic heterogeneity and tumor extent in glioblastoma. PLoS One 2015;10(11):e0141506.

69. Kotrotsou A, Thomas G, Abrol S, et al. Determining tumor infiltration in the normal appearing white matter using radioman characterization. American Society of Neuroradiology 54th Annual Meeting, Washington, DC, May 23–26, 2016.

70. Mahmoud-Ghoneim D, Toussaint G, Constans JM, et al. Three dimensional texture analysis in MRI: a preliminary evaluation in gliomas. Magn Reson Imaging 2003;21(9):983–7.

71. Mahmoud-Ghoneim D, Alkaabi MK, de Certaines JD, et al. The impact of image dynamic range on texture classification of brain white matter. BMC Med Imaging 2008;8:18.

72. Brynolfsson P, Nilsson D, Henriksson R, et al. ADC texture: an imaging biomarker for high-grade glioma? Med Phys 2014;41(10):101903.

73. Lee J, Jain R, Khalil K, et al. Texture feature ratios from relative CBV maps of perfusion MRI are associated with patient survival in glioblastoma. AJNR Am J Neuroradiol 2016;37(1):37–43.

74. Hegi ME, Diserens AC, Gorlia T, et al. MGMT gene silencing and benefit from temozolomide in glioblastoma. N Engl J Med 2005;352:997–1003.

75. Levner I, Drabycz S, Roldan G, et al. Predicting MGMT methylation status of glioblastomas from MRI texture. Med Image Comput Assist Interv 2009;12(Pt 2):522–30.

76. Drabycz S, Roldan G, de Robles P, et al. An analysis of image texture, tumor location, and MGMT promoter methylation in glioblastoma using magnetic resonance imaging. Neuroimage 2010;49(2):1398–405.

77. Eoli M, Menghi F, Bruzzone MG, et al. Methylation of O6-methylguanine DNA methyltransferase and loss of heterozygosity on 19q and/or 17p are overlapping features of secondary glioblastomas with prolonged survival. Clin Cancer Res 2007;13(9):2606–13.

78. Graham-Rowe D, Goldston D, Doctorow C, et al. Big data: Science in the petabyte era. Nature 2008; 455(7209):8–9.

79. Science. Dealing with data. Science 2011;331:639–806. http://www.sciencemag.org/content/331/6018.toc#SpecialIssue.

80. Thomson R, Lebiere C, Bennati S. Human, model and machine: a complementary approach to big data. Workshop in Human Centered Big Data Research. Raleigh, NC, April 1–3, 2014.

81. Big data. 2014. Available at: https://en.wikipedia.org/wiki/Big_data. Accessed August 10, 2016.

82. G.E. Opens its big data platform. 2014. Available at: http://bits.blogs.nytimes.com/2014/10/09/ge-opens-its-big-data-platform/. Accessed October 9, 2014.

83. A.C. Privacy and security of big data: current challenges and future research perspectives. Proceedings of the first international workshop on Privacy and Security of Big Data. Shanghai, China, November 3–7, 2015.

84. IBM scores weather data deal and starts Internet of things unit. 2015. Available at: http://bits.blogs.nytimes.com/2015/03/31/ibm-scores-a-weather-data-deal-and-starts-an-internet-of-things-unit/?version=meter+at+0&module=meter-Links&pgtype=Blogs&contentId=&mediaId=&referrer=https%3A%2F%2Fwww.google.com%2F&priority=true&action=click&contentCollection=meter-links-click;. Accessed March 31, 2015.

85. Using patient data to democratize medical discovery. 2015. Available at: http://bits.blogs.nytimes.com/2015/04/02/using-patient-data-to-democratize-medical-discovery/?version=meter+at+0&module=meter-Links&pgtype=Blogs&contentId=&mediaId=&referrer=https%3A%2F%2Fwww.google.com%2F&priority=true&action=click&contentCollection=meter-links-click;. Accessed April 2, 2015.

86. Omics. Available at: https://en.wikipedia.org/wiki/Omics. Accessed August 9, 2016.

87. Big data: The next frontier for innovation, competition and productivity. 2011. Available at: http://www.mckinsey.com/business-functions/business-technology/our-insights/big-data-the-next-frontier-for-innovation. Accessed May, 2011.

88. Watson JD, Crick FH. Molecular structure of nucleic acids; a structure for deoxyribose nucleic acid. Nature 1953;171:737–8.

89. Drmanac R, Sparks AB, Callow MJ, et al. Human genome sequencing using unchained base reads on self-assembling DNA nanoarrays. Science 2010;327(5961):78–81.

90. Schadt EE, Linderman MD, Sorenson J, et al. Computational solutions to large-scale data management and analysis. Nat Rev Genet 2010;11(9): 647–57.

91. Bibault JE, Giraud P, Burgun A. Big data and machine learning in radiation oncology: state of the art and future prospects. Cancer Lett 2016. [Epub ahead of print].

92. Siegel R, Ma J, Zou Z, et al. Cancer statistics, 2014. CA Cancer J Clin 2014;64(1):9–29.

93. Colen R, Hatami M, Kotrotsou A, et al. Radiomic subclassifications of glioblastoma. Neuro Oncol 2015;17(suppl 5):v155.

Imaging Genomics in Glioblastoma Multiforme
A Predictive Tool for Patients Prognosis, Survival, and Outcome

Rahul Anil, MBBS, Rivka R. Colen, MD*

KEYWORDS

• Imaging • Genomics • Glioblastoma • Prognosis • Survival • Outcome

KEY POINTS

• The integration of imaging characteristics and genomic data has started a new trend in the approach toward management of glioblastoma multiforme (GBM).
• Recently many ongoing studies are investigating imaging phenotypical signatures that could explain more about the behavior of the GBM and its outcome decisively.
• The discovery of biomarkers has played an adjuvant role in treating and predicting the outcome of patients with GBM.
• Discovering these imaging phenotypical signatures and dysregulated pathways/genes is the need of the hour and is a prerequisite to engineer treatment based on specific GBM manifestations.
• Characterizing these parameters will lay terra firma and establish well-defined criteria so researchers can build on and revolutionize the treatment of GBM through personal medicine.

INTRODUCTION

Among several forms of brain malignancies, glioblastoma (GBM) is the most common malignant brain neoplasm, accounting for 29.5% of all primary brain tumors.[1] In the United States alone more than 10,000 patients are newly diagnosed with GBM every year.[2] Current treatment is aggressive multimodal therapy with targeted surgical resection followed by radiation therapy and temozolomide.[3] Despite the prevailing standards of treatment, GBM still has an appalling prognosis with an overall median duration of survival ranging from 12.2 to 15.9 months.[4]

The largest cause of failure in GBM therapy is attributed to the inherent heterogeneity existing in intratumoral tissues. This heterogeneity, in turn, leads to a varying response to treatment and poor patient prognosis.[5] Using molecular techniques to understand the underlying cause for GBM would aid greatly in tackling this multifaceted tumor. Relying merely on histopathologic evidence would be detrimental to successful treatment of GBM, and a dependable genetic characteristic needs to be identified to improve accuracy and ensure effective therapy. The genetic heterogeneity of the tumor translates to different expression patterns within the neoplasm, which influences the magnetic resonance (MR) image.[6] To develop personalized targeted therapy it is critical to identify these patterns of genetic alterations in GBM.

Given the nascent nature of imaging genomics, it still does not have a standard definition. It can be thought of as an integration of medical imaging data and -omics data, which represents chiefly MR imaging on one hand and gene, protein, or metabolite expressions on the other.[7–9] Thus, imaging genomics has a lot of potential in identifying

The authors have nothing to disclose.
Department of Neuroradiology, The University of Texas MD Anderson Cancer Center, 1400 Pressler Street, Houston, TX 77030, USA
* Corresponding author.
E-mail address: RColen@mdanderson.org

mri.theclinics.com

morphologic and expressional profiles of the tumor with a holistic view while drawing parallels with the visible phenotypical results obtained from MR images.[10]

MICROARRAY TECHNIQUES

With the advent of breakthrough molecular biology techniques, the microarray has gained importance in its ability to detect mRNA expression levels and analyze whole genomes and individual genes.[11,12] Using microarrays can help discover new targets[13,14] of therapy for treatment of GBM, and there is currently an ongoing effort to find such targets. Micro-RNAs (mRNAs) are small-chain RNAs that do not code for any protein. Their mode of operation is different from regular RNAs in a way that they can regulate the expression of several target genes simultaneously. They carry the code to match the upstream 3′ UTR sequences of genes and can bind there to knockdown their expression.[15] mRNAs have been used as a powerful gene-silencing tool to discover new pathways and determine protein interactions in a cell. This technique could be the answer to the problem of lack of targets for treating GBM. Using mRNAs to alter the expression of oncogenes and tumor suppressors seems a promising strategy to find novel therapy by regulating proliferation, apoptosis, neovascularization, invasion, and migration.[16–18]

All said and done, microarray does have its shortcomings. The source of tissues for running such microarray assays is the resected tumor (or biopsy) from patients. These tissues are not only composed of tumor tissue but also the adjoining healthy cells, stroma, and so forth. So the microarray is not a perfect representation of the gene profile of the tumor. Secondly, the accuracy of the microarray depends largely on the availability of a specific probe, varying sensitivity of multiple probes, among other parameters. The lack of specific probes can result in skewing of the outcome of the assay and paint a different picture of mRNA expression. Thirdly, mRNA expression measurements from different parts of the tumor only reflect the level of transcription, whereas measurement of protein levels would serve as more reliable data to assess the tumor's subtype.[19,20] Also, microarrays performed of different systems are coherent with different standards and cannot be compared directly, hence, mandating the need for normalization.[21,22]

MOLECULAR CLASSIFICATION

Traditionally, GBM has been classified as primary and secondary: primary is composed of advance cancer with no evidence of low-grade lesions before diagnosis, and those tumors that have been detected at an earlier stage and subsequent evidence of progression (radiological or histopathologic) into a high-grade tumor was classified as a secondary tumor.[23]

In recent years, based on genetic aberrations, Phillips and colleagues[24] and Verhaak and colleagues[5] independently classified GBM into differing subtypes. Phillips and colleagues[24] emphasized the variations in expression levels of epidermal growth factor receptor (EGFR) and phosphatase and tensin homolog (PTEN). Accordingly, GBM was subdivided as proliferative (PTEN loss and increased/normal EGFR), proneural (normal PTEN and EGFR levels, notch pathway activation), and mesenchymal (increased neural stem cell markers, Akt activation, PTEN loss, and occasional EGFR activation). The proneural type of GBM had shown better survival rates in comparison with the mesenchymal and proliferative subgroups.

In a similar fashion, Verhaak and colleagues[5] also classified GBM into 4 subtypes based on genetic variations in genes, such as tumor suppressor p53 (TP53), EGFR, PTEN, isocitrate dehydrogenase-1 (IDH1), neurofibromatosis type-1 (NF1), and platelet-derived growth factor receptor A (PDGFRA). Classic GBM was predicted to have the longest survival when subject to vigorous treatment among all classes. Besides having common mutations in the TP53 gene, the proneural and mesenchymal subgroups differed in their genetic background indicated chiefly by variations in the PDGFRA, PTEN, IDH1, and NF1 genes. Lastly, there also existed a neural subtype of GBM that commonly affected elderly patient groups; it shared common mutations with other subgroups with no specific gene dysregulation.

BIOMARKERS

The genetic aberrations or their varying phenotypic expression levels in tumor cells, blood, or urine can be used as a potential prognostic and diagnostic parameter, also called a biomarker. These biomarkers may reliably help in determining the prognosis, response to treatment, and survival and also allow identification of a resistance mechanism in patients with GBM undergoing treatment.

O-6-methylguanine-DNA Methyltransferase

The O-6-methylguanine-DNA methyltransferase (MGMT) gene is located at 10q26 and is responsible for DNA repair mechanisms in cells. This enzyme removes alkylating agents that are attached to the guanosine bases in DNA. At times, the expression of this enzyme is silenced because of the methylation of its promoter region. In such patients, not only is the DNA repair mechanism impaired but also treatment with alkylating agents is far more effective as the MGMT enzyme is absent, thus improving response to therapy. It has been shown clinically in a randomized phase III trial involving 206 subjects (hazard ratio = 0.45 and 95% confidence interval [CI] [0.32–0.61] P<.001) that patients who have an epigenetic silencing of this MGMT gene (by methylation) have responded better with temozolomide, radiotherapy, and showed a good prognosis.[3,13] The median survival in the patients having the methylated MGMT gene with concomitant therapy with temozolomide and radiotherapy was 23.4 months as compared with normal individuals with active MGMT genes whose survival was only 15.3 months.[25] MGMT methylation status was the first biomarker that indicated GBM prognosis and since then has been predominantly important in predicting the response to alkylating agents.[26–28] However, it was not useful in aiding the diagnosis and designing treatment strategies for affected individuals.[29]

Isocitrate Dehydrogenase–1

IDH is the rate-limiting enzyme that acts on the substrate isocitrate and converts it into α-ketoglutarate. This in turn protects the cell from oxidative damage as this reaction also reduces NADP to NADPH as a byproduct. Among the isoforms of IDH, the cytosolic IDH1 is of pertinence to GBM.[30] IDH1 has been known to have mutations at the 132nd amino acid (arginine to histidine). This mutation increases its affinity to 2-oxaloglutarate and produces an oncometabolite: 2-hydroxyglutarate (2-HG).[31] 2-HG in turn acts on hypoxia inducible factor 1α (HIF-1α) and hydroxylates it. An increase in HIF-1α activation is believed to be instrumental in progression of tumor in the case of GBM.[32]

Janson and colleagues[33] made a noteworthy clinical observation in 149 patients with GBM, of which 12% (n = 18) were found to have IDH1 mutations and showed increased overall survival (OS) of 31 months in patients who were IDH1 mutant versus 15 months in patients with normal IDH1.[34] It is recently reported that the 5-year survival rate in patients with IDH1 mutations was 93%, which is significantly higher than 51% as seen in their IDH1-negative counterparts.[31] Thus, these findings strongly imply that improved outcome, reduced aggressiveness, and better prognosis in high-grade glioma cases have been associated with mutations in the IDH1 gene. In recent years, studies highlight the potential application of IDH1

in determining therapy outcome. Song Tao and colleagues[35] reported that the median progression-free survival rate for patients with both IDH1 and MGMT mutations in response to temozolomide treatment was 13.4 months, whereas those who had only IDH1 mutation showed a median survival rate of 10.2 months. Patients who lack any mutations in the aforementioned biomarkers had the least median survival rate of 6.1 months.

Deletion of 1p/19q (Loss of Heterozygosity)

Deletion of 1p/19q (loss of heterozygosity [LOH]) has been found to be a significant biomarker in cases of oligodendromas. The 1p/19q deletions in GBM are found to be uncommon (<10%) in diffuse astrocytic gliomas.[34] Contrastingly, the most common genetic mutations (40%–90%) in the oligodendroglioma component of GBM is 1p and 19q codeletion, which is associated with a favorable response to chemotherapy, radiation, and survival.[36] These tumors with 1p/19q codeletion have a greater propensity to occur in the frontal lobe as compared with insular tumors that rarely show deletion or alteration in neither 1p nor 19q.[37] In a trial study by the European Organization for Research and Treatment of Cancer/National Cancer Information Center, 360 subjects with GBM were studied for their differential response to chemo-radiotherapy with temozolomide, whereby the particular focus was on the presence of an oligodendromalike component (GBM-O). It was reported that 15% of the total population were positive for the presence of GBM-O. Another key finding of this study was that this 15% of patients with GBM-O had an ominous outcome. But codeletion of 1p/19q was found in only 1 case.[38] There is some ambiguity associated with the correlation of 1p/19q codeletions and prognosis of GBM. In one study performed by Hill and colleagues[39] it was reported that there was an improvement in prognosis of GBM cases with 1p/19q deletion. Conversely, in another study, despite the presence of an oligodendroma component there was no apparent improvement in prognosis.[40] Jesionek-Kupnicka and colleagues,[41] however, reported that there was no reciprocity between LOH of 1p/19q codeletion and patient survival.

A study conducted by Homma and colleagues[42] of 209 patients with GBM sought to find parallels between 1p deletions and prognosis. Interestingly, the results showed that patients (21% of population) with 1p LOH had significantly longer duration of survival (13.1 ± 10.8 months) than the patients without the LOH (9.6 ± 7.4 months; P<.05). These results were conclusive even after further adjustments were made for age and sex in a multivariate analysis; survival in patients with LOH of 1p had a hazard ratio of 0.7 (with 95% CI; 0.5–1.0).

Epidermal Growth Factor Receptor

EGFR is a tyrosine kinase–linked receptor that is present on epidermal cells.[43] It dimerizes on activation to switch on signaling and increase phosphoinositide 3 kinase (PI3K) and subsequently *PTEN*. This aids in increasing neovascularization, cell proliferation, and survival in tumors.[44,45] It is observed that EGFR is overexpressed in about 50% to 60% of patients with GBM.[46] The most common variant of EGFR seen in these cases is the EGFRvIII (24%–67%)[47] that activates the EGFR-PI3K pathway constitutively. A genetic sense-mutation leading to the deletion of exons 2 to 7 results in premature truncation of the extracellular ligand binding domain of EGFR, hence, resulting in expression of EGFRvIII.[48]

Several studies have been conducted to screen for correlations of wild-type-EGFR (wtEGFR) as a prognostic factor in patients with GBM; and results showed wtEGFR as not an independent favorable prognostic factor.[49–51] However, these results depict only a skewed image of reality as one study had a limited sample size; another study used ill-defined resection of surgical cavity and variations in postoperative treatment. Although tumor invasion seems to be more profound in the EGFRvIII as compared with wtEGFR, EGFRvIII expression levels have not been used as an independent factor for determining prognosis in patients with GBM. A heterogeneous study by Shinojima and colleagues[52] conveyed EGFRvIII overexpression in the presence of EGFR amplification as a potent indicator of negative prognosis. However, a homogenous study by Heimberger and colleagues[53] concluded that EGFRvIII is as an independent negative prognostic predictor in patients with GBM who survived greater than 1 year.

Besides being a potential negative prognostic factor of GBM, EGFR can also be a potential target for therapy, as a reported 97% of patients with primary classic GBM show EGFR amplification.[5] So, use of an EGFR inhibitor could be useful in treating this subtype of GBM. Hence, therapy can be tailored better by determining the EGFR amplification/overexpression in patients.

Vascular Endothelial Growth Factor

VEGF is an important proangiogenic factor that is highly regulated by HIF-1α. Hypoxia is commonly seen in tumors whereby the core is starved of oxygen. VEGF mediates this response to hypoxia by inducing growth of new blood vessels, which have a higher permeability, thus, causing local edema.[54] Nearly 64.1% of GBM cases have been found to have increased VEGF.[55] Further, a study that was conducted by Carlson and colleagues[56] in 2007 whereby they studied the relationship between VEGF expression and edema revealed that VEGF expression levels correlated well with tumor grade. GBM showed a 4-fold increase in VEGF expression when compared with grade 3 tumors. They outlined 2 groups of patients: no edema and little or abundant edema based on imaging characteristics. Interestingly, the group that had no edema showed no VEGF overexpression; on the other hand, the group with little or abundant edema showed higher VEGF levels, which correlated with survival.[56]

Subsequently, Pope and colleagues[57] reported another study in 2008 that considered completely enhancing (CE) and incompletely enhancing (IE) tumors of GBM based on MR images. Gene analyses were then conducted on these two groups, and the disparity in gene expression was studied. CE tumors were characterized by an increase in VEGF among other genes when compared with IE tumors, and a conclusion was drawn that targeting VEGF in these cases could be very important to improve response to therapy. VEGF is not a solitary factor that orchestrates the neovascularization and progression of tumor in GBM. It works in conjunction with other proteins, such as interleukin-8 and matrix metalloproteinase 7, to further tumor progression and cell survival.[57] This finding is shown by the clinical study whereby monotherapy using bevacizumab (a VEGF-targeting monoclonal antibody) has not been very successful in prolonging tumor-free survival and patient survival.[58] A global view of GBM can be obtained using MR imaging to track edema in tumors, and correlations can be made to monitor effectiveness of therapy and predict prognosis.

QUANTITATIVE ANALYSIS OF IMAGING GENOMICS

Quantitative measurement parameters have been recently studied for possible clues of expected survivability in patients with GBM, which could not have been accomplished without the aid of the qualitative imaging analyses performed over the last decade. A pioneering study using volumetric MR imaging by Zinn and colleagues[59] in conjunction with molecular biology techniques show some very interesting results. The study focused on analysis of gene expression in high versus low FLAIR patients. In the ingenuity pathway analysis of the 53 genes that were screened, 29 genes were shown to have a significant part in cancer, whereas another 20 genes were shown to play a role in cell migration and invasion and 16 genes played a common role in cancer and invasion. However, the gene periostin (POSTN) seemed to have the largest increase in expression in high versus low fluid-attenuated inversion recovery (FLAIR) patients (about a 7.5–mean fold increase). Furthermore, reports stated that POSTN was upregulated in the mesenchymal versus proneural subtype ($P<.0001$). POSTN expression has been shown to increase under TWIST-1 induction and modulate the migratory response in vitro.[60] The switch from the epithelial type to the mesenchymal type (called EMT) is one of the critical ways of cell invasion and treatment failure, which implies POSTN in some way responsible for influencing the migratory character of the tumor in vivo, which could explain the outcome of Zinn and colleagues'[59] study. The classic method of distinguishing patients with GBM into proneural and mesenchymal is a relatively poor indicator of patient survival with a P value of .202. However, when POSTN expression levels were considered as an independent determining factor for survival, its correlation with survival was found to be statistically significant ($P = .03$) in a Cox proportional hazards model. There have been parallels showing the existence of overlaps between tumor invasiveness and tumor resistance; because POSTN is a viable marker for tumor invasiveness, it could also serve as a marker for predicting response to therapy in patients with GBM.

In 2012 Zinn and colleagues[61] published another study using quantitative analysis and built a preoperative prognostic predictive model in patients with GBM. The variables of their predictive models were (1) volume of the tumor, (2) patient age, and (3) Karnofsky performance status (KPS); hence, they presented a new clinically applicable VAK classification. The VAK classification used a simple 3-point scoring system that would allow bisection of patients with GBM into VAK-A (score of 0 or 1) and VAK-B (score of 2 or 3). It was reported that patients with larger tumor volumes showed decreased survival compared with patients with smaller lesions ($P = .14$, survival 12.0 vs 18.5 months) when the median cutoff (30,000 mm^3) was considered as previously described in the literature.[62] Although KPS and age did not hold much significance independently, when combined with the tumor volume parameter, the prognostic value of the aforementioned variables was enhanced (age, KPS, and tumor volume) and dividing the patient population was aided, with $P = .007$, survival 12 versus 20 months

(VAK-B vs VAK-A). The patient data from The Cancer Genome Atlas (TCGA) and Rembrandt's database were used in validating the VAK model; the resulting VAK classification was more significant in predicting patient survival when corrected for age and KPS. Such innovative methods for predicting patient prognosis preoperatively is made possible because of the ability to accurately quantify tumor volume in lesions using MR imaging. The investigators also furthered their study by examining variations in patterns of genetic expression (TP53 and MGMT methylation) and incorporated it into the VAK classification with better correlation to patient survival.

An interesting recent study was conducted by Colen and colleagues[63] involving a sex-specific prediction of cell death by alternative mechanisms of apoptotic pathways using imaging genomics. Female patients were found to have smaller volumes of necrosis when compared with their male counterparts (6821 vs 11,050 mm^3, $P = .03$). Female patients (n = 30) who showed a lower volume of necrosis on imaging had significantly higher benefit of survival of 11.5 months when compared with the female patients with higher necrosis volumes ($P = .01$). Male patients (n = 69) of high and low necrosis groups did not show any change in survival. Although male patients with low necrosis volumes did not show any significant benefit in survival when compared with female patients with low necrosis volumes (n = 50, $P = .9$), the male patients with high necrosis volumes showed significantly higher survival benefit (8 months) when compared with female patients with high necrosis volumes (14.5 vs 6.5 months; $P = .01$, n = 49).

In an effort to understand this phenomenon, the investigators examined the mechanisms of apoptosis in both groups and arrived at the conclusion that the TP53-mediated apoptosis in male patients was the reason for increased necrosis, whereas the female patients had a differing mechanism of MYC oncogene dysregulation mediating necrosis. This finding opens a new avenue of potential therapeutic targets to treat sex-specific and sex-nonspecific mediation of necrosis in patients with GBM.

Gevaert and colleagues[64] conducted a study to extract quantitative features from MR images of the regions of interest (ROI) (enhancing necrotic zones and the surrounding peritumoral edematous areas) that characterize the radiographic phenotype of GBM lesions to create a radiogenomic map that correlates quantitative imaging features with molecular data.

A part of their study concentrated on correlating robust quantitative image features with survivability (OS and progression-free survival). Interestingly,

3 noteworthy correlations for enhancement image features were reported (P<.05): (1) OS was shown to highly correlate with variance of the radial distance signal of the enhancement of the ROI feature (P = .017; hazard ratio = 0.67). This feature defines the irregularity of the border of the ROI, and a smaller value would imply good prognosis. (2) The sharpness of the edge was also shown to correlate with OS, the smoother indicating better prognosis (P = .023; hazard ratio = 1.43). (3) In a similar fashion, a lesser blurriness of the edge was reported to have correlated with progression-free survival (P = .028; hazard ratio = 0.48). By this study the investigators highlighted the emphasis of quantitative image analysis in GBM and reported significant correlations with survival.

A study by Naeini and colleagues[65] demonstrates a simple method to potentially predict the mesenchymal (MES) subtype of GBM in patients and their survival using various ratios of quantified zones in MR images. The quantifiable parameters are (1) volume of contrast enhancement, (2) volume of central necrosis, (3) hyperintensity of T2/FLAIR, and (4) ratio of T2/FLAIR hyperintense volume to the volume of contrast enhancement and necrosis.

Among the different parameters that were calculated, the one the authors are interested in is the ratio of T2/FLAIR hyperintense volume to contrast enhancing and necrosis volume. A ratio of more than 3 had a sensitivity of 71% and a specificity of 100% for predicting the MES subtype. The investigators then classified patients based on the T2/FLAIR hyperintense volume to contrast enhancing and necrosis volume ratio into long (ratio >3.0) and short (ratio <3.0) OS groups (P = .0064). Then a multivariate Cox proportional hazards ratio analysis was performed to confirm that the ratio is able to independently classify the patients into short- and long-term survival groups when age and KPS are taken into consideration (Cox regression; ratio >3.0 vs ratio <3.0 covariate, P = .05; age covariate, P = .9617; KPS covariate = 0.1410). Thus, this study shows that the ratio of T2/FLAIR hyperintense volume to contrast enhancing and necrosis volume could be potentially a straightforward and influential marker for predicting the MES subtype of GBM from other phenotypes and their survival.

Hirai and colleagues[66] in 2008 came up with an unconventional yet radical study (n = 49) that correlated high-grade gliomas (GBM and astrocytoma) and prognosis to MR imaging features using relative cerebral blood volume (rCBV). The investigators used receiver operating characteristic analysis to establish an rCBV cutoff of 2.3, which showed a sensitivity of 98% and specificity of 98% (positive predictive value = 66%; negative predictive value = 90%). When the investigators correlated the maximum rCBV and survival time, they found the 2-year survival to be significantly lower in patients with GBM (4 of 31 individuals) with high rCBV ($\geq$2.3) when compared with patients with astrocytoma (16 of 18 individuals; P<.001). In patients with high-grade gliomas exhibiting low rCBV (18 of 27), the 2-year survival was shown to be significantly higher when compared with patients with a high rCBV (2 of 22; P<.001).[66]

In 2013 Jain and colleagues[67] performed a study along similar lines as Hirai and colleagues[66] whereby they used perfusion CT to measure rCBV and permeability surface area-product (PS) in patients with high-grade glioma retrospectively and correlated it with patient OS. When they concentrated on grade 4 gliomas, the rCBV was statistically significant (P = .019) between high and low rCBV with a 2-year survival rate being 24% (median OS = 14.2 months) for high rCBV when compared with low being 86% (median OS not reached). The investigators reported that contrastingly when only PS was considered for the correlation, there was no statistical relationship between PS (high vs low) and OS. However, the median OS was significantly higher in the high rCBV + PS group when compared with the low rCBV + PS group (39.5 months vs 13.6 months; P = .004). Thus, rCBV and PS together served as a much better indicator of patient survival than the two parameters considered independently. This finding promises the capacity of the use of vascular imaging parameters as prognostic biomarkers in high-grade gliomas.

FUTURE DIRECTIONS

There is a lot of scope for improvement in imaging genomics, especially with respect to GBM. Owing to the limited number of cases that are reported in several hospitals and medical centers world over, it is important to collect and maintain patient data so meaningful inferences can be drawn from statistical analysis. Currently, the scope of research is limited by the number of patients involved in a study; this bottleneck can be released by the use of computer and networking strategies, such as big data. Although publicly available databases, such as the TCGA, TCIA (The Cancer Imaging Archive), and Rembrandt's database, provide a unified platform for multiple institutions to record and share patient data in a secured fashion, the process needs to be streamlined further so common parameters are recorded and notified, hence, improving the usability of available data.

Translating the function of genes from cell to animals (in vivo) and further to humans is perplexing. There is often overlap between pathways, and involvement of one gene in modulating multiple molecular signals is inevitable. Although most of the biomarkers pertaining to GBM have been established based on screening clinical samples derived from patients, tumor heterogeneity and accuracy of resection/biopsy plays a crucial role in determining the validity of the genetic screens performed. Improvements in image-guided biopsy procedures in the last couple of decades has helped locating and isolating tumors with increased accuracy and, hence, validity of the sample.

There is a large unmet medical need in GBM, and one of the most promising strategies is personalized medicine. The general approach of treating patients with standardized therapy has proven mostly unsuccessful thus far with poor patient survival. Given the recent identification and characterization of several genetic biomarkers and the trends associated therewith, it is but apt to tailor therapies directed toward individual patients and target the underlying genes and molecular pathways involved in tumorigenesis and disease progression. Thus, the departure from the more traditional approach of treatment is a challenge worth overcoming. To aid this transition, there exists a plethora of techniques at the disposal of a clinician, namely, RNA sequencing, gene methylation studies, and databases, not to mention the innumerable articles that correlate patient prognosis and survival to molecular biomarkers. In this manner, we could apply known prognostic markers to treat patients and define new predictive biomarkers that can in turn help developing novel strategies for personalized treatment. The outcomes obtained from such targeted therapies can yield much valuable information about tumor biology, mechanisms of resistance, migration, and tumorigenesis, so newer therapies can be designed. Standard therapy for GBM would reveal information about how a specific type of tumor reacts to it. However, by implementing gene-targeted therapy, many other questions would arise: How effective has gene silencing been? How long does it take a tumor to develop resistance to the gene-targeted therapy? How has the cancer managed to acquire resistance? Which new pathway is subsequently modulating cancer growth, proliferation, and invasion? Such questions can be answered using the current methods practiced in clinics and hospitals today. This could not only improve patients' OS but also help clinicians design newer strategies and drugable targets to tackle this multifaceted problem. Not to mention, the currently abysmal patient outcomes would potentially improve significantly if personalized therapies are adopted at least as a pilot study.

A fine example of this kind of revolutionary drug discovery and patient treatment can be seen in the case of Kalydeco. Vertex Pharmaceuticals harnessed the power of big data and computerized modeling to characterize and design this molecule that could successfully treat cystic fibrosis (CF), a niche group of patients with CF who have a G155D mutation, which only accounts for about 4% of all reported CF cases[68,69]; however, it highlights the potency of new-age techniques to design personalized therapy. Targeted therapy using imaging genomics can reap the benefits of big data provided software is optimized for this particular purpose. The first step toward such integration has been taken by IBM in developing an artificially intelligent machine prototype called Watson that aims at dramatically shortening the time involved in diagnoses and choosing appropriate treatment, thereby giving physicians a head start with their patients. To take matters another step further, Watson also has the capability to assess a patients genomic mutations and tailoring therapy to cater their specific DNA profile. Remarkably Watson updates itself based on current developments, constantly increasing its data pool.[70] Larger strides toward such developments in GBM should also occur in the upcoming decade with much anticipation.

SUMMARY

The integration of imaging characteristics and genomic data has started a new trend in approach toward the management of GBM. Recently many ongoing studies are investigating into imaging phenotypical signatures that could explain more about the behavior of the GBM and its outcome decisively. The discovery of biomarkers has played an adjuvant role in treating and predicting the outcome of patients with GBM. Discovering these imaging phenotypical signatures and dysregulated pathways/genes is the need of the hour and is a prerequisite to engineer treatment based on specific GBM manifestations. Characterizing these parameters will lay terra firma and establish well-defined criteria so researchers can build on and revolutionize the treatment of GBM through personal medicine.

REFERENCES

1. International Radiosurgery Association. Available at: http://www.irsa.org/glioblastoma.html. Accessed June 1, 2016.

2. Central Brain Tumor Registry of the United States. Available at: http://www.cbtrus.org/. Accessed April 31, 2015.

3. Stupp R, Mason WP, van den Bent MJ, et al. Radiotherapy plus concomitant and adjuvant temozolomide for glioblastoma. N Engl J Med 2005;352(10):987–96.

4. Young RJ, Gupta A, Shah AD, et al. Potential role of preoperative conventional MRI including diffusion measurements in assessing epidermal growth factor receptor gene amplification status in patients with glioblastoma. AJNR Am J Neuroradiol 2013;34(12):2271–7.

5. Verhaak RG, Hoadley KA, Purdom E, et al. Integrated genomic analysis identifies clinically relevant subtypes of glioblastoma characterized by abnormalities in PDGFRA, IDH1, EGFR, and NF1. Cancer Cell 2010;17(1):98–110.

6. Barajas RF Jr, Phillips JJ, Parvataneni R, et al. Regional variation in histopathologic features of tumor specimens from treatment-naive glioblastoma correlates with anatomic and physiologic MR Imaging. Neuro Oncol 2012;14(7):942–54.

7. Aerts HJ, Velazquez ER, Leijenaar RT, et al. Decoding tumour phenotype by noninvasive imaging using a quantitative radiomics approach. Nat Commun 2014;5:4006.

8. Kim N, Choi J, Yi J, et al. An engineering view on megatrends in radiology: digitization to quantitative tools of medicine. Korean J Radiol 2013;14(2):139–53.

9. Kuo MD, Jamshidi N. Behind the numbers: decoding molecular phenotypes with radiogenomics–guiding principles and technical considerations. Radiology 2014;270(2):320–5.

10. Zinn PO, Colen RR. Imaging genomic mapping in glioblastoma. Neurosurgery 2013;60(Suppl 1):126–30.

11. Rickman DS, Bobek MP, Misek DE, et al. Distinctive molecular profiles of high-grade and low-grade gliomas based on oligonucleotide microarray analysis. Cancer Res 2001;61(18):6885–91.

12. Mischel PS, Cloughesy TF, Nelson SF. DNA-microarray analysis of brain cancer: molecular classification for therapy. Nat Rev Neurosci 2004;5(10):782–92.

13. Hegi ME, Diserens AC, Gorlia T, et al. MGMT gene silencing and benefit from temozolomide in glioblastoma. N Engl J Med 2005;352(10):997–1003.

14. Quant EC, Wen PY. Novel medical therapeutics in glioblastomas, including targeted molecular therapies, current and future clinical trials. Neuroimaging Clin N Am 2010;20(3):425–48.

15. Esquela-Kerscher A, Slack FJ. Oncomirs - microRNAs with a role in cancer. Nat Rev Cancer 2006;6(4):259–69.

16. Gaziel-Sovran A, Segura MF, Di Micco R, et al. miR-30b/30d regulation of GalNAc transferases enhances invasion and immunosuppression during metastasis. Cancer Cell 2011;20(1):104–18.

17. Rothe F, Ignatiadis M, Chaboteaux C, et al. Global microRNA expression profiling identifies MiR-210 associated with tumor proliferation, invasion and poor clinical outcome in breast cancer. PLoS One 2011;6(6):e20980.

18. Kwak HJ, Kim YJ, Chun KR, et al. Downregulation of Spry2 by miR-21 triggers malignancy in human gliomas. Oncogene 2011;30(21):2433–42.

19. Vogel C, Marcotte EM. Insights into the regulation of protein abundance from proteomic and transcriptomic analyses. Nat Rev Genet 2012;13(4):227–32.

20. Chen G, Gharib TG, Huang CC, et al. Discordant protein and mRNA expression in lung adenocarcinomas. Mol Cell Proteomics 2002;1(4):304–13.

21. De Cecco L, Dugo M, Canevari S, et al. Measuring microRNA expression levels in oncology: from samples to data analysis. Crit Rev Oncog 2013;18(4):273–87.

22. Butte A. The use and analysis of microarray data. Nat Rev Drug Discov 2002;1(12):951–60.

23. Ohgaki H, Kleihues P. The definition of primary and secondary glioblastoma. Clin Cancer Res 2013;19(4):764–72.

24. Phillips HS, Kharbanda S, Chen R, et al. Molecular subclasses of high-grade glioma predict prognosis, delineate a pattern of disease progression, and resemble stages in neurogenesis. Cancer Cell 2006;9(3):157–73.

25. Stupp R, Hegi ME, Mason WP, et al. Effects of radiotherapy with concomitant and adjuvant temozolomide versus radiotherapy alone on survival in glioblastoma in a randomised phase III study: 5-year analysis of the EORTC-NCIC trial. Lancet Oncol 2009;10(5):459–66.

26. Esteller M, Garcia-Foncillas J, Andion E, et al. Inactivation of the DNA-repair gene MGMT and the clinical response of gliomas to alkylating agents. N Engl J Med 2000;343(19):1350–4.

27. Hegi ME, Diserens AC, Godard S, et al. Clinical trial substantiates the predictive value of O-6-methylguanine-DNA methyltransferase promoter methylation in glioblastoma patients treated with temozolomide. Clin Cancer Res 2004;10(6):1871–4.

28. Weller M, Felsberg J, Hartmann C, et al. Molecular predictors of progression-free and overall survival in patients with newly diagnosed glioblastoma: a prospective translational study of the German Glioma Network. J Clin Oncol 2009;27(34):5743–50.

29. Mason S, McDonald K. MGMT testing for glioma in clinical laboratories: discordance with methylation analyses prevents the implementation of routine immunohistochemistry. J Cancer Res Clin Oncol 2012;138(11):1789–97.

30. Frezza C, Tennant DA, Gottlieb E. IDH1 mutations in gliomas: when an enzyme loses its grip. Cancer Cell 2010;17(1):7–9.

31. Cohen AL, Holmen SL, Colman H. IDH1 and IDH2 mutations in gliomas. Curr Neurol Neurosci Rep 2013;13(5):345.
32. Tan WL, Huang WY, Yin B, et al. Can diffusion tensor imaging noninvasively detect IDH1 gene mutations in astrogliomas? A retrospective study of 112 cases. AJNR Am J Neuroradiol 2014;35(5):920–7.
33. Jansen M, Yip S, Louis DN. Molecular pathology in adult gliomas: diagnostic, prognostic, and predictive markers. Lancet Neurol 2010;9(7):717–26.
34. Riemenschneider MJ, Jeuken JW, Wesseling P, et al. Molecular diagnostics of gliomas: state of the art. Acta Neuropathol 2010;120(5):567–84.
35. SongTao Q, Lei Y, Si G, et al. IDH mutations predict longer survival and response to temozolomide in secondary glioblastoma. Cancer Sci 2012;103(2):269–73.
36. Gladson CL, Prayson RA, Liu WM. The pathobiology of glioma tumors. Annu Rev Pathol 2010;5:33–50.
37. Goze C, Rigau V, Gibert L, et al. Lack of complete 1p19q deletion in a consecutive series of 12 WHO grade II gliomas involving the insula: a marker of worse prognosis? J Neurooncol 2009;91(1):1–5.
38. Hegi ME, Janzer RC, Lambiv WL, et al. Presence of an oligodendroglioma-like component in newly diagnosed glioblastoma identifies a pathogenetically heterogeneous subgroup and lacks prognostic value: central pathology review of the EORTC_26981/NCIC_CE.3 trial. Acta Neuropathol 2012;123(6):841–52.
39. Hill C, Hunter SB, Brat DJ. Genetic markers in glioblastoma: prognostic significance and future therapeutic implications. Adv Anat Pathol 2003;10(4):212–7.
40. Pinto LW, Araujo MB, Vettore AL, et al. Glioblastomas: correlation between oligodendroglial components, genetic abnormalities, and prognosis. Virchows Arch 2008;452(5):481–90.
41. Jesionek-Kupnicka D, Szybka M, Potemski P, et al. Association of loss of heterozygosity with shorter survival in primary glioblastoma patients. Pol J Pathol 2013;64(4):268–75.
42. Homma T, Fukushima T, Vaccarella S, et al. Correlation among pathology, genotype, and patient outcomes in glioblastoma. J Neuropathol Exp Neurol 2006;65(9):846–54.
43. Fan QW, Cheng CK, Gustafson WC, et al. EGFR phosphorylates tumor-derived EGFRvIII driving STAT3/5 and progression in glioblastoma. Cancer Cell 2013;24(4):438–49.
44. Jura N, Endres NF, Engel K, et al. Mechanism for activation of the EGF receptor catalytic domain by the juxtamembrane segment. Cell 2009;137(7):1293–307.
45. Zadeh G, Bhat KP, Aldape K. EGFR and EGFRvIII in glioblastoma: partners in crime. Cancer Cell 2013;24(4):403–4.
46. Ekstrand AJ, James CD, Cavenee WK, et al. Genes for epidermal growth factor receptor, transforming growth factor alpha, and epidermal growth factor and their expression in human gliomas in vivo. Cancer Res 1991;51(8):2164–72.
47. Wikstrand CJ, McLendon RE, Friedman AH, et al. Cell surface localization and density of the tumor-associated variant of the epidermal growth factor receptor, EGFRvIII. Cancer Res 1997;57(18):4130–40.
48. Ekstrand AJ, Longo N, Hamid ML, et al. Functional characterization of an EGF receptor with a truncated extracellular domain expressed in glioblastomas with EGFR gene amplification. Oncogene 1994;9(8):2313–20.
49. Galanis E, Buckner J, Kimmel D, et al. Gene amplification as a prognostic factor in primary and secondary high-grade malignant gliomas. Int J Oncol 1998;13(4):717–24.
50. Newcomb EW, Cohen H, Lee SR, et al. Survival of patients with glioblastoma multiforme is not influenced by altered expression of p16, p53, EGFR, MDM2 or Bcl-2 genes. Brain Pathol 1998;8(4):655–67.
51. Waha A, Baumann A, Wolf HK, et al. Lack of prognostic relevance of alterations in the epidermal growth factor receptor-transforming growth factor-alpha pathway in human astrocytic gliomas. J Neurosurg 1996;85(4):634–41.
52. Shinojima N, Tada K, Shiraishi S, et al. Prognostic value of epidermal growth factor receptor in patients with glioblastoma multiforme. Cancer Res 2003;63(20):6962–70.
53. Heimberger AB, Hlatky R, Suki D, et al. Prognostic effect of epidermal growth factor receptor and EGFRvIII in glioblastoma multiforme patients. Clin Cancer Res 2005;11(4):1462–6.
54. Plate KH. Mechanisms of angiogenesis in the brain. J Neuropathol Exp Neurol 1999;58(4):313–20.
55. McNamara MG, Sahebjam S, Mason WP. Emerging Biomarkers in Glioblastoma. Cancers 2013;5(3):1103–19.
56. Carlson MR, Pope WB, Horvath S, et al. Relationship between survival and edema in malignant gliomas: role of vascular endothelial growth factor and neuronal pentraxin 2. Clin Cancer Res 2007;13(9):2592–8.
57. Pope WB, Chen JH, Dong J, et al. Relationship between gene expression and enhancement in glioblastoma multiforme: exploratory DNA microarray analysis. Radiology 2008;249(1):268–77.
58. Gilbert MR, Dignam JJ, Armstrong TS, et al. A randomized trial of bevacizumab for newly diagnosed glioblastoma. N Engl J Med 2014;370(8):699–708.
59. Zinn PO, Mahajan B, Sathyan P, et al. Radiogenomic mapping of edema/cellular invasion MRI-phenotypes

in glioblastoma multiforme. PLoS One 2011;6(10): e25451.

60. Mikheeva SA, Mikheev AM, Petit A, et al. TWIST1 promotes invasion through mesenchymal change in human glioblastoma. Mol Cancer 2010;9:194.

61. Zinn PO, Sathyan P, Mahajan B, et al. A novel volume-age-KPS (VAK) glioblastoma classification identifies a prognostic cognate microRNA-gene signature. PLoS One 2012;7(8):e41522.

62. Iliadis G, Selviaridis P, Kalogera-Fountzila A, et al. The importance of tumor volume in the prognosis of patients with glioblastoma: comparison of computerized volumetry and geometric models. Strahlenther Onkol 2009;185(11):743–50.

63. Colen RR, Wang J, Singh SK, et al. Glioblastoma: imaging genomic mapping reveals sex-specific oncogenic associations of cell death. Radiology 2015;275(1):215–27.

64. Gevaert O, Mitchell LA, Achrol AS, et al. Glioblastoma multiforme: exploratory radiogenomic analysis by using quantitative image features. Radiology 2014;273(1):168–74.

65. Naeini KM, Pope WB, Cloughesy TF, et al. Identifying the mesenchymal molecular subtype of glioblastoma using quantitative volumetric analysis of anatomic magnetic resonance images. Neuro Oncol 2013;15(5):626–34.

66. Hirai T, Murakami R, Nakamura H, et al. Prognostic value of perfusion MR imaging of high-grade astrocytomas: long-term follow-up study. AJNR Am J Neuroradiol 2008;29(8):1505–10.

67. Jain R, Narang J, Griffith B, et al. Prognostic vascular imaging biomarkers in high-grade gliomas: tumor permeability as an adjunct to blood volume estimates. Acad Radiol 2013;20(4):478–85.

68. Smolan RaE, J. The human face of big data. Against all odds productions2012.

69. Barrett PM, Alagely A, Topol EJ. Cystic fibrosis in an era of genomically guided therapy. Hum Mol Genet 2012;21(R1):R66–71.

70. Jeelani M. WATSON Watson, Come here. I want you. Johnson & Johnson's CEO enlists IBM's big-data service to find new drugs. Fortune 2014; 170(6):36.

Shedding Light on the 2016 World Health Organization Classification of Tumors of the Central Nervous System in the Era of Radiomics and Radiogenomics

CrossMark

Rivka R. Colen, MD[a],*, Islam Hassan, MD[a],
Nabil Elshafeey, MD[a], Pascal O. Zinn, MD, PhD[b]

KEYWORDS

• Tumors • Central nervous system • WHO Classification • Radiogenomic • Radiomics

KEY POINTS

• The new World Health Organization (WHO) classification has been recently released where integration of genotype and phenotype was done to achieve a more accurate and clinically relevant classification of different brain tumors.
• The new classification depends on combining the histologic light microscopy features of central nervous system tumors with key canonical genetic alterations.
• This new integrated diagnosis is redrawing the pedigree chart of brain tumors with rearrangement of tumor groups on basis of geno-phenotypical behaviors into clinically meaningful groups.

INTRODUCTION

Neoplasm of the central nervous system (CNS) represent a wide range of tumors.[1–3] Each tumor is characterized by a set of unique features that are translated in the form of specific clinical presentations, different treatment approaches, and distinct outcomes.[2] Therefore, accurate and precise classification and grading of brain tumors become essential steps in management of such tumors, which are expected to affect over 23,000 patients in 2016.[1] Historically, brain tumor grading and classifications depended solely on their microscopic picture, where similarities with putative cells of origin and the degree of differentiation were the key classifiers.[4] Tumors were grouped on the basis of light microscopic features in hematoxylin and eosin-stained sections, immunohistochemical detection of specific protein expression, or characteristic ultrastructure features.[4]

Confining tumor classification to structural similarities was limiting, as sharing similar structural appearance did not fully reflect on clinical features or tumor behavior.[4] For instance, astrocytic tumors that share similar microscopic features can behave distinctly from each other.[5,6] Therefore, a more comprehensive classification is essential. In the effort to reach such clinically relevant classification, several studies in the past decade identified key genetic alterations that contribute to the

The authors have nothing to disclose.
[a] Department of Diagnostic Radiology, The University of Texas MD Anderson Cancer Center, 1400 Pressler Street, Unit 1482, Room # FCT 16.5037, Houston, TX 77030, USA; [b] Department of Neurosurgery, Baylor College of Medicine, 1 Baylor Plaza, Houston, TX 77030, USA
* Corresponding author.
E-mail address: rcolen@mdanderson.org

mri.theclinics.com

tumorigenesis process of distinct tumors.[6,7] These canonical genetic alterations were recently implemented in the new 2016 World Health Organization (WHO) classification of brain tumors.[4]

The new WHO classification combined both the phenotypic and the genotypic key features for CNS tumor classification.[4] Combining both features resulted in a more clinically relevant grouping of tumors, which would reflect on diagnostic accuracy with direct impact on management plans.[4,8,9] This linking of both phenotypic and genotypic parameters is another step to an integrated efficient classification of brain tumors. However, it still faces multiple challenges, including:

- Economic challenges of availability of genotyping.
- Technical challenges involving the choice of genotyping techniques as well as standardization of such techniques to ensure universality of results.
- Communication challenges on how such integrated diagnoses should be reported.[4]

Recently, many studies have focused on creating a bridge between the imaging gross appearance of CNS tumors and the underlying key genetic and molecular features.[10,11] These radiogenomic correlation between the imaging phenotype and genetic profile of tumor can play a pivotal role in a more comprehensive tumor classification that integrates histologic appearance of the tumor with canonical genetic alterations in addition to imaging phenotypes of the tumor observed on different imaging modalities.[10,11] In addition, an exponential amount of imaging features can be extracted to detect the trivial and minute voxel-by-voxel changes occurring in the context of CNS tumors.[12] The term radiomics is used to describe such high throughput extraction of imaging features.[12,13] These features can be correlated with clinical outcomes to create robust prognostic predictive markers and can be further correlated to genetic and epigenetic alterations occurring in different tumors.[14–20] This exponential amount of data can be easily integrated into big data analytics for a more precise and accurate prediction of tumor type, grade, and more importantly its genetic features.[12] Such advances in the field of medical imaging and imaging analytics are anticipated to become cornerstone of future classifications of brain tumors.

THE NEW 2016 CENTRAL NERVOUS SYSTEM TUMOR CLASSIFICATION

Multiple studies have been deployed in the past decade to unveil and decode the genetic encryption of different CNS tumors.[5,6,21–24] These studies have revealed sets of key genetic alterations that direct and harmonize the development of specific tumors and represent efficient prognostic biomarkers.[4] Therefore, the new 2016 CNS tumor classification incorporated these canonical genetic alterations with light microscopy features to refine tumor grading and improve diagnostic precision.[4] Such integration paved the way for a more clinically sound grouping of clinically analogous tumors, as tumors that share the similar genetic drivers are expected to follow a common, if not similar, pathway with overlapping treatment response and subsequently common patient outcome.[4,8,9] Although it is still unclear if tumor grouping and classification can depend solely on the basis of genotypical features,[4] the new integrated phenotypic–genotypic diagnostic parameters are reflected as a number of newly recognized entities, variants, and patterns that will be discussed in the following sections.

DIFFUSE GLIOMAS

On previous classifications, all astrocytic tumors were believed to share the same behavioral hierarchy and growth patterns and were thus grouped together.[4] However, this grouping was modified on basis of IDH1 and IDH2 mutations, key driver mutations noticed in all diffusely infiltrating gliomas, including those with oligodendroglial phenotypical appearance and those with astrocytic phenotypical appearance.[4–6,9,11,21–25] Such integrated grouping reflects on the variable aspects of better care via incorporation of both phenotypic and genotypic features, eventually leading to proper categorization of tumors with similar prognostic biomarkers and shepherding therapeutic plans for biogenetically analogous entities.[4]

According to the new classification, diffuse gliomas include WHO grade II and III astrocytic tumors; WHO grade II and III oligodendroglioma; the grade IV glioblastoma (GBM), and diffuse gliomas of childhood.[4] This reformatted pedigree chart of tumor classification (Fig. 1) clearly distinguishes diffuse gliomas from other gliomas that are characterized by a circumscribed pattern of growth, including pilocytic astrocytoma, pleomorphic xanthrocytoma, as well as the subependymal giant cell astrocytoma.[4] This highlights the fact that sharing a common progenitor cannot be the sole grouping variable in CNS Tumors, as one can see that a diffusely growing grade III astrocytoma would share more clinically meaningful features with grade III oligodendroglioma than a more circumscribed pilocytic astrocytoma.[4,6]

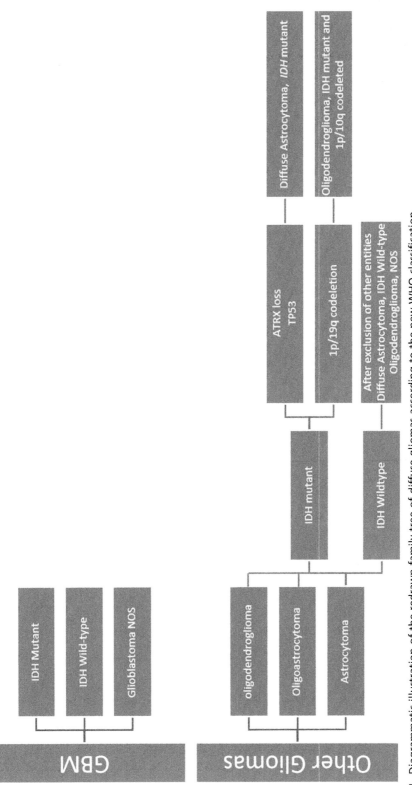

Fig. 1. Diagrammatic illustration of the redrawn family tree of diffuse gliomas according to the new WHO classification.

DIFFUSE ASTROCYTOMAS AND ANAPLASTIC ASTROCYTOMAS

According to the new WHO classification, 3 categories of astrocytoma are adopted depending on the key driver mutation of the *IDH* family of genes (*IDH1, IDH2*): *IDH*-wild type, *IDH*-mutant and not otherwise specific (NOS).[4] Most diffuse astrocytomas and anaplastic astrocytomas are expected to belong to the *IDH*-mutant category.[4,9] According to the WHO guidelines, mutation in the *IDH* family of genes requires immunohistochemical (IHC) staining for the R132H IDH1 protein in addition to sequencing for *IDH1* codon 132 and *IDH2* codon 172.[4] Diagnosis of *IDH*-wild-type astrocytoma requires either tests to come back negative or at least negative gene sequencing. These testing check-points are essential to ensure accurate diagnosis of the uncommon diffuse astrocytoma and anaplastic astrocytoma with *IDH*-wild type genetic annotation.[4] In cases of unavailable Genetic testing or indeterminate testing results (eg, negative IHC staining for *IDH* with unavailable sequencing), WHO classification opts toward a diagnosis of diffuse astrocytoma or anaplastic astrocytoma NOS.[4]

Currently, the WHO classification limits the variants of diffuse astrocytomas to gemistocytic astrocytoma, removing both the protoplasmic astrocytoma and fibrillary astrocytoma from its diagnostic glossary.[4] In addition, gliomatosis cerebri is no longer considered a distinct entity in the new classification but rather a growth pattern seen across *IDH* mutant astrocytic and oligodendroglial tumors as well as the *IDH* wild-type GBM.[4]

GLIOBLASTOMA

A schematic classification of glioblastoma was proposed previously, in which key genetic mutations in *PDGFRA, IDH1, EGFR*, and *NF1* stratified GBM into clinically relevant subtypes.[8] However, the new WHO classification addressed only the *IDH* family mutation in its classification of GBM.[4] The grade IV lethal tumor was classified into a majority of *IDH* wild-type GBM, representing 90% of cases with a minority that falls under *IDH*-mutant GBM category (**Fig. 2**).[4,23,26,27] *IDH* wild-type GBM was mostly associated with an older age of incidence and a predilection toward de novo or primary GBM.[4,23] On the other hand, *IDH*-mutant GBM was closely associated with younger age (**Fig. 3**) and the diagnosis of secondary GBM that arises on top of previous lower-grade glioma.[4,23]

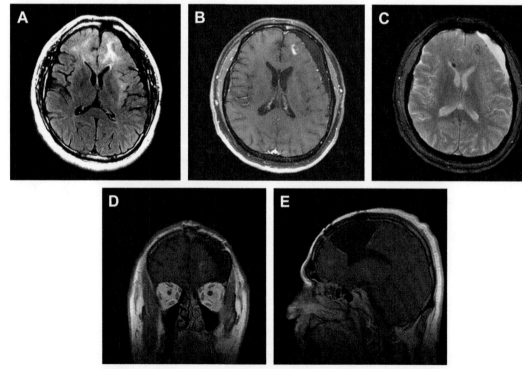

Fig. 2. A case of secondary glioblastoma, *IDH*-mutant. A 50-year-old man with prior history of WHO III anaplastic astrocytoma, NOS. The tumor sample showed positive sequence testing for codon 132 *IDH1* mutation. (*A*) Axial fluid attenuation inversion recovery (FLAIR) WIs. (*B*) Axial T1 postcontrast WIs. (*C*) Axial T2*WIs. (*D*) Coronal T1 postcontrast WIs. (*E*) Sagittal T1 postcontrast WIs.

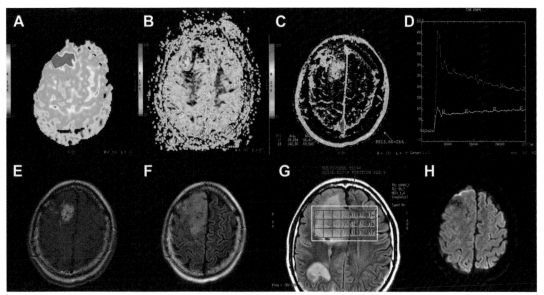

Fig. 3. Advanced MRI of a case of secondary glioblastoma, *IDH* mutant. A 20-year-old man with prior history of diffuse anaplastic astrocytoma grade III who developed glioblastoma. (*A*) Arterial spin labeling. (*B*) Dynamic susceptibility contrast. (*C*) Dynamic contrast enhancement. (*D*) Dynamic contrast enhancement curve. (*E*) Axial T1 postcontrast WIs. (*F*) Axial T2 FLAIR WIs. (*G*) MRS. (*H*) Diffusion WIs.

Testing for the *IDH* family mutation in GBM is slightly different from what was proposed for diffuse astrocytoma and anaplastic astrocytoma, as a negative IHC test of R132H *IDH1* protein in patients older than 55 years of age is deemed sufficient for diagnosis of *IDH* wild-type GBM without the need for further sequencing.[4]

Multiple variants were included under the flag of *IDH* wild-type GBM including gliosarcoma, giant cell glioblastoma, and a new variant of GBM epithelioid glioblastoma.[4,28,29] This newly proposed variant is more common in children and young adults.[4] Epithelioid GBM is characterized by an IHC-positive stain for *BRAF* V600E mutation in addition to the loss INI1 expression that differentiates it from the microscopically analogous rhabdoid GBM.[28,29] However, epithelioid GBM lacks some characteristic genotypical features of *IDH* wild-type GBM including EGFR amplification and chromosome 10 losses.[4] GBM patterns currently include GBM/astrocytoma and granular cell glioblastoma in addition to a newly added pattern named glioblastoma with primitive neural component.[4]

OLIGODENDROGLIOMA

The new WHO classification for oligodendroglioma requires the presence of a mutation of *IDH* gene family in addition to 1p/19q codeletion.[4,6,9,30–32] Such classification is concordant with the findings of the cancer genome atlas research network that resulted from the integration of genome-wide data from multiple platforms of 293 lower-grade gliomas in adults.[9] The Cancer Genome Atlas Research Network also demonstrated that a strong correlation exists between the histologic class of oligodendroglioma and the presence of *IDH* mutation together with a combined whole-arm loss of 1p and 19q.[9] In this context, a positive mutant R132H IDH1 IHC stain is sufficient for diagnosis.[4] In case the result of IHC comes back negative, sequencing of *IDH1* codon 132 and *IDH2* codon 172 is recommended.[4]

OLIGOASTROCYTOMA

According to the new WHO classification, genetic testing should provide the basis for accurate classification of tumors that have a mixed histologic pattern (ie, oligodendroglial and astrocytic components).[4,33] As such, diagnosis of oligoastrocytoma would be rather limited, and the WHO classification assigned a NOS genetic status to both grade II oligoastrocytoma and grade III anaplastic oligoastrocytomas.[4,33] This is mainly due to the rarity of true oligoastrocytoma tumors, which limits the available samples for accurate genetic profiling and determination of their key genetic alteration.[2,4]

PEDIATRIC DIFFUSE GLIOMA AND MEDULLOBLASTOMA

Prior to the new WHO classification, pediatric gliomas were usually identified in the same lexicon as adult gliomas.[4,34] However, such grouping was inaccurate, as the clinical behavior of pediatric gliomas differs from their counterparts in adults.[4,35,36] With the continuous revelation of genetic landscape of pediatric tumors, a more accurate classification of these tumors can be achieved.[36] According to the new WHO classification, a new entity is defined as diffuse midline glioma, *H3 K27M*-mutant, which includes the previously described diffuse intrinsic pontine gliomas (DIPGs).[4,35,37] These tumors are characterized by a mutation of the histone H3 gene *H3F3A* and a characteristic midline location.[4]

Classification of medulloblastoma is relatively more complicated, as histologic diagnostic entities that have a clinical relevance were already established, and different genetic studies classified medulloblastoma into 4 subgroups according to genetic pathways activated.[4,36] Merging histologic and genetic parameters in this context will entirely depend on the reporting pathologist who can provide accurate integrated diagnosis that would include both phenotype and genotype into a clinically relevant diagnosis from multiple different possible combinations.[4]

EPENDYMOMA AND NEURONAL AND MIXED NEURONAL–GLIAL TUMORS

Currently there is no prognostic classification available for ependymomas. Ependymoma with RELA fusion-positive is the only currently identified subtype that was included in the new classification and is characteristic of supratentorial tumors in children.[4,38–40] Also, a new entity was included in the new classification under the title of diffuse leptomeningeal glioneural tumor; this entity is characterized by absent *IDH1* mutation and a combination *BRAF* fusion and a deletion of chromosome arm 1p.[4]

OTHER EMBRYONAL TUMORS, MENINGIOMA, AND NERVE SHEATH TUMORS

The diagnosis of embryonal tumors other than medulloblastoma is now revolving around a key genetic alteration in the form of amplification of the C19MC region on chromosome 19 (19q13.42).[4,41] Tumors showing this amplification were coined the annotation of embryonal tumor with multilayered rosettes (ETMR), *C19MC*-altered.[4,41] On the other hand, absence of such amplification will change the diagnosis to become ETMR, NOS.[4] In addition, previously described primitive neuroectodermal tumor (PNET) was removed from the diagnostic glossary.[4] On the

other hand, diagnosis of meningioma and nerve sheath tumors was not changed dramatically.[4]

FUTURE ROLE OF ADVANCED MRI, RADIOMICS, AND RADIOGENOMICS

It is now clear that the new WHO classification of CNS tumors is leaning toward a more comprehensive description of phenotype and genotype of the tumors.[4,9] Tumor phenotype depends on the light microscopy features of tumor, while IHC staining as well as sequencing are the current tools for disclosing tumor genotype.[4] Although these tools remain the diagnostic gold standard, availability of these techniques is relatively limited due to logistic and economic factors.[4] On the other hand, the first large-scale imaging–genomic study performed in GBM demonstrated a probable role of both qualitative and quantitative MRI as discovery tools for tumor genetic profile and microRNA expression.[10] This potential correlation between imaging features and histologic patterns of tumors as well as tumor genetic profile can enhance the accuracy of tumor classification through an integrated radio-histo-genomic interpretation.[10,14,16,20]

Radiomics was also introduced as a tool for postprocessing of conventional and advanced MRI aiming at extraction of an exponential amount of data points that can be further correlated with derive both diagnostic and prognostic imaging biomarkers.[12,15,16,20] This high throughput analysis method is providing a robust platform for tumor imaging genomic studies as a potential discovery tool.[10,12,17] Recently, mutliple studies have been implemented to discover the potential correlation between radiomic imaging features and tumor pathology.[15,17,19] Upon reaching a consensus understanding for standardization of radiomic techniques, radiomic imaging features can play multiple roles; initially, they can provide a relatively accurate and early prediction of tumor genotype when genetic sequencing is not available. Also, an integrated radio-histo-genomic classification can be applied and may result in further refinement of current pathologic entities, variants, and patterns or even cause a paradigm shift in the understanding of the pathologic process of common and rare tumors.

One of the striking examples is the role that magnetic resonance spectroscopy (MRS) can play in determining the mutation status of *IDH1* and *IDH2* genes,[42,43] a key mutation that plays a significant role in the new WHO classification of CNS tumors.[4,9,24,25,30,31] Mutations of the *IDH1* and *IDH2* genes result in over-reduction of α-ketoglutarate to 2-hydroxyglutarate (2HG) metabolite.[42] Accumulation of 2HG can be detected using advanced optimized MRS post-processing steps that can provide noninvasive qualitative (eg, binomial annotation of presence or absence of significant 2HG concentration) and quantitative parameters (eg, actual concentration of 2HG in tumor tissue).[42] These parameters can be used as a diagnostic imaging biomarker for the status of the *IDH* family gene mutations.[42,43] Furthermore, detection of such metabolite is also of prognostic value, as it is capable of capturing treatment response.[42] As such, MRS results of 2HG concentrations can be integrated along with sequencing data for *IDH1* and *IDH2* as well as results of IHC for R132H to overcome any inconsistent results of both techniques.[4,42,43]

Furthermore, imaging features of conventional MRI can also play a role in the radio-histo-genomic classification. For instance, location of tumor has been proposed as one of the key classifiers of tumors and their genetic profile.[10,11,44] For example, the combined whole-arm deletion of chromosome 1p and 19q, a landmark for oligodendrogliomas, is usually absent in tumors occupying the insula.[44] Also, *IDH1*-mutant tumors are more likely frontal.[44] In addition to location, the vascular behavior of the tumor can also be used to predict genetic profile of tumors (eg, noncontrast enhancing tumors are mostly *IDH1* mutant).[11] Multiple studies have also suggested that imaging features extracted from conventional MRI can predict the status of *IDH* family gene mutation with an overall accuracy of 97.5%.[44–46] However, further studies must be done to validate these results both in-vitro and in-vivo using Mouse models as well as image-guided spatially labeled tumor samples to achieve a comprehensive spatial profile of the tumor landscape that can be further used to accomplish the goal of precision medicine.[44]

To this end, the new WHO classification is another substantial step taken toward a more precise and accurate classification of CNS tumors.[4] This step is a keystone that will significantly augment our understanding of cancer. Yet, it would require further enrichment effort that can address every prospect of diagnosis, prognosis, and therapeutic planning, where every aspect of tumor assessment is combined and integrated to reach a comprehensive understanding of different CNS tumors.

REFERENCES

1. Siegel RL, Miller KD, Jemal A. Cancer statistics, 2016. CA Cancer J Clin 2016;66:7–30.
2. Ostrom QT, Gittleman H, Fulop J, et al. CBTRUS statistical report: primary brain and central nervous system tumors diagnosed in the United States in 2008-2012. Neuro Oncol 2015;17(Suppl 4):iv1–62.
3. Vescovi AL, Galli R, Reynolds BA. Brain tumour stem cells. Nat Rev Cancer 2006;6:425–36.
4. Louis DN, Perry A, Reifenberger G, et al. The 2016 World Health Organization classification of tumors of the central nervous system: a summary. Acta Neuropathol 2016;131:803–20.
5. Mellai M, Piazzi A, Caldera V, et al. IDH1 and IDH2 mutations, immunohistochemistry and associations in a series of brain tumors. J Neurooncol 2011;105:345–57.
6. Li S, Yan C, Huang L, et al. Molecular prognostic factors of anaplastic oligodendroglial tumors and its relationship: a single institutional review of 77 patients from China. Neuro Oncol 2012;14:109–16.
7. Kandoth C, McLellan MD, Vandin F, et al. Mutational landscape and significance across 12 major cancer types. Nature 2013;502:333–9.
8. Verhaak RG, Hoadley KA, Purdom E, et al. Integrated genomic analysis identifies clinically relevant subtypes of glioblastoma characterized by abnormalities in PDGFRA, IDH1, EGFR, and NF1. Cancer Cell 2010;17:98–110.
9. Brat DJ, Verhaak RG, Aldape KD, et al. Comprehensive, integrative genomic analysis of diffuse lower-grade gliomas. N Engl J Med 2015;372:2481–98.
10. Zinn PO, Mahajan B, Sathyan P, et al. Radiogenomic mapping of edema/cellular invasion MRI-phenotypes in glioblastoma multiforme. PLoS One 2011;6:e25451.
11. Baldock AL, Yagle K, Born DE, et al. Invasion and proliferation kinetics in enhancing gliomas predict IDH1 mutation status. Neuro Oncol 2014;16:779–86.
12. Gillies RJ, Kinahan PE, Hricak H. Radiomics: images are more than pictures, they are data. Radiology 2016;278:563–77.
13. Huang Y, Liu Z, He L, et al. Radiomics signature: a potential biomarker for the prediction of disease-free survival in early-stage (i or ii) non-small cell lung cancer. Radiology 2016;152234. http://dx.doi.org/10.1148/radiol.2016152234.
14. Chang K, Zhang B, Guo X, et al. Multimodal imaging patterns predict survival in recurrent glioblastoma patients treated with bevacizumab. Neuro Oncol 2016. http://dx.doi.org/10.1093/neuonc/now086.
15. Coroller TP, Agrawal V, Narayan V, et al. Radiomic phenotype features predict pathological response in non-small cell lung cancer. Radiother Oncol 2016;119(3):480–6.
16. Gnep K, Fargeas A, Gutiérrez-Carvajal RE, et al. Haralick textural features on T2-weighted MRI are associated with biochemical recurrence following radiotherapy for peripheral zone prostate cancer. J Magn Reson Imaging 2016. http://dx.doi.org/10.1002/jmri.25335.
17. Kickingereder P, Burth S, Wick A, et al. Radiomic profiling of glioblastoma: identifying an imaging

predictor of patient survival with improved perfor-mance over established clinical and radiologic risk models. Radiology 2016;160845. http://dx.doi.org/10.1148/radiol.2016160845.

18. Li H, Zhu Y, Burnside ES, et al. MR imaging radio-mics signatures for predicting the risk of breast can-cer recurrence as given by research versions of Mammaprint, Oncotype DX, and PAM50 Gene As-says. Radiology 2016;152110. http://dx.doi.org/10.1148/radiol.2016152110.

19. Liu Y, Kim J, Balagurunathan Y, et al. Radiomic fea-tures are associated with EGFR mutation status in lung adenocarcinomas. Clin Lung Cancer 2016. http://dx.doi.org/10.1016/j.cllc.2016.02.001.

20. Wu J, Gong G, Cui Y, et al. Intratumor partitioning and texture analysis of dynamic contrast-enhanced (DCE)-MRI identifies relevant tumor subregions to predict pathological response of breast cancer to neoadjuvant chemotherapy. J Magn Reson Imaging 2016. http://dx.doi.org/10.1002/jmri.25279.

21. Watanabe T, Vital A, Nobusawa S, et al. Selective acquisition of IDH1 R132C mutations in astrocy-tomas associated with Li-Fraumeni syndrome. Acta Neuropathol 2009;117:653–6. http://dx.doi.org/10.1007/s00401-009-0528-x.

22. Jha P, Suri V, Sharma V, et al. IDH1 mutations in gli-omas: first series from a tertiary care centre in India with comprehensive review of literature. Exp Mol Pathol 2011;91:385–93. http://dx.doi.org/10.1016/j.yexmp.2011.04.017.

23. Ichimura K, Pearson DM, Kocialkowski S, et al. IDH1 mutations are present in the majority of common adult gliomas but rare in primary glioblastomas. Neuro Oncol 2009;11:341–7. http://dx.doi.org/10.1215/15228517-2009-025.

24. Horbinski C, Kelly L, Nikiforov YE, et al. Detection of IDH1 and IDH2 mutations by fluorescence melting curve analysis as a diagnostic tool for brain bi-opsies. J Mol Diagn 2010;12:487–92. http://dx.doi.org/10.2353/jmoldx.2010.090228.

25. Horbinski C, Kofler J, Kelly LM, et al. Diagnostic use of IDH1/2 mutation analysis in routine clinical testing of formalin-fixed, paraffin-embedded glioma tissues. J Neuropathol Exp Neurol 2009;68:1319–25. http://dx.doi.org/10.1097/NEN.0b013e3181c391be.

26. Lu Z, Zhou L, Killela P, et al. Glioblastoma proto-oncogene SEC61gamma is required for tumor cell survival and response to endoplasmic reticulum stress. Cancer Res 2009;69:9105–11.

27. Mangiola A, Saulnier N, De Bonis P, et al. Gene expression profile of glioblastoma peritumoral tissue: an ex vivo study. PLoS One 2013;8:e57145.

28. Sugimoto K, Ideguchi M, Kimura T, et al. Epithe-lioid/rhabdoid glioblastoma: a highly aggressive subtype of glioblastoma. Brain Tumor Pathol 2016;33:137–46.

29. Matsumura N, Nakajima N, Yamazaki T, et al. Con-current TERT promoter and BRAF V600E mutation in epithelioid glioblastoma and concomitant low-grade astrocytoma. Neuropathology 2016. http://dx.doi.org/10.1111/neup.12318.

30. Rajmohan KS, Sugur HS, Shwetha SD, et al. Prognostic significance of histomolecular subgroups of adult anaplastic (WHO Grade III) gliomas: applying the 'integrated' diagnosis approach. J Clin Pathol 2016. http://dx.doi.org/10.1136/jclinpath-2015-203456.

31. Zacher A, Kaulich K, Stepanow S, et al. Molecular diagnostics of gliomas using next generation sequencing of a glioma-tailored gene panel. Brain Pathol 2016. http://dx.doi.org/10.1111/bpa.12367.

32. Osswald M, Solecki G, Wick W, et al. A malignant cellular network in gliomas: potential clinical implica-tions. Neuro Oncol 2016;18:479–85. http://dx.doi.org/10.1093/neuonc/now014.

33. Pentsova EI, Reiner AS, Panageas KS, et al. Anaplastic astrocytoma and non-1p/19q co-deleted anaplastic oligoastrocytoma: long-term survival, employment, and performance status of survivors. Neurooncol Pract 2016;3:71–6.

34. Louis DN, Ohgaki H, Wiestler OD, et al. The 2007 WHO classification of tumours of the cen-tral nervous system. Acta Neuropathol 2007;114:97–109.

35. Wu G, Broniscer A, McEachron TA, et al. Somatic histone H3 alterations in pediatric diffuse intrinsic pontine gliomas and non-brainstem glioblastomas. Nat Genet 2012;44:251–3.

36. Ramaswamy V, Remke M, Bouffet E, et al. Risk strat-ification of childhood medulloblastoma in the molec-ular era: the current consensus. Acta Neuropathol 2016;131:821–31.

37. Castel D, Philippe C, Calmon R, et al. Histone H3F3A and HIST1H3B K27M mutations define two subgroups of diffuse intrinsic pontine gliomas with different prognosis and phenotypes. Acta Neuropa-thol 2015;130:815–27.

38. Pajtler KW, Witt H, Sill M, et al. Molecular classifica-tion of ependymal tumors across All CNS compart-ments, histopathological grades, and age groups. Cancer Cell 2015;27:728–43.

39. Nambirajan A, Malgulwar PB, Sharma MC, et al. C11orf95-RELA fusion present in a primary intracra-nial extra-axial ependymoma: report of a case with literature review. Neuropathology 2016. http://dx.doi.org/10.1111/neup.12299.

40. Wu J, Armstrong TS, Gilbert MR. Biology and man-agement of ependymomas. Neuro Oncol 2016;18:902–13.

41. Korshunov A, Jakobiec FA, Eberhart CG, et al. Comparative integrated molecular analysis of intra-ocular medulloepitheliomas and central nervous system embryonal tumors with multilayered rosettes

confirms that they are distinct nosologic entities. Neuropathology 2015;35:538–44.

42. Alkhalili K, Zenonos GA, Fernandez-Miranda JC. 2-hydroxy-glutarate 3-dimensional functional spectroscopy in the evaluation of isocitrate dehydrogenase-mutant glioma response to therapy. Neurosurgery 2016;78:N9.

43. Choi C, Ganji SK, DeBerardinis RJ, et al. 2-hydroxy-glutarate detection by magnetic resonance spectroscopy in IDH-mutated patients with gliomas. Nat Med 2012;18:624–9.

44. Carrillo JA, Lai A, Nghiemphu PL, et al. Relationship between tumor enhancement, edema, IDH1 mutational status, MGMT promoter methylation, and survival in glioblastoma. AJNR Am J Neuroradiol 2012;33:1349–55.

45. Wasserman JK, Nicholas G, Yaworski R, et al. Radiological and pathological features associated with IDH1-R132H mutation status and early mortality in newly diagnosed anaplastic astrocytic tumours. PLoS One 2015;10:e0123890.

46. Wang K, Wang Y, Fan X, et al. Radiological features combined with IDH1 status for predicting the survival outcome of glioblastoma patients. Neuro Oncol 2016;18:589–97.

Molecular Imaging of Brain Tumors Using Liposomal Contrast Agents and Nanoparticles

Arnav Mehta, PhD[a,b], Ketan Ghaghada, PhD[c,d],
Srinivasan Mukundan Jr, MD, PhD[e,*]

KEYWORDS

- Molecular imaging • Molecular targeting • Brain tumor • Liposomes • Iron oxide nanoparticle
- Gold nanoparticle

KEY POINTS

- The advent of genomic, proteomic, and high-throughput screening technologies has made available many new targets for brain tumor imaging; however, target availability and accessibility need to be carefully considered when designing imaging probes.
- Nanoparticles, although largely still only used in preclinical studies, are a versatile tool for targeted imaging of physiologic and molecular aspects of brain tumors through many clinically used modalities.
- Liposomes can be used to transport diverse payloads in vivo, including contrast agents and drugs, and may be functionalized to increase circulation half-life and achieve targeting specificity.
- Polymeric, gold, and iron oxide nanoparticles have been used for diverse applications in preclinical studies; however, the utility of other methods, such as quantum dots and self-assembling DNA molecules, is yet to be established.

INTRODUCTION

The development of nanoparticles involves manipulating a variety of molecular constructs, including metals, lipids, polymers, proteins, and nucleic acids.[1–14] These particles typically range from 1 to 100 nm (although some may be as large as 400 nm) and may enhance imaging contrast through their intrinsic molecular properties or by serving as a scaffold for carrying imaging agents.[12,15] Importantly, nanoparticles have been used therapeutically as well for targeted drug delivery and during surgical resection of tumors.[13,15–19] Several approaches have been developed to functionalize nanoparticles to enable transport of water-soluble drugs, increase the half-life of the particles and their cargo in vivo, and minimize the side effect profile of toxic free agents.[12,20–22]

This article provides an overview of the molecular targets available for brain tumor imaging, then focuses on the use of liposomal contrast agents

Disclosure: The authors have nothing to disclose.
[a] Medical Scientist Training Program, David Geffen School of Medicine at UCLA, 757 Westwood Plaza, Los Angeles, CA 90095, USA; [b] Division of Biology and Biological Engineering, California Institute of Technology, 1200 East California Boulevard, Pasadena, CA 91125, USA; [c] Edward B. Singleton Department of Pediatric Radiology, Texas Children's Hospital, 1102 Bates Street, Suite 850, Houston, TX 77030, USA; [d] Department of Radiology, Baylor College of Medicine, One Baylor Plaza, Houston, TX 77030, USA; [e] Division of Neuroradiology, Department of Radiology, Brigham and Woman's Hospital, Harvard Medical School, 75 Francis Street, Boston, MA 02115, USA
* Corresponding author.
E-mail address: smukundan@partners.org

Magn Reson Imaging Clin N Am 24 (2016) 751–763
http://dx.doi.org/10.1016/j.mric.2016.06.004
1064-9689/16/© 2016 Elsevier Inc. All rights reserved.

mri.theclinics.com

for imaging some of these targets. It next discusses other classes of nanoparticles, including those that show potential in preclinical studies, such as gold nanoparticles, quantum dots, and self-assembling DNA molecules, and others that have been used in clinical studies, such as iron oxide nanoparticles.

MOLECULAR TARGETING OF BRAIN TUMORS

The molecular properties and availability of cellular and molecular targets dramatically influences the type of imaging modality and the nanoparticle platform used for detection. The flow of detectable biological information is amplified by transcription and translation, starting with 2 copies of a gene in DNA, which is transcribed to 10^2 to 10^3 copies of messenger RNA (mRNA), which is then in turn translated into 10^2 to 10^6 polypeptides. These polypeptides may assemble to form enzymatic proteins, whose function can be further used to amplify signals from target detection.[23] Several methods have been developed for the discovery of new targets and for the design of efficient, high-affinity probes for them. These approaches include genomic and transcriptomic sequencing to identify differentially expressed genes in brain tumors, high-throughput robotic screening, phage display, rational design, and combinatorial approaches.[5–7,24–26]

Barriers to Nanoparticle and Probe Entry

Despite the rapid discovery of new targets and probes, the accessibility of cellular targets can limit their detection by nanoparticles because these molecules do not cross lipid bilayers and diffuse through cytoplasm easily (**Fig. 1**). On entering the vasculature, the nanoparticles have to cross the endothelial layer to encounter the appropriate target cell. In the case of brain tumor targeting, the presence of the blood-brain barrier (BBB) presents an additional, significant challenge for the entry of nanoparticles.[27–30] Once the nanoparticles gain entry into the brain parenchyma, the most accessible cellular targets are cell surface proteins. An additional barrier, the cell membrane, needs to be traversed for detection of most RNAs and cytosolic proteins. In contrast, both the cell and nuclear membranes must be crossed to reach DNA targets, making them the most difficult to detect. The localization of a particular target is therefore critical when considering the material properties and design of a nanoparticle.

To circumvent the physiologic barriers that prevent nanoparticle and probe binding to their targets, several approaches have been used for brain tumor imaging. Surface chemical modifications are often used, such as polyethylene glycol (PEG) coating, and result in longer circulatory half-lives caused by decreased uptake by the

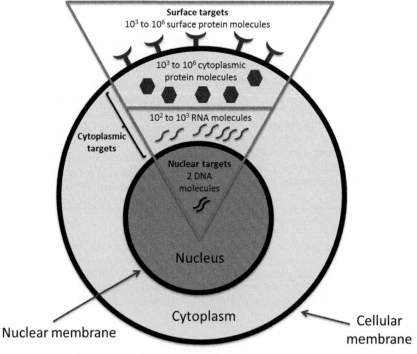

Fig. 1. The accessibility and distribution of molecular targets in a cell.

reticuloendothelial system, which helps to achieve a uniform distribution of nanoparticles to increase distribution to all cellular targets.[31] In certain circumstances, if the location of a tumor is known, localized delivery of nanoparticles may enhance detection of the desired target.[32] Another approach allows cellular tracking through the detection of internalized nanoparticles into the cytoplasm from cell surface proteins.[33] To gain entry into the brain, the use of ligand-bearing targeted nanoparticles for penetrating the BBB has also been extensively studied.[28,34,35]

Signal Amplification

Given the difficulty of traversing cellular barriers and the low abundance of DNA and mRNA in cells, these are seldom targeted because significant signal amplification would be needed for appreciable detection. A few successful attempts have been made to tether nucleic acids to gold, carbon, and platinum nanoparticles.[36–38] Several recent efforts have also enabled better detection of nucleic acid targets by exponential signal amplification. These approaches include nanosensors for specific DNA or RNA base pairing, rolling circle amplification, branched DNA amplification, hybridization chain reaction, and single-molecule RNA fluorescence in-situ hybridization.[39–43] The applicability of these approaches to tumor imaging in clinical settings has yet to be established.

Unlike nucleic acids, proteins are abundant and accessible targets in living cells. As such, several approaches have been developed to amplify signal from protein detection. These approaches include manipulating the physiochemical behavior of a probe after target binding, harnessing unique cellular biochemistry to trap probes, and augmenting probe kinetics to increase effective target concentration.[44–47]

Probe Classifications

Nanoparticles are in 3 classes of probes when used for brain tumor imaging: (1) compartment probes, (2) targeted probes, and (3) smart probes. Compartment probes are used to measure physiologic parameters, such as flow and perfusion.[48] In this case, the properties of this probe force its compartmentalization to a specific region in the body, and allows an indirect measure of a particular process. Targeted probes contain a target-recognition moiety, which binds to the target molecule, and a contrast moiety, which is the signal being detected during imaging.[48] An example of a targeted probe includes $\alpha_v\beta_3$ antibodies conjugated to gadolinium(III) [Gd(III)]–containing liposomes, which have been used for preclinical imaging of blood vessels.[49] Smart probes require a trigger to activate, and in this way have an enhanced signal/background ratio compared with other probes. An example of a smart probe is EgadMe, a Gd chelating agent that occupies 7 of 8 Gd(III) coordination sites conjugated to a galactopyranose residue that blocks the remaining Gd(III) coordinate site. In the presence of a β-galactosidase, the blocked Gd(III) site is freed, allowing access to water for contrast enhancement.[50] Calcium-activated and zinc-activated MR contrast agents have also been used in smart probes to detect activation of biochemical pathways in cells.[51,52]

LIPOSOMAL CONTRAST AGENTS

Liposomes have been used as a particularly versatile class of nanoparticles for both diagnostic and therapeutic use in the central nervous system. They are composed either of a single bilayer, known as unilamellar vesicles, or multiple bilayers, known as multilamellar vesicles (MLVs). The approaches to fabricate liposomes and the ways in which they can be designed for targeting cellular and molecular processes for brain tumor imaging are discussed later.

Design and Functional Properties of Liposomes

Liposomes can vary in size depending on the method used to synthesize them. These methods include high-pressure extrusion and sonication. High-pressure extrusion is used for the synthesis of MLVs greater than 100 nm in diameter and large unilamellar vesicles (LUVs) 50 to 400 nm in diameter with remarkable consistency. Sonication is mostly used for the synthesis of small unilamellar vesicles (SUVs) of less than 30 to 50 nm.[53]

The clearance of liposomes is predominantly mediated by the reticuloendothelial system, which consists of macrophages and other phagocytes in the hepatic and splenic compartments.[54] This clearance depends on the size and surface properties of each liposome; traditional liposomes usually have half-lives of around minutes to hours, whereas liposomes larger than 200 nm have shorter half-lives because of more efficient immune clearance.[55] These half-lives can be prolonged to more than 18 hours by coating the surface of liposomes with hydrophilic biopolymers such as PEG, creating so-called stealth liposomes that are better equipped to evade the immune system.[56–58]

Liposomes have hydrophilic cores that may encapsulate imaging contrast agents or other compounds, such as drugs. As such, they have been used for diverse applications in both diagnostic imaging and therapeutics. Several trials have successfully shown the use of liposomes in delivering chemotherapeutic agents, including cytarabine,[59] doxorubicin,[15,60,61] and daunorubicin,[62] as well as nucleic acids for gene therapy.[63,64] They have further been used in image-guided therapeutic delivery by inclusion of both an imaging agent and a drug.[65,66]

These nanoparticles have also been used for physiologic and molecular imaging using MR imaging and computed tomography (CT) by serving as carriers of gadolinium-based and iodine-based contrast agents.[67–70] Liposomal contrast agents encapsulating a high payload of conventional iodine contrast agent molecules ($\sim$1 million iodine atoms per liposome) have enabled ultrahigh-resolution CT imaging of rodent cerebrovasculature[71] (**Fig. 2**). Significant effort has been made to develop liposome-based MR imaging contrast agents.[72–75] These nanoparticles have been successfully used as blood-pool contrast agents[68] and for imaging neurovasculature[72] and monitoring convection-enhanced drug delivery[73] in vivo. As targeted probes,[74,76,77] liposomes have been used to enhance targeting of brain tumors,[78,79] for convection-enhanced delivery (CED),[80,81] and to deliver boron for neutron-capture therapy.[82,83]

Targeting of Tumors Using Liposomes

Delivery of nanoparticles to tumors may involve passive diffusion or active targeting. The ability to create small liposome nanoparticles allows passive targeting of liposomes to brain tumors by means of diffusion through leaky vasculature surrounding tumor cells.[84,85] Through this mechanism, referred to as the enhanced permeation and retention effect, liposomes carrying therapeutics or contrast agents can pool in the interstitial space of a tumor.[86–89] The use of liposomes for molecular targeting of brain tumors involves conjugation of cell surface receptor recognizing antibodies to PEG chains on the liposome outer coat.[79,90] Approaches to target multiple surface receptors using a single liposome have also been described.[91] Liposomes can thus be targeted to the tumor microenvironment or to the endothelium of blood vessels within it. These approaches have been used to increase specificity of drug delivery by targeting the folate, transferrin, and epidermal growth factor receptors.[78,79,82,90,92] In addition, triggered release liposomes have also been developed. These nanoparticles are designed to release contents, such as chemotherapeutics, in response to environmental changes such as temperature and pH.[93–96]

Liposomes as MR Imaging–based Contrast Agents for Brain Tumors

The use of Gd core-encapsulated (CE-Gd) and surface-conjugated (SC-Gd) liposomes as T1-based MR imaging contrast agents has been validated extensively in animal models[67,69,74,75,97,98] (**Fig. 3**). Liposomes that use both core and surface

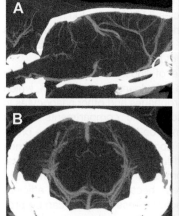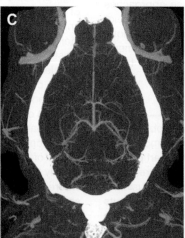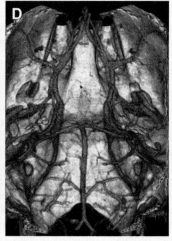

Fig. 2. Ultrahigh resolution in vivo CT imaging of mouse cerebrovasculature using a long-circulating liposomal-iodine contrast agent. Thick-slab maximum intensity projection (MIP) images in (*A*) sagittal, (*B*) axial, and (*C*) coronal planes showing the arterial and venous circulatory system in the mouse brain. (*D*) Three-dimensional (3D) volume-rendered image of the mouse circle of Willis. The CT images were acquired on a micro-CT scanner at 19-μm isotropic spatial resolution. (*Adapted from* Starosolski Z, Villamizar CA, Rendon D, et al. Ultra high-resolution in vivo computed tomography imaging of mouse cerebrovasculature using a long circulating blood pool contrast agent. Sci Rep 2015;5:10178; with permission.)

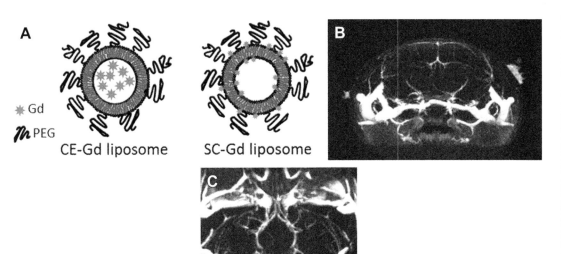

Fig. 3. Liposomes as MR imaging contrast agents. (A) Gadolinium (Gd) core-encapsulated (CE-Gd) or surface-conjugated (SC-Gd) liposomal MR imaging contrast agents coated with PEG. (B, C) High-resolution in vivo MR angiography of mouse cerebrovasculature using a long-circulating liposomal-Gd contrast agent (SC-Gd). Thick-slab MIP images in (B) sagittal and (C) coronal planes showing the arterial and venous circulatory system in the mouse brain. The mouse circle of Willis is shown in the coronal image. The images were acquired using a 3D gradient recalled echo sequence at 100-μm isotropic spatial resolution on a permanent 1.0-T MR scanner. (Courtesy of Z. Starosolski, K. Ghaghada, A. Annapragada.)

Gd stores are referred to as dual-Gd liposomes.[97] Of note, liposome cores encapsulated with ultrasmall superparamagnetic iron oxide particles (USPIOs) may be used for enhanced signal in T2-weighted MR imaging.[99] These contrast agents have prolonged circulation, which provides uniform signal intensity and enhancement compared with traditional Gd chelates, thus making them ideal for steady-state imaging like MR angiography.[100]

Thus, in preclinical studies, CE-Gd liposomes have been shown to result in lower background signal and increased vessel clarity in the spine and heart compared with conventional contrast agents.[101–103] SC-Gd liposomes show higher T1 relaxivities compared with CE-Gd liposomes because water molecules do not have to diffuse through the lipid bilayer to interact with Gd atoms. As such, these agents have been used for higher-resolution imaging of both arterial and venous central nervous system vasculature, including the circle of Willis.[72] Dual-Gd contrast agents afford the advantage of signal amplification from both modes of Gd pooling.[97]

Unlike extracranial tumors, the presence of the BBB presents significant challenges to the entry of liposomes and other nanoparticle contrast agents into the brain.[29,30] Focused ultrasonography-mediated enhancement of BBB permeability for augmenting intratumoral transport of liposomes has been studied.[104] Active targeting of liposomes has also been examined for imaging of brain tumors.[105–107] Importantly, although most nanoparticles are able to localize to brain tumors by extravasation through blood vessels, they are still large enough that this diffusion is limited by slow kinetics. Other smaller contrast agents are able to traverse the tumor microenvironment more rapidly through diffusion via brownian motion.[87] CED is an approach whereby a burr hole is drilled into the brain, and a therapeutic or contrast agent is infused via a catheter directly into the tumor site.[108] The positive pressure gradient of the infusion process reliably distributes the agent over the entire tumor volume, and, when the gradient normalizes, the distribution of the agent becomes diffusion limited. However, this approach has several limitations, including its invasive nature, limited versatility in terms of the shape and distribution of agent delivery, and often overtreatment, although overtreatment may be beneficial when trying to ensure tumor removal outside the expected margins.[108–110]

Several preclinical studies have shown the safe and effective administration of liposome-encapsulated therapeutics to brain tumors using

CED. These studies were limited in that they were unable to track the extent of nanoparticle delivery. Other studies in primate brains have used CE-Gd liposomes to monitor in real time the distribution of therapeutic nanoparticles infused into brain tumors by CED.[66,111] The coencapsulation of both Gd contrast agents and therapeutics has enabled more accurate tracking of CED-mediated treatment of brain tumors.[80,112]

NONLIPOSOMAL NANOPARTICLES FOR BRAIN TUMOR IMAGING

In addition to liposomes, several other types of nanoparticles have been used for brain tumor imaging, including other lipid-based nanoparticles, such as micelles, as well as polymeric, gold, and iron oxide nanoparticles. Recently, semiconductor nanocrystals, or quantum dots, that have tunable optical properties have also been used during surgery and in tumor imaging. A brief discussion of nucleic acid nanoparticles and their potential future application in molecular imaging is provided here.

Lipid-based Nanoparticles

Like liposomes, micelles and lipid-coated perfluorocarbon (PFC) nanoparticles are lipid-based nanoparticles. Micelles are approximately 10 to 50 nm in diameter. They are composed of several self-assembling amphiphilic molecules, which aggregate to form spherical particles that have a hydrophilic outer surface and a hydrophobic core. These nanoparticles can be used for imaging by tethering contrast moieties to the amphiphilic components.[113] Often these micelles are PEGylated, which allows better immune evasion and prolonged circulation in the body.[114] In addition, their surfaces can be further modified with proteins that facilitate cell-surface receptor binding in order to achieve tumor-specific targeting.[114] An advantage of the hydrophobic core is that it may be used to deliver water-insoluble payloads.[115]

PFC nanoparticles tend to be much larger than micelles, usually around 250 nm in diameter. They are composed of a lipid monolayer encapsulating a hydrophobic PFC core.[116] The lipid monolayer can be used to carry contrast or therapeutic agents, or molecules to facilitate tumor targeting.[117] PFC nanoparticles have been investigated preclinically for molecular imaging of brain tumors and the cardiovascular system.[118] These nanoparticles may be used in both proton-based and ^{19}F-based MR imaging, because of the presence of fluorine atoms (perfluorocarbon) in the core interior.[118] In addition to their use in MR imaging, PFCs along with porphysomes, which are liposomelike

nanoparticles, have been used in photoacoustic imaging in the brain.[119]

Polymeric Nanoparticles

Many years of investigation have gone into the synthesis and customization of biodegradable polymers, and this has been harnessed for molecular imaging. Dendrimers build the backbone of perhaps the most well-described class of polymeric nanoparticles.[120] Dendrimers are highly branched, synthetic polymers that are effectively functionalized by conjugation to contrast moieties[121,122] and may also be used for therapeutics.[123–127] These nanoparticles have been used effectively for brain tumor imaging with both MR imaging and CT.[128] Importantly, antibody-conjugated dendrimers can be used for increased target specificity to brain tumors.[123,127]

Biodegradable polymers including polylysine, polylactic acid, polylactic coglycolyic acid, and PEG-based polymers can be used to generate a homogeneous preparation of nanoparticles from 10 nm to 10^3 nm. These biopolymers can be effectively functionalized by fine-tuned control of nanoparticle size and structure, and by the conjugation of functional molecules or contrast agents.[129–132] In particular, such polymeric nanoparticles have been used to effectively deliver chemotherapeutics to brain tumors.[130,133]

Iron Oxide Nanoparticles

Perhaps the most widely described MR imaging contrast agents to date are iron oxide nanoparticles.[134] These particles are composed of an iron oxide core that is stabilized with a coating of dextran or another hydrophilic polymer.[135–137] They are developed either as USPIOs or supermagnetic iron oxide particles (SPIOs). USPIOs are less than 50 nm in diameter and have lower T2 relaxivities during MR imaging, thus they have been used as blood pool contrast agents.[135,138,139] In contrast, SPIOs range between 50 and 200 nm in diameter, and have high T2 relaxivites.[135,140] Therefore, they are used predominantly for T2-weighted MR imaging.[135,140]

To date, these nanoparticles are the only ones approved for use as a contrast agent in humans,[141] although several have been withdrawn by the manufacturers. They have a plasma half-life of more than 18-hours, which is significantly longer than traditional Gd-based contrast agents. They have been used as a contrast agent for brain tumor imaging and for visualizing blood vessels in the tumor microenvironment.[142–146] When coated with dextran, these nanoparticles are rapidly taken up by T lymphocytes; as such, they can be effectively used to image the immune response in inflammatory diseases, tumors, and lymph nodes, such as for cancer staging.[147,148] Given their long half-life and rapid uptake by dividing cells, these nanoparticles have been further used for MR imaging tracking of stem cells and microglia.[149–152]

Gold Nanoparticles

A variety of gold nanoparticles have been developed and tested in preclinical imaging.[153–155] The high attenuation of gold, compared with iodine, makes gold nanoparticles attractive for radiograph and CT imaging.[153,156] Spectral CT imaging using a combination of gold nanoparticles and liposomal-iodine contrast agents has been investigated to simultaneously visualize tumor vasculature and intratumoral uptake of nanoparticles.[157,158] Gold nanoparticles have a silica core covered by an extremely thin gold shell and have been investigated for multimodality imaging.[159] These particles are extremely versatile because the core dimensions and shell thickness can be varied to impart the ability either absorb or scatter light,[160–162] or x-rays.[157,158] As a result, gold nanoparticles can be used in optical imaging[162,163] and for highly sensitive surface-enhanced Raman scattering, which has been used for real-time visualization of tumor margins during surgical resection.[163,164] Gold particles synthesized to absorb in the near-infrared spectrum have been used as a cancer therapeutic in certain animal models by means of photothermal ablation of cells.[165–168] In humans, a similar approach has been used in trials for treatment of head and neck cancers. In addition, these nanoparticles are the most commonly used inorganic nanoparticle, along with quantum dots, in photoacoustic imaging.[119]

Quantum Dots

As with gold nanoparticles, quantum dots have unique, flexible optical properties that can be modulated by altering their size. They are composed of a core made of a semiconductor material, usually a cadmium derivative, covered by an inert metallic layer.[169] These nanoparticles have been used for optical imaging of the molecular properties of various tumors and may be helpful for guiding neurosurgical resection of brain tumors.[170–173] Transferrin-conjugated quantum dots have been used for brain tumor targeting by virtue of binding to the transferrin receptor. The utility of these nanoparticles may be limited because they contain cadmium, which can be cytotoxic.

Self-assembling Nucleic Acid Nanoparticles

Recent advances in DNA origami have led to the development of self-assembling nucleic acid nanoparticles, which have the potential to be highly customizable in size and shape, and also able to carry a wide variety of payloads.[174] Although still far away from practical use for clinical imaging, these nanoparticles have been used for small interfering RNA delivery to cells[18] and may be conjugated to other nanoparticles, such as quantum dots and gold nanoparticles.[175]

SUMMARY

The promise of in vivo characterization of the attributes of brain tumors is becoming closer to reality each day. Although primarily in the preclinical realm, many of the technologies described in this article are being used in vivo. It is hoped that these technologies will continue to mature over the coming decade to more widespread clinical use in the same way as advanced functional approaches have come to fruition over the past decade.

REFERENCES

1. Davis KR, Taveras JM, New PF, et al. Cerebral infarction diagnosis by computerized tomography. Analysis and evaluation of findings. Am J Roentgenol Radium Ther Nucl Med 1975;124:643–60.
2. Eastwood JD, Lev MH, Wintermark M, et al. Correlation of early dynamic CT perfusion imaging with whole-brain MR diffusion and perfusion imaging in acute hemispheric stroke. AJNR Am J Neuroradiol 2003;24:1869–75.
3. Cancer Genome Atlas Research Network. Comprehensive genomic characterization defines human glioblastoma genes and core pathways. Nature 2008;455:1061–8.
4. Geiger T, Cox J, Ostasiewicz P, et al. Super-SILAC mix for quantitative proteomics of human tumor tissue. Nat Methods 2010;7:383–5.
5. Parsons DW, Jones S, Zhang X, et al. An integrated genomic analysis of human glioblastoma multiforme. Science 2008;321:1807–12.
6. Pugh TJ, Weeraratne SD, Archer TC, et al. Medulloblastoma exome sequencing uncovers subtype-specific somatic mutations. Nature 2012; 488:106–10.
7. Rausch T, Jones DT, Zapatka M, et al. Genome sequencing of pediatric medulloblastoma links catastrophic DNA rearrangements with TP53 mutations. Cell 2012;148:59–71.
8. Cai W, Chen X. Multimodality molecular imaging of tumor angiogenesis. J Nucl Med 2008;49(Suppl 2): 113s–28s.

9. Gambhir SS. Molecular imaging of cancer with positron emission tomography. Nat Rev Cancer 2002;2:683–93.

10. Weissleder R. Scaling down imaging: molecular mapping of cancer in mice. Nature reviews. Cancer 2002;2:11–8.

11. Weissleder R, Moore A, Mahmood U, et al. In vivo magnetic resonance imaging of transgene expression. Nat Med 2000;6:351–5.

12. Gao X, Li C. Nanoprobes visualizing gliomas by crossing the blood brain tumor barrier. Small 2014;10:426–40.

13. Leary SP, Liu CY, Yu C, et al. Toward the emergence of nanoneurosurgery: part I–progress in nanoscience, nanotechnology, and the comprehension of events in the mesoscale realm. Neurosurgery 2005;57:606–34 [discussion: 606–34].

14. Zhang L, Zhao D. Applications of nanoparticles for brain cancer imaging and therapy. J Biomed Nanotechnol 2014;10:1713–31.

15. Bertrand N, Wu J, Xu X, et al. Cancer nanotechnology: the impact of passive and active targeting in the era of modern cancer biology. Adv Drug Deliv Rev 2014;66:2–25.

16. Leary SP, Liu CY, Apuzzo ML. Toward the emergence of nanoneurosurgery: part II–nanomedicine: diagnostics and imaging at the nanoscale level. Neurosurgery 2006;58:805–23 [discussion: 805–23].

17. Barnaby SN, Sita TL, Petrosko SH, et al. Therapeutic applications of spherical nucleic acids. Cancer Treat Res 2015;166:23–50.

18. Lee H, Lytton-Jean AK, Chen Y, et al. Molecularly self-assembled nucleic acid nanoparticles for targeted in vivo siRNA delivery. Nat Nanotechnol 2012;7:389–93.

19. Lee TJ, Haque F, Vieweger M, et al. Functional assays for specific targeting and delivery of RNA nanoparticles to brain tumor. Methods Mol Biol 2015;1297:137–52.

20. Iv M, Telischak N, Feng D, et al. Clinical applications of iron oxide nanoparticles for magnetic resonance imaging of brain tumors. Nanomedicine (Lond) 2015;10:993–1018.

21. Kaluzova M, Bouras A, Machaidze R, et al. Targeted therapy of glioblastoma stem-like cells and tumor non-stem cells using cetuximab-conjugated iron-oxide nanoparticles. Oncotarget 2015;6:8788–806.

22. Li J, Cai P, Shalviri A, et al. A multifunctional polymeric nanotheranostic system delivers doxorubicin and imaging agents across the blood-brain barrier targeting brain metastases of breast cancer. ACS Nano 2014;8:9925–40.

23. Mehta AG, Ghaghada KB, Mukundan S Jr. Future clinical applications of molecular imaging: nanoparticles, cellular probes, and imaging of gene expression. In: Pillai JJ, editor. Functional brain tumor imaging. New York: Springer; 2014. p. 225–37.

24. Rudin M, Weissleder R. Molecular imaging in drug discovery and development. Nat Rev Drug Discov 2003;2:123–31.

25. Loi M, Di Paolo D, Soster M, et al. Novel phage display-derived neuroblastoma-targeting peptides potentiate the effect of drug nanocarriers in preclinical settings. J Control Release 2013;170:233–41.

26. Staquicini FI, Sidman RL, Arap W, et al. Phage display technology for stem cell delivery and systemic therapy. Adv Drug Deliv Rev 2010;62:1213–6.

27. Toy R, Bauer L, Hoimes C, et al. Targeted nanotechnology for cancer imaging. Adv Drug Deliv Rev 2014;76:79–97.

28. Cheng Y, Morshed RA, Auffinger B, et al. Multifunctional nanoparticles for brain tumor imaging and therapy. Adv Drug Deliv Rev 2014;66:42–57.

29. Doolittle ND, Muldoon LL, Culp AY, et al. Delivery of chemotherapeutics across the blood-brain barrier: challenges and advances. Adv Pharmacol 2014;71:203–43.

30. Meyers JD, Doane T, Burda C, et al. Nanoparticles for imaging and treating brain cancer. Nanomedicine (Lond) 2013;8:123–43.

31. Suk JS, Xu Q, Kim N, et al. PEGylation as a strategy for improving nanoparticle-based drug and gene delivery. Adv Drug Deliv Rev 2016;99(Pt A):28–51.

32. Neuwelt EA, Weissleder R, Nilaver G, et al. Delivery of virus-sized iron oxide particles to rodent CNS neurons. Neurosurgery 1994;34:777–84.

33. Lewin M, Carlesso N, Tung CH, et al. Tat peptide-derivatized magnetic nanoparticles allow in vivo tracking and recovery of progenitor cells. Nat Biotechnol 2000;18:410–4.

34. Karathanasis E, Ghaghada KB. Crossing the barrier: treatment of brain tumors using nanochain particles. Wiley Interdiscip Rev Nanomed Nanobiotechnol 2016. http://dx.doi.org/10.1002/wnan.1387.

35. van der Meel R, Vehmeijer LJ, Kok RJ, et al. Ligand-targeted particulate nanomedicines undergoing clinical evaluation: current status. Adv Drug Deliv Rev 2013;65:1284–98.

36. Li H, Zhang Y, Wang L, et al. Nucleic acid detection using carbon nanoparticles as a fluorescent sensing platform. Chem Commun (Camb) 2011;47:961–3.

37. Polsky R, Gill R, Kaganovsky L, et al. Nucleic acid-functionalized Pt nanoparticles: catalytic labels for the amplified electrochemical detection of biomolecules. Anal Chem 2006;78:2268–71.

38. Thaxton CS, Georganopoulou DG, Mirkin CA. Gold nanoparticle probes for the detection of nucleic acid targets. Clin Chim Acta 2006;363:120–6.

39. Choi HM, Chang JY, Trinh le A, et al. Programmable in situ amplification for multiplexed imaging

of mRNA expression. Nat Biotechnol 2010;28: 1208–12.

40. Collins ML, Irvine B, Tyner D, et al. A branched DNA signal amplification assay for quantification of nucleic acid targets below 100 molecules/ml. Nucleic Acids Res 1997;25:2979–84.

41. Perez JM, O'Loughin T, Simeone FJ, et al. DNA-based magnetic nanoparticle assembly acts as a magnetic relaxation nanoswitch allowing screening of DNA-cleaving agents. J Am Chem Soc 2002; 124:2856–7.

42. Raj A, van den Bogaard P, Rifkin SA, et al. Imaging individual mRNA molecules using multiple singly labeled probes. Nat Methods 2008;5:877–9.

43. Smolina IV, Demidov VV, Cantor CR, et al. Real-time monitoring of branched rolling-circle DNA amplification with peptide nucleic acid beacon. Anal Biochem 2004;335:326–9.

44. Barbet J, Peltier P, Bardet S, et al. Radioimmunodetection of medullary thyroid carcinoma using indium-111 bivalent hapten and anti-CEA x anti-DTPA-indium bispecific antibody. J Nucl Med 1998;39:1172–8.

45. Gambhir SS, Barrio JR, Phelps ME, et al. Imaging adenoviral-directed reporter gene expression in living animals with positron emission tomography. Proc Natl Acad Sci U S A 1999;96:2333–8.

46. Hu S, Shively L, Raubitschek A, et al. Minibody: a novel engineered anti-carcinoembryonic antigen antibody fragment (single-chain Fv-CH3) which exhibits rapid, high-level targeting of xenografts. Cancer Res 1996;56:3055–61.

47. Weissleder R, Tung CH, Mahmood U, et al. In vivo imaging of tumors with protease-activated near-infrared fluorescent probes. Nat Biotechnol 1999; 17:375–8.

48. Dzik-Jurasz AS. Molecular imaging in vivo: an introduction. Br J Radiol 2003;76(Spec No 2): S98–109.

49. Schmieder AH, Winter PM, Williams TA, et al. Molecular MR imaging of neovascular progression in the Vx2 tumor with alphavbeta3-targeted paramagnetic nanoparticles. Radiology 2013;268:470–80.

50. Louie AY, Hüber MM, Ahrens ET, et al. In vivo visualization of gene expression using magnetic resonance imaging. Nat Biotechnol 2000;18:321–5.

51. Li WH, Parigi G, Fragai M, et al. Mechanistic studies of a calcium-dependent MRI contrast agent. Inorg Chem 2002;41:4018–24.

52. Major JL, Parigi G, Luchinat C, et al. The synthesis and in vitro testing of a zinc-activated MRI contrast agent. Proc Natl Acad Sci U S A 2007; 104:13881–6.

53. Szoka F Jr, Papahadjopoulos D. Comparative properties and methods of preparation of lipid vesicles (liposomes). Annu Rev Biophys Bioeng 1980; 9:467–508.

54. Yan X, Scherphof GL, Kamps JA. Liposome opsonization. J Liposome Res 2005;15:109–39.

55. Senior JH. Fate and behavior of liposomes in vivo: a review of controlling factors. Crit Rev Ther Drug Carrier Syst 1987;3:123–93.

56. Allen TM, Hansen C, Martin F, et al. Liposomes containing synthetic lipid derivatives of poly(ethylene glycol) show prolonged circulation half-lives in vivo. Biochim Biophys Acta 1991;1066:29–36.

57. Klibanov AL, Maruyama K, Torchilin VP, et al. Amphipathic polyethyleneglycols effectively prolong the circulation time of liposomes. FEBS Lett 1990;268:235–7.

58. Woodle MC, Newman MS, Cohen JA. Sterically stabilized liposomes: physical and biological properties. J Drug Target 1994;2:397–403.

59. Lassaletta A, Lopez-Ibor B, Mateos E, et al. Intrathecal liposomal cytarabine in children under 4 years with malignant brain tumors. J Neurooncol 2009;95:65–9.

60. Marina NM, Cochrane D, Harney E, et al. Dose escalation and pharmacokinetics of pegylated liposomal doxorubicin (Doxil) in children with solid tumors: a pediatric oncology group study. Clin Cancer Res 2002;8:413–8.

61. Fabel K, Dietrich J, Hau P, et al. Long-term stabilization in patients with malignant glioma after treatment with liposomal doxorubicin. Cancer 2001;92: 1936–42.

62. Lippens RJ. Liposomal daunorubicin (DaunoXome) in children with recurrent or progressive brain tumors. Pediatr Hematol Oncol 1999;16:131–9.

63. Yoshida J, Mizuno M. Clinical gene therapy for brain tumors. Liposomal delivery of anticancer molecule to glioma. J Neurooncol 2003;65:261–7.

64. Delac M, Motaln H, Ulrich H, et al. Aptamer for imaging and therapeutic targeting of brain tumor glioblastoma. Cytometry A 2015;87:806–16.

65. Karathanasis E, Chan L, Balusu SR, et al. Multifunctional nanocarriers for mammographic quantification of tumor dosing and prognosis of breast cancer therapy. Biomaterials 2008;29: 4815–22.

66. Saito R, Bringas JR, McKnight TR, et al. Distribution of liposomes into brain and rat brain tumor models by convection-enhanced delivery monitored with magnetic resonance imaging. Cancer Res 2004; 64:2572–9.

67. Ghaghada K, Hawley C, Kawaji K, et al. T1 relaxivity of core-encapsulated gadolinium liposomal contrast agents–effect of liposome size and internal gadolinium concentration. Acad Radiol 2008; 15:1259–63.

68. Mukundan S Jr, Ghaghada KB, Badea CT, et al. A liposomal nanoscale contrast agent for preclinical CT in mice. AJR Am J Roentgenol 2006;186: 300–7.

69. Tilcock C, Unger E, Cullis P, et al. Liposomal Gd-DTPA: preparation and characterization of relaxivity. Radiology 1989;171:77–80.

70. Annapragada AV, Hoffman E, Divekar A, et al. High-resolution CT vascular imaging using blood pool contrast agents. Methodist Debakey Cardiovasc J 2012;8:18–22.

71. Starosolski Z, Villamizar CA, Rendon D, et al. Ultra high-resolution in vivo computed tomography imaging of mouse cerebrovasculature using a long circulating blood pool contrast agent. Sci Rep 2015;5:10178.

72. Howles GP, Ghaghada KB, Qi Y, et al. High-resolution magnetic resonance angiography in the mouse using a nanoparticle blood-pool contrast agent. Magn Reson Med 2009;62:1447–56.

73. Krauze MT, Forsayeth J, Park JW, et al. Real-time imaging and quantification of brain delivery of liposomes. Pharm Res 2006;23:2493–504.

74. Mulder WJ, Strijkers GJ, van Tilborg GA, et al. Lipid-based nanoparticles for contrast-enhanced MRI and molecular imaging. NMR Biomed 2006;19:142–64.

75. Unger EC, Shen DK, Fritz TA. Status of liposomes as MR contrast agents. J Magn Reson Imaging 1993;3:195–8.

76. Mulder WJ, Strijkers GJ, Griffioen AW, et al. A liposomal system for contrast-enhanced magnetic resonance imaging of molecular targets. Bioconjug Chem 2004;15:799–806.

77. Mulder WJ, Strijkers GJ, Habets JW, et al. MR molecular imaging and fluorescence microscopy for identification of activated tumor endothelium using a bimodal lipidic nanoparticle. FASEB J 2005;19:2008–10.

78. Madhankumar AB, Slagle-Webb B, Wang X, et al. Efficacy of interleukin-13 receptor-targeted liposomal doxorubicin in the intracranial brain tumor model. Mol Cancer Ther 2009;8:648–54.

79. Mamot C, Drummond DC, Noble CO, et al. Epidermal growth factor receptor-targeted immunoliposomes significantly enhance the efficacy of multiple anticancer drugs in vivo. Cancer Res 2005;65:11631–8.

80. Grahn AY, Bankiewicz KS, Dugich-Djordjevic M, et al. Non-PEGylated liposomes for convection-enhanced delivery of topotecan and gadodiamide in malignant glioma: initial experience. J Neurooncol 2009;95:185–97.

81. Krauze MT, Nobel CO, Kawaguchi T, et al. Convection-enhanced delivery of nanoliposomal CPT-11 (irinotecan) and PEGylated liposomal doxorubicin (Doxil) in rodent intracranial brain tumor xenografts. Neuro Oncol 2007;9:393–403.

82. Doi A, Kawabata S, Lida K, et al. Tumor-specific targeting of sodium borocaptate (BSH) to malignant glioma by transferrin-PEG liposomes: a modality for boron neutron capture therapy. J Neurooncol 2008;87:287–94.

83. Nakamura H. Boron lipid-based liposomal boron delivery system for neutron capture therapy: recent development and future perspective. Future Med Chem 2013;5:715–30.

84. Ishida O, Maruyama K, Sasaki K, et al. Size-dependent extravasation and interstitial localization of polyethyleneglycol liposomes in solid tumor-bearing mice. Int J Pharm 1999;190:49–56.

85. McDonald DM, Choyke PL. Imaging of angiogenesis: from microscope to clinic. Nat Med 2003;9:713–25.

86. Alberts DS, Muggia FM, Carmichael J, et al. Efficacy and safety of liposomal anthracyclines in phase I/II clinical trials. Semin Oncol 2004;31:53–90.

87. Jain RK. Transport of molecules, particles, and cells in solid tumors. Annu Rev Biomed Eng 1999;1:241–63.

88. Jain RK. Delivery of molecular and cellular medicine to solid tumors. Adv Drug Deliv Rev 2012;64:353–65.

89. Maeda H. Vascular permeability in cancer and infection as related to macromolecular drug delivery, with emphasis on the EPR effect for tumor-selective drug targeting. Proc Jpn Acad Ser B Phys Biol Sci 2012;88:53–71.

90. Madhankumar AB, Slagle-Webb B, Mintz A, et al. Interleukin-13 receptor-targeted nanovesicles are a potential therapy for glioblastoma multiforme. Mol Cancer Ther 2006;5:3162–9.

91. Saul JM, Annapragada AV, Bellamkonda RV. A dual-ligand approach for enhancing targeting selectivity of therapeutic nanocarriers. J Control Release 2006;114:277–87.

92. Mamot C, Drummond DC, Greiser U, et al. Epidermal growth factor receptor (EGFR)-targeted immunoliposomes mediate specific and efficient drug delivery to EGFR- and EGFRvIII-overexpressing tumor cells. Cancer Res 2003;63:3154–61.

93. Kale AA, Torchilin VP. Environment-responsive multifunctional liposomes. Methods Mol Biol 2010;605:213–42.

94. Momekova D, Rangelov S, Lambov N. Long-circulating, pH-sensitive liposomes. Methods Mol Biol 2010;605:527–44.

95. Momekova D, Rangelov S, Yanev S, et al. Long-circulating, pH-sensitive liposomes sterically stabilized by copolymers bearing short blocks of lipid-mimetic units. Eur J Pharm Sci 2007;32:308–17.

96. Ponce AM, Vujaskovic Z, Yuan F, et al. Hyperthermia mediated liposomal drug delivery. Int J Hyperthermia 2006;22:205–13.

97. Ghaghada KB, Ravoori M, Sabapathy D, et al. New dual mode gadolinium nanoparticle contrast agent for magnetic resonance imaging. PLoS One 2009; 4:e7628.

98. Tilcock C, Ahknog QF, Koeing SH, et al. The design of liposomal paramagnetic MR agents: effect of vesicle size upon the relaxivity of surface-incorporated lipophilic chelates. Magn Reson Med 1992;27:44–51.

99. Bulte JW, De Cuyper M. Magnetoliposomes as contrast agents. Methods Enzymol 2003;373: 175–98.

100. Ayyagari AL, Zhang X, Ghaghada KB, et al. Long-circulating liposomal contrast agents for magnetic resonance imaging. Magn Reson Med 2006;55: 1023–9.

101. Bucholz E, Ghaghada K, Qi Y, et al. Four-dimensional MR microscopy of the mouse heart using radial acquisition and liposomal gadolinium contrast agent. Magn Reson Med 2008; 60:111–8.

102. Bucholz E, Ghaghada K, Qi Y, et al. Cardiovascular phenotyping of the mouse heart using a 4D radial acquisition and liposomal Gd-DTPA-BMA. Magn Reson Med 2010;63:979–87.

103. Ghaghada KB, Bockhorst KH, Mukundan S Jr, et al. High-resolution vascular imaging of the rat spine using liposomal blood pool MR agent. AJNR Am J Neuroradiol 2007;28:48–53.

104. Aryal M, Park J, Vykhodtseva N, et al. Enhancement in blood-tumor barrier permeability and delivery of liposomal doxorubicin using focused ultrasound and microbubbles: evaluation during tumor progression in a rat glioma model. Phys Med Biol 2015;60:2511–27.

105. Flament J, Geffroy F, Medina C, et al. In vivo CEST MR imaging of U87 mice brain tumor angiogenesis using targeted LipoCEST contrast agent at 7 T. Magn Reson Med 2013;69:179–87.

106. Liu X, Madhankumar AB, Miller PA, et al. MRI contrast agent for targeting glioma: interleukin-13 labeled liposome encapsulating gadolinium-DTPA. Neuro Oncol 2016;18(5):691–9.

107. Winter PM, Pearce J, Chu Z, et al. Imaging of brain tumors with paramagnetic vesicles targeted to phosphatidylserine. J Magn Reson Imaging 2015; 41:1079–87.

108. Morrison PF, Laske DW, Bobo H, et al. High-flow microinfusion: tissue penetration and pharmacodynamics. Am J Physiol 1994;266:R292–305.

109. Ferguson S, Lesniak MS. Convection enhanced drug delivery of novel therapeutic agents to malignant brain tumors. Curr Drug Deliv 2007;4: 169–80.

110. Kaiser MG, Parsa AT, Fine RL, et al. Tissue distribution and antitumor activity of topotecan delivered by intracerebral clysis in a rat glioma model. Neurosurgery 2000;47:1391–8 [discussion: 1398–9].

111. Saito R, Krauze MT, Bringas JR, et al. Gadolinium-loaded liposomes allow for real-time magnetic resonance imaging of convection-enhanced delivery in the primate brain. Exp Neurol 2005;196: 381–9.

112. Dickinson PJ, LeCounter RA, Higgins RJ, et al. Canine model of convection-enhanced delivery of liposomes containing CPT-11 monitored with real-time magnetic resonance imaging: laboratory investigation. J Neurosurg 2008;108: 989–98.

113. Amirbekian V, Lipinski MJ, Briley-Saebo KC, et al. Detecting and assessing macrophages in vivo to evaluate atherosclerosis noninvasively using molecular MRI. Proc Natl Acad Sci U S A 2007;104: 961–6.

114. Dabholkar RD, Sawant RM, Mongayt DA, et al. Polyethylene glycol-phosphatidylethanolamine conjugate (PEG-PE)-based mixed micelles: some properties, loading with paclitaxel, and modulation of P-glycoprotein-mediated efflux. Int J Pharm 2006;315:148–57.

115. Torchilin VP. Lipid-core micelles for targeted drug delivery. Curr Drug Deliv 2005;2:319–27.

116. Kaneda MM, Caruthers S, Lanza GM, et al. Perfluorocarbon nanoemulsions for quantitative molecular imaging and targeted therapeutics. Ann Biomed Eng 2009;37:1922–33.

117. Tran TD, Caruthers SD, Huqhes M, et al. Clinical applications of perfluorocarbon nanoparticles for molecular imaging and targeted therapeutics. Int J Nanomedicine 2007;2:515–26.

118. Lanza GM, Caruthers SD, Hughes M, et al. 1H/19F magnetic resonance molecular imaging with perfluorocarbon nanoparticles. Curr Top Dev Biol 2005;70:57–76.

119. Wang D, Wu Y, Xia J. Review on photoacoustic imaging of the brain using nanoprobes. Neurophotonics 2016;3:010901.

120. Cheng CJ, Tietjen GT, Saucier-Sawyer JK, et al. A holistic approach to targeting disease with polymeric nanoparticles. Nat Rev Drug Discov 2015;14: 239–47.

121. Tan M, Wu X, Jeong EK, et al. Peptide-targeted nanoglobular Gd-DOTA monoamide conjugates for magnetic resonance cancer molecular imaging. Biomacromolecules 2010;11:754–61.

122. Wiener EC, Brechbiel MW, Brother H, et al. Dendrimer-based metal chelates: a new class of magnetic resonance imaging contrast agents. Magn Reson Med 1994;31:1–8.

123. Boswell CA, Eck PK, Regino CA, et al. Synthesis, characterization, and biological evaluation of integrin alphavbeta3-targeted PAMAM dendrimers. Mol Pharm 2008;5:527–39.

124. Han L, Zhang A, Wang H, et al. Tat-BMPs-PAMAM conjugates enhance therapeutic effect of small interference RNA on U251 glioma cells in vitro and in vivo. Hum Gene Ther 2010;21:417–26.

125. Sarin H, Kanevsky AS, Wu H, et al. Effective transvascular delivery of nanoparticles across the blood-brain tumor barrier into malignant glioma cells. J Transl Med 2008;6:80.

126. Singh P, Gupta U, Asthana A, et al. Folate and folate-PEG-PAMAM dendrimers: synthesis, characterization, and targeted anticancer drug delivery potential in tumor bearing mice. Bioconjug Chem 2008;19:2239–52.

127. Yang W, Wu G, Barth RF, et al. Molecular targeting and treatment of composite EGFR and EGFRvIII-positive gliomas using boronated monoclonal antibodies. Clin Cancer Res 2008;14:883–91.

128. Regino CA, Walbridge S, Bernardo M, et al. A dual CT-MR dendrimer contrast agent as a surrogate marker for convection-enhanced delivery of intracerebral macromolecular therapeutic agents. Contrast Media Mol Imaging 2008;3:2–8.

129. Danson S, Ferry D, Alakhov V, et al. Phase I dose escalation and pharmacokinetic study of pluronic polymer-bound doxorubicin (SP1049C) in patients with advanced cancer. Br J Cancer 2004;90: 2085–91.

130. Kuroda J, Kuratsu J, Yasunaga M, et al. Antitumor effect of NK012, a 7-ethyl-10-hydroxycamptothecin-incorporating polymeric micelle, on U87MG orthotopic glioblastoma in mice compared with irinotecan hydrochloride in combination with bevacizumab. Clin Cancer Res 2010;16:521–9.

131. Torchilin VP. Polymeric contrast agents for medical imaging. Curr Pharm Biotechnol 2000;1:183–215.

132. Torchilin VP. PEG-based micelles as carriers of contrast agents for different imaging modalities. Adv Drug Deliv Rev 2002;54:235–52.

133. Inoue T, Yamashita Y, Nishihara M, et al. Therapeutic efficacy of a polymeric micellar doxorubicin infused by convection-enhanced delivery against intracranial 9L brain tumor models. Neurooncol 2009;11:151–7.

134. Weissleder R, Elizondo G, Wittenberg J, et al. Ultrasmall superparamagnetic iron oxide: characterization of a new class of contrast agents for MR imaging. Radiology 1990;175:489–93.

135. Laurent S, Boutry S, Mahieu I, et al. Iron oxide based MR contrast agents: from chemistry to cell labeling. Curr Med Chem 2009;16:4712–27.

136. Laurent S, Forge D, Port M, et al. Magnetic iron oxide nanoparticles: synthesis, stabilization, vectorization, physicochemical characterizations, and biological applications. Chem Rev 2008;108:2064–110.

137. Thorek DL, Chen AK, Czupryna J, et al. Superparamagnetic iron oxide nanoparticle probes for molecular imaging. Ann Biomed Eng 2006;34:23–38.

138. Li W, Tutton S, Vu AT, et al. First-pass contrast-enhanced magnetic resonance angiography in humans using ferumoxytol, a novel ultrasmall superparamagnetic iron oxide (USPIO)-based blood pool agent. J Magn Reson Imaging 2005; 21:46–52.

139. Tombach B, Reimer P, Bremer C, et al. First-pass and equilibrium-MRA of the aortoiliac region with a superparamagnetic iron oxide blood pool MR contrast agent (SH U 555 C): results of a human pilot study. NMR Biomed 2004;17:500–6.

140. Wang YX, Hussain SM, Krestin GP. Superparamagnetic iron oxide contrast agents: physicochemical characteristics and applications in MR imaging. Eur Radiol 2001;11:2319–31.

141. Ros PR, Freeny PC, Harms SE, et al. Hepatic MR imaging with ferumoxides: a multicenter clinical trial of the safety and efficacy in the detection of focal hepatic lesions. Radiology 1995;196:481–8.

142. Christoforidis GA, Yang M, Kontzialis MS, et al. High resolution ultra high field magnetic resonance imaging of glioma microvascularity and hypoxia using ultra-small particles of iron oxide. Invest Radiol 2009;44:375–83.

143. Gambarota G, Leenders W. Characterization of tumor vasculature in mouse brain by USPIO contrast-enhanced MRI. Methods Mol Biol 2011; 771:477–87.

144. Neuwelt EA, Várallayay CG, Manninger S, et al. The potential of ferumoxytol nanoparticle magnetic resonance imaging, perfusion, and angiography in central nervous system malignancy: a pilot study. Neurosurgery 2007;60:601–11 [discussion: 611–2].

145. Varallyay CG, Muldoon LL, Gahramanov S, et al. Dynamic MRI using iron oxide nanoparticles to assess early vascular effects of antiangiogenic versus corticosteroid treatment in a glioma model. J Cereb Blood Flow Metab 2009;29:853–60.

146. Weinstein JS, Varallyay CG, Dosa E, et al. Superparamagnetic iron oxide nanoparticles: diagnostic magnetic resonance imaging and potential therapeutic applications in neurooncology and central nervous system inflammatory pathologies, a review. J Cereb Blood Flow Metab 2010;30:15–35.

147. Harisinghani MG, Barentsz J, Hahn PF, et al. Noninvasive detection of clinically occult lymph-node metastases in prostate cancer. N Engl J Med 2003;348:2491–9.

148. Lahaye MJ, Engelen SM, Kessels AG, et al. USPIO-enhanced MR imaging for nodal staging in patients with primary rectal cancer: predictive criteria. Radiology 2008;246:804–11.

149. Fleige G, Nolte C, Synowitz M, et al. Magnetic labeling of activated microglia in experimental gliomas. Neoplasia 2001;3:489–99.

150. Thu MS, Najbauer J, Kendall SE, et al. Iron labeling and pre-clinical MRI visualization of therapeutic human neural stem cells in a murine glioma model. PLoS One 2009;4:e7218.

151. Valable S, Barbier EL, Bernaudin M, et al. In vivo MRI tracking of exogenous monocytes/macrophages targeting brain tumors in a rat model of glioma. Neuroimage 2008;40:973–83.

152. Wu X, Hu J, Zhou L, et al. In vivo tracking of superparamagnetic iron oxide nanoparticle-labeled mesenchymal stem cell tropism to malignant gliomas using magnetic resonance imaging. Laboratory investigation. J Neurosurg 2008;108:320–9.

153. Cole LE, Ross RD, Tilley JM, et al. Gold nanoparticles as contrast agents in x-ray imaging and computed tomography. Nanomedicine (Lond) 2015;10:321–41.

154. Li W, Chen X. Gold nanoparticles for photoacoustic imaging. Nanomedicine (Lond) 2015;10:299–320.

155. Vo-Dinh T, Liu Y, Fales AM, et al. SERS nanosensors and nanoreporters: golden opportunities in biomedical applications. Wiley Interdiscip Rev Nanomed Nanobiotechnol 2015;7:17–33.

156. Ashton JR, West JL, Badea CT. In vivo small animal micro-CT using nanoparticle contrast agents. Front Pharmacol 2015;6:256.

157. Ashton JR, Clark DP, Moding EJ, et al. Dual-energy micro-CT functional imaging of primary lung cancer in mice using gold and iodine nanoparticle contrast agents: a validation study. PLoS One 2014;9:e88129.

158. Clark DP, Ghaghada K, Moding EJ, et al. In vivo characterization of tumor vasculature using iodine and gold nanoparticles and dual energy micro-CT. Phys Med Biol 2013;58:1683–704.

159. Hirsch LR, Gobin AM, Lowery AR, et al. Metal nanoshells. Ann Biomed Eng 2006;34:15–22.

160. Loo C, Hrisch L, Lee MH, et al. Gold nanoshell bioconjugates for molecular imaging in living cells. Opt Lett 2005;30:1012–4.

161. West JL, Halas NJ. Engineered nanomaterials for biophotonics applications: improving sensing, imaging, and therapeutics. Annu Rev Biomed Eng 2003;5:285–92.

162. Lin AW, Lewinski NA, West JL, et al. Optically tunable nanoparticle contrast agents for early cancer detection: model-based analysis of gold nanoshells. J Biomed Opt 2005;10:064035.

163. Talley CE, Jackson JB, Oubre C, et al. Surface-enhanced Raman scattering from individual au nanoparticles and nanoparticle dimer substrates. Nano Lett 2005;5:1569–74.

164. Harmsen S, Huang R, Wall MA, et al. Surface-enhanced resonance Raman scattering nanostars for high-precision cancer imaging. Sci Transl Med 2015;7:271ra7.

165. Hirsch LR, Stafford RJ, Bankson JA, et al. Nanoshell-mediated near-infrared thermal therapy of tumors under magnetic resonance guidance. Proc Natl Acad Sci U S A 2003;100:13549–54.

166. Loo C, Lowery A, Halas N, et al. Immunotargeted nanoshells for integrated cancer imaging and therapy. Nano Lett 2005;5:709–11.

167. O'Neal DP, Hirsch LR, Halas NJ, et al. Photo-thermal tumor ablation in mice using near infrared-absorbing nanoparticles. Cancer Lett 2004;209:171–6.

168. Schwartz JA, Shetty AM, Price RE, et al. Feasibility study of particle-assisted laser ablation of brain tumors in orthotopic canine model. Cancer Res 2009;69:1659–67.

169. Reiss P, Protiere M, Li L. Core/shell semiconductor nanocrystals. Small 2009;5:154–68.

170. Jackson H, Muhammad O, Daneshvar H, et al. Quantum dots are phagocytized by macrophages and colocalize with experimental gliomas. Neurosurgery 2007;60:524–9 [discussion: 529–30].

171. Khalessi AA, Liu CY, Apuzzo ML. Neurosurgery and quantum dots: part I–state of the art. Neurosurgery 2009;64:1015–27 [discussion: 1027–8].

172. Popescu MA, Toms SA. In vivo optical imaging using quantum dots for the management of brain tumors. Expert Rev Mol Diagn 2006;6:879–90.

173. Smith AM, Duan H, Mohs AM, et al. Bioconjugated quantum dots for in vivo molecular and cellular imaging. Adv Drug Deliv Rev 2008;60:1226–40.

174. Zhang Y, Lu F, Yager KG, et al. A general strategy for the DNA-mediated self-assembly of functional nanoparticles into heterogeneous systems. Nat Nanotechnol 2013;8:865–72.

175. Chou LY, Zagorovsky K, Chan WC. DNA assembly of nanoparticle superstructures for controlled biological delivery and elimination. Nat Nanotechnol 2014;9:148–55.

Perfusion Imaging in Neuro-Oncology
Basic Techniques and Clinical Applications

Brent Griffith, MD[a],*, Rajan Jain, MD[b]

KEYWORDS

- MR perfusion • CT perfusion • DCE-T1 • DSC-T2* • ASL • Cerebral blood volume

KEY POINTS

- Perfusion imaging allows for assessment of changes occurring at the tumor microvasculature level.
- Perfusion-based parameters have the potential to serve as important quantitative imaging biomarkers, providing information not routinely available with standard morphologic imaging.
- Perfusion imaging is increasingly used for neuro-oncologic applications, including brain tumor grading, directing biopsies or targeted therapy, and evaluation of treatment response and disease progression.
- Perfusion-based quantitative biomarkers, when used in conjunction with standard morphologic imaging, have the potential to provide early indication of treatment failure or treatment response.
- Increased use of perfusion MR in the routine surveillance imaging of brain tumors allows for evaluation of relative cerebral blood volume (rCBV) trends, which may bolster its effectiveness as an imaging biomarker.

WHAT IS PERFUSION IMAGING?

Perfusion imaging is a method for assessing the flow of blood occurring at the tissue level.[1] Depending on the modality (eg, MR, CT) and method (eg, dynamic contrast enhanced [DCE], arterial spin labeled) used, several perfusion parameters can be evaluated, both qualitatively and quantitatively. These parameters include those related to the volume of blood within a given region of tissue, as well as those describing the movement of blood through that region over time. In addition to assessing blood volume and flow, these techniques also allow for the quantitative assessment of vessel leakiness through the measurement of vascular permeability.

WHAT IS MEASURED AND HOW IS IT USED?
Blood Volume and Blood Flow

Blood volume (BV), mean transit time (MTT), and blood flow (BF) are all parameters used to describe the flow of blood within a particular region of tissue.

- BV refers to the total volume of blood flowing within a given area of tissue and is measured in milliliters of blood per 100 g of tissue (mL/100 g).
- BF refers to the volume of blood flowing within a given area of tissue per unit time and is measured in milliliters of blood per 100 g of tissue per minute (mL/100 g/min).
- MTT refers to the average time blood takes to traverse through a given area of tissue and is measured in seconds (s).

Measuring the volume and flow of blood in a particular region of brain can have important clinical implications. In the setting of acute ischemia, measurement of CBV, MTT, and CBF helps in differentiating the "core" of irreversibly infarcted brain tissue from the ischemic, but potentially salvageable, brain tissue (ie, penumbra).[1] Similarly, CBV

This article originally appeared in Radiologic Clinics of North America, Volume 53, Issue 3, May 2015.
[a] Department of Radiology, Henry Ford Health System, Detroit, MI, USA; [b] NYU School of Medicine, NYU Langone Medical Center, New York, NY, USA
* Corresponding author.
E-mail address: brentg@rad.hfh.edu

Magn Reson Imaging Clin N Am 24 (2016) 765–779
http://dx.doi.org/10.1016/j.mric.2016.07.004

has also been used successfully to identify patients with hemodynamic impairment in the setting of major arterial occlusive disease,[2] as well as in evaluating cerebrovascular reserve in patients with Moya-Moya.[3] In addition, assessment of CBV has been used extensively in neuro-oncologic applications, including for brain tumor grading and directing biopsies or targeted therapy, as well as for the evaluation of treatment response and disease progression.[4,5] These neuro-oncologic applications of perfusion imaging are the focus of this article.

Vessel Permeability

In addition to parameters describing the volume and flow of blood within a particular region of brain, perfusion imaging also allows for assessment of vessel permeability. This is particularly important for applications involving the brain, given the role of the blood–brain barrier (BBB), which serves as a physical barrier to the entry of lipophobic substances into the brain and can be disrupted by a number of disease processes, including brain tumors. This breakdown of the BBB, which accounts for the contrast enhancement seen on standard imaging, also provides a potential surrogate imaging marker. Various methods have been developed to quantify this vessel "leakiness," most notably by measurement of the permeability surface-area product (PS), which characterizes the diffusion of contrast agent from the blood vessels into the interstitial space, or by the transfer constant (K_{trans}).[6]

METHODS
CT Perfusion

CT perfusion (CTP) allows for the assessment of CBV and permeability with a single acquisition. The greatest advantage of CT perfusion is the linear relationship between iodine concentration and attenuation on CT. This easy conversion allows for a direct measurement of vascular parameters.

CTP protocols vary depending on the manufacturer and scanner model used, as well as depending on the reason for the examination (eg, tumor volume protocol vs acute stroke imaging). However, as a general concept, CTP is based on the principle of sequential acquisition of CT images during the washin and washout of iodinated contrast material from brain parenchyma (**Fig. 1**)[7] with the goal being to observe the distribution of contrast agent within tissues over time.

How Is It Done?

- Before obtaining the perfusion scan, a low radiation dose noncontrast CT head study can be performed.
- For the perfusion scan at our institution, 50 mL of nonionic contrast is injected at a rate of 4 to 5 mL/s through an intravenous line using an automatic power injector.
- A cine scan is then initiated at 5 seconds into the injection, using the following parameters: 80 kV (peak), 100 to 120 mÅ, and 1 second per rotation for a duration of 50 seconds. After the initial 50-s cine scan, 8 additional axial images are acquired, 1 image every 15 seconds for an additional 2 minutes, resulting in a total acquisition time of 170 seconds to assess delayed permeability.[8]
- Perfusion maps can then be obtained through the use of a number of commercially available software applications with the superior sagittal sinus generally used as the venous output function and the artery with the greatest peak and slope on the time–attenuation curves as the arterial input function.[8]

MR Perfusion

The measurement of vascular parameters with MR perfusion can be accomplished with both contrast-enhanced and non–contrast-enhanced (arterial spin labeling [ASL]) techniques. Dynamic contrast-enhanced MRI utilizes 2 techniques—a T1-weighted acquisition (DCE MR) and a T2*-based acquisition (DSC MR). Although the methods used by these techniques in quantifying cerebral perfusion differ, both rely on a trace of contrast agent concentration over time to estimate blood volume and permeability.[9] In contrast to these contrast-enhanced methods, evaluation of perfusion with ASL is accomplished through the use of magnetically labeled arterial blood water as a freely diffusible tracer.

In contrast with CT perfusion, which directly images the iodinated contrast agent, contrast agents utilized in MR perfusion are not imaged directly and instead rely on signal intensity to provide an estimate of CBV. However, regardless of the technique used, MR perfusion offers 2 major advantages over CT perfusion. First, MR perfusion requires no radiation, which is very important in oncologic imaging, because patients often require frequent imaging for tumor surveillance. Second, particularly in neuro-oncologic imaging, MR is the standard of care for assessing treatment response or progression of disease. Therefore, the acquisition of perfusion parameters with MR perfusion requires only additional sequences to be obtained rather than an entirely separate examination as in the case of CT perfusion.

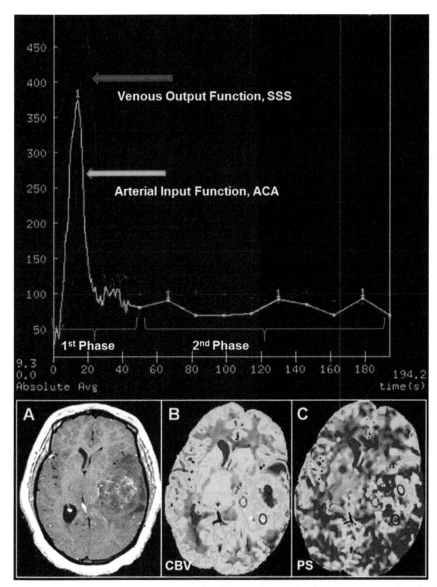

Fig. 1. (*Top*) CT perfusion time concentration curves for the anterior cerebral artery, representing the input artery (*green arrow*) and the superior sagittal sinus, representing the output vein (*red arrow*). (*Bottom row*) Postcontrast axial T1-weighted image shows a heterogeneously enhancing WHO grade III glioma centered in the left temporal region (*A*). CT perfusion maps show regions of interest placed in various regions of the tumor on both the cerebral blood volume map (*B*) and permeability surface area product map (*C*) showing heterogeneous areas of both increased CBV and permeability surface-area product (PS), suggesting a high-grade neoplasm.

Dynamic Contrast Enhanced-T1 Imaging

DCE-T1 imaging is based on the fact that an increase in the concentration of contrast agent results in a proportional increase in the rate of T1 relaxation from which a time–concentration curve can be generated and is tracked over a longer time period (5–10 minutes; **Fig. 2**).

DCE-T1 MR allows characterization of the vascular microenvironment through the measurement of a number of different parameters, including K_{trans} (influx transfer constant), K_b (reverse transfer constant), V_e (volume of the extravascular extracellular space), and V_P (blood plasma volume). The clinical application of these parameters, however, is often limited by the complicated, multicompartment physiologic models required to obtain the quantitative metrics. To improve the clinical utility, model-free "semiquantitative" indices have been developed to assess tissue perfusion.[10] These methods have been used to both assess the shape of the uptake and washout of contrast (ie, curveology), as well as to provide objective indices for

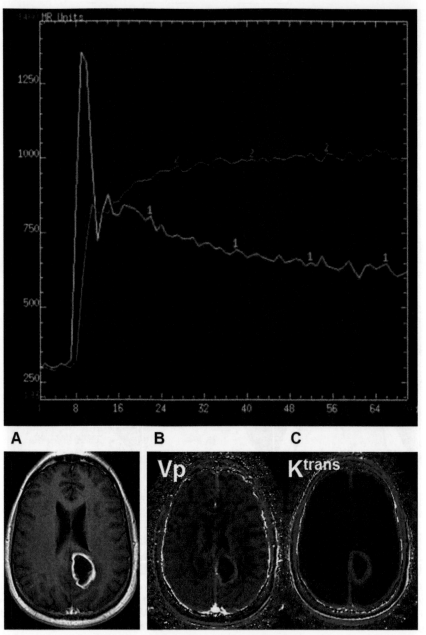

Fig. 2. (*Top*) DCE T1 time concentration curves from the arterial input function (*green*) and the tumor tissue (*red*). (*Bottom Row*) Post-contrast axial T1-weighted image shows a heterogeneously ring enhancing WHO grade IV glioma centered in the left medial occipital lobe (*A*). Plasma volume map (*B*) and K_{trans} map (*C*) showing markedly increased Vp and K_{trans} in the peripheral component of the tumor suggesting a high-grade neoplasm.

evaluation. These indices include maximum slope of enhancement in the initial vascular phase (MSIVP), which assesses change of signal intensity per second; normalized slope of the delayed equilibrium phase (nSDEP), which is the slope of the fitted linear curve to final 25% samples; as well as the initial area under the time–intensity curve (IAUC) at 60 and 120 seconds (IAUC$_{60}$ and IAUC$_{120}$).[10]

How Is It Done?

- At our institution DCE-MRI studies are performed on a 3T MR system using a standard 8-channel phased array radiofrequency (RF) coil and receiver with the following sequence parameters: TE/TR ∼ 0.84/5.8 ms; flip angles, θi, of 2, 5, 10, 15, 20, and 25°; asset number = 2; matrix of 256 × 128; field of view, 240 mm; 16 slices of 5 mm; no gap.

- The precontrast T1 maps are used to establish baseline T1 values before the administration of contrast.

Dynamic Susceptibility Contrast T2* Imaging

DSC-T2* MRI is based on rapid imaging of the first pass of gadolinium-based contrast material through the tumor vasculature and utilizes susceptibility weighted imaging to generate a time–concentration curve after contrast administration. The contrast agent results in an initial drop in signal intensity owing to the T2* shortening effects, which in turn leads to loss and then recovery of signal in the tumor bed as the agent is redistributed or diluted (**Fig. 3**). This drop in signal intensity, also known as "negative enhancement," is proportional to the concentration of the contrast agent. As such, the area under the time concentration curve can be calculated and used to derive the rCBV map, which is the most widely used quantitative variable derived from DSC imaging.[11]

Because the bolus transit time for DSC-T2* imaging is so short, a fast acquisition technique, such as echo planar imaging (EPI) is typically performed, which provides the necessary temporal resolution to adequately characterize the transient drop in signal intensity.[12] Although both spin echo (SE) and gradient echo (GRE) techniques are used, GRE is most commonly used because it has been shown to be more sensitive to broader ranges of vessel size, an important feature when evaluating the morphologically abnormal vessels commonly seen in tumors undergoing neovascularization.[12] This finding is in contrast with the SE technique, which is more sensitive to capillary-sized vessels. The downside, of course, to the use of GRE DSC-MRI technique is its susceptibility to artifacts related to adjacent bony structures, air, or blood products, which is commonly encountered in the setting of brain tumors, particularly in the postoperative follow-up period.

In addition to these limitations related to susceptibility artifacts, DSC-T2* methods are also prone to errors related to contrast leakage, a common problem in high-grade gliomas owing to the leakiness of the BBB owing to significant neovascularization. The leakiness of the vessels, coupled with the use of low-molecular-weight extravascular contrast agents (eg, gadolinium-DTPA), results in rapid extravasation of contrast from the vascular compartment into the interstitium. This leakage results in both enhanced T1 relaxation effects, as well as increased or decreased T2* effects.[12] These effects can either result in overestimation or underestimation of rCBV, depending on the relative magnitude of the T2* or T1 effects, respectively.[12]

How Is It Done?

- At our institution, studies are performed on either a 1.5-T or 3-T MR system. Routine unenhanced MRIs are performed before the perfusion portion of the study.
- Perfusion images are performed during the injection of contrast agent, which is infused via a power injector at a constant rate of 5 mL/s.
- Perfusion images include the acquisition of a series of 95 phases of T2*-weighted GRE-EPI (repetition time ms/echo time ms, 1900/40; flip angle, 90°) with an acquisition matrix of 128 × 128 with a 26-cm field of view and 5-mm section thickness. The temporal resolution is 2.0 s. The number of sections obtained varies according to tumor size with the goal of including the entire tumor in the acquisition.
- T1-weighted contrast-enhanced images are then acquired after the perfusion study.

Arterial Spin Labeling

MR perfusion with ASL utilizes the magnetic labeling of arterial blood water through the use of an RF pulse.[13] After this proton labeling, a period of time referred to as the postlabeling delay is necessary to give the labeled blood time to reach the brain parenchyma.[14] In addition to the labeled images, all ASL techniques require the acquisition of control, or unlabeled, images. The signal remaining after subtraction of the labeled and control images can then be used to provide information regarding the CBF. Owing to the low signal-to-noise ratio between the labeled and control images, multiple control and label image pairs must be obtained.[14]

Different methods are used for labeling arterial water, including continuous ASL (CASL), pseudo-continuous ASL (PCASL), pulsed ASL (PASL), and velocity-selective ASL methods.[15] In CASL, a prolonged RF pulse continuously labels arterial blood water below the imaging slab.[13,14,16] The major advantage of CASL compared with the other labeling methods is its higher perfusion sensitivity.[14,15] The downside, however, to the prolonged RF pulse is 2-fold. First, the prolonged pulse lead to magnetization transfer effects that, if not appropriately balanced in the control acquisition, can lead to overestimation of perfusion.[13,16] In addition, these prolonged RF pulses result in greater energy deposition to the patient, which can exceed US Food and Drug Administration guidelines.[14,15] Finally, continuous RF transmit hardware is not available commonly on commercial MR scanners, which limits its widespread application in clinical practice.[14] In contrast with CASL, PASL utilizes a short RF pulse to label a thick slab of arterial blood at a single point in

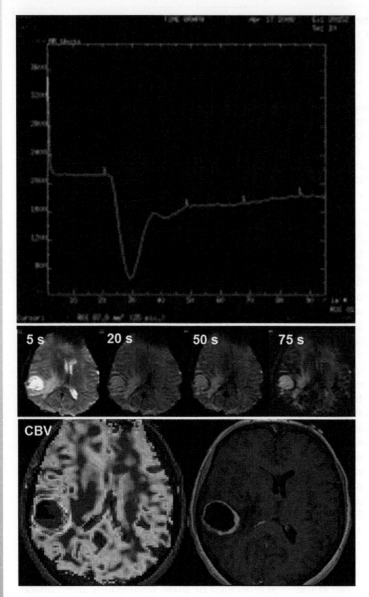

Fig. 3. (*Top*) Time concentration curve for a dynamic susceptibility contrast (DSC) T2* MR demonstrating the initial drop in signal intensity owing to the T2* shortening effects, which leads to signal loss and then recovery of signal as the contrast agent is redistributed (*green curve*). (*Second row*) Serial axial gradient echo images showing progressive signal drop through the brain as well as peripheral part of a necrotic tumor in right cerebral hemisphere, which was proven to be a GBM. (*Third row*) Cerebral blood volume map shows increased blood volume (*left*) corresponding with the enhancing rim of the tumor shown on the axial post-contrast T1-weighted image (*right*), suggesting a high-grade neoplasm.

time.[14,16] There are various methods of PASL differing in the labeling plane location and magnetic state of the labeled blood; however, this is beyond the scope of this article.[14] Whereas PASL offers a high labeling efficiency with lesser RF power deposition, its perfusion sensitivity is less when compared with CASL.[14] The third technique to discuss briefly is PCASL, which mimics CASL through the use of a train of RF pulses in addition to a synchronous gradient field.[14] PCASL offers high inversion efficiency, but with reduced magnetization transfer effects and RF power deposition when compared with CASL. Despite these advantages, however, PCASL is susceptible to both B0 inhomogeneity and eddy currents.[14,17]

Finally, once the blood has been labeled appropriately, ASL imaging is performed typically using an EPI technique, allowing for a fast acquisition speed. Unfortunately, as with DSC-T2* perfusion images, EPI is also sensitive to susceptibility artifacts caused by adjacent bony structures, air, or blood products, which are frequently encountered, particularly in neuro-oncologic applications.

Aside from the advantages of the various labeling methods described, in general there are several advantages to using ASL versus other perfusion imaging methods. First, as with contrast-enhanced MR perfusion techniques, ASL requires no radiation and requires only an additional sequence to the standard of care surveillance MRI, which provides important advantages over CT perfusion. Second, contrary to the other perfusion methods described, ASL does not rely on the use of an exogenous tracer, such as iodinated contrast material or gadolinium-based contrast material as is required for CT perfusion and contrast-enhanced MR perfusion techniques, respectively.[15] This is particularly advantageous in patients with chronic renal failure, given concerns regarding nephrogenic systemic fibrosis.[14,16]

CLINICAL UTILITY IN NEURO-ONCOLOGIC IMAGING

Although the regular use of perfusion imaging in oncologic imaging has been a more recent trend, its importance, particularly in the arena of tumor physiology, has been well-recognized for many years. In 1992, Folkman[18] discussed the role of angiogenesis in tumor growth, describing the neovascularization of a tumor as it moves from a prevascular to vascular phase, a phase that has the potential for rapid cell population expansion and a propensity for metastasis. This correlation between neovascularization and increasing aggressiveness of tumors has been well-documented in the brain tumor perfusion literature with both CT and MR perfusion methods, demonstrating a correlation between higher CBVs and permeability in higher grade tumors.[4,19–21]

Tumor Grading

The standard for grading of brain tumors is histopathologic assessment of tissue, for which a variety of classification systems are available, the most common being the World Health Organization (WHO) grading system. However, grading systems based on histopathology are plagued by a number of limitations, particularly sampling error and interobserver variation.[8] This is especially true in the case of gliomas, particularly high-grade gliomas, owing to their significant heterogeneity, which can lead to inaccurate grading and classification.[8]

Both MR and CT perfusion have been successfully used to grade gliomas on the basis of perfusion parameters. Previous studies by Shin and colleagues[21] and Jackson and colleagues[19] found that higher grade tumors demonstrated statistically significant higher mean values than lower grade tumors. By using an rCBV threshold value of 1.75, Law and colleagues[5] were able to differentiate low- and high-grade tumors with a sensitivity of 95% and specificity of 57.5%. In addition, Provenzale and colleagues[20] in 2002 found that permeability values for high-grade tumors obtained using a T2*-weighted method were significantly greater than those for low-grade tumors.

Similar to MR perfusion, CT perfusion has also demonstrated the ability to differentiate low grade and high grade tumors. A 2006 study by Ellika and colleagues[4] found that CT perfusion with a CBV normalized relative to a normal-appearing contralateral white matter threshold of 1.92 was able to differentiate low- and high-grade gliomas with a sensitivity of 85.7% and specificity of 100% (**Fig. 4**). Furthermore, Jain and colleagues[22] showed that in addition to differentiating low- and high-grade gliomas, PS measurements also enabled the differentiation of high-grade tumors into grades III and IV on the basis of PS measurements.

Differentiating Primary Gliomas from Tumefactive Demyelinating Lesions

In addition to tumor grading, perfusion imaging has also shown the ability to differentiate brain tumors from other masslike enhancing lesions, most notably from tumefactive demyelinating lesions (TDLs). TDLs have been described on imaging to demonstrate larger sizes with associated mass effect and edema, as well as atypical enhancement patterns, including ring enhancement.[23] This imaging appearance can make differentiation from primary gliomas, in particular glioblastoma multiforme (GBM), difficult, oftentimes requiring surgical biopsy for definitive diagnosis. However, not only can TDLs mimic an intracranial neoplasm on morphologic imaging, but these lesions can also simulate gliomas on histopathologic examination.[24] Given these similarities, preoperative suspicion of a demyelinating process can be helpful to ensure appropriate management.

One important difference that can be exploited by MR perfusion in differentiating these entities relates to differences in vascularity.[25] Whereas high-grade gliomas demonstrate neoangiogenesis and vascular endothelial proliferation, TDLs are characterized by inflamed vessels with mild inflammatory angiogenesis.[25,26] Given the lack of significant neoangiogenesis seen within TDLs, these lesions have been shown to demonstrate lower PS and CBV when compared with high-grade gliomas on CT perfusion, offering a potential in vivo means of differentiating the 2 entities (**Fig. 5**).[25] Similarly, rCBV measurements on MR perfusion have also

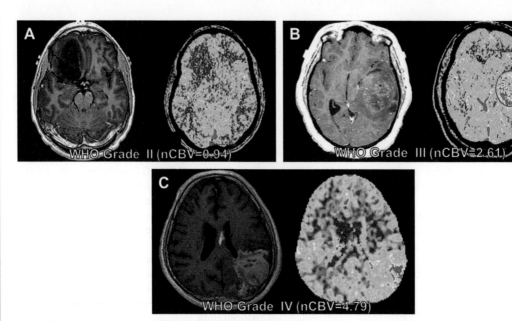

Fig. 4. (*A*) Postcontrast T1-weighted axial image (*left*) and CT perfusion CBV map (*right*) in a patient with a WHO grade II glioma showing a nonenhancing mass in the right frontal lobe with low CBV (nCBV = 0.94). (*B*) Postcontrast T1-weighted axial image (*left*) and CT perfusion CBV map (*right*) in a patient with a WHO grade III glioma showing a large, heterogeneously enhancing left temporal mass with significant mass effect and a nCBV of 2.61. (*C*) Postcontrast T1-weighted axial image (*left*) and CT perfusion CBV map (*right*) in a patient with a WHO grade IV glioma showing an enhancing mass in the left parietal region with very high CBV (nCBV = 4.79). (*From* Ellika S, Jain R, Patel SC, et al. Role of perfusion CT in glioma grading and comparison with conventional MRI features. AJNR Am J Neuroradiol 2007;28(10):1984; with permission.)

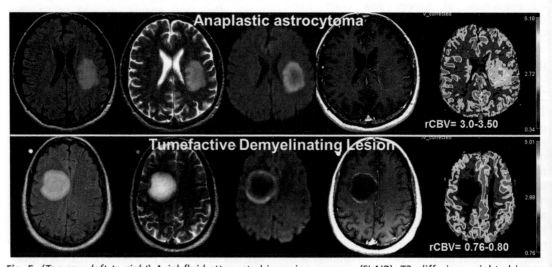

Fig. 5. (*Top row, left to right*) Axial fluid-attenuated inversion recovery (FLAIR), T2, diffusion-weighted image (DWI), T1 postcontrast, and rCBV map demonstrates a T2 FLAIR hyperintense lesion within the left hemispheric white matter, which demonstrates patchy enhancement and bright signal on DWI at its periphery. The lesion demonstrates an rCBV of 3.0 to 3.5, suggestive of a neoplastic process, proven to be a WHO grade III glioma with surgery and histopathology. (*Bottom row, left to right*) Axial FLAIR, T2, DWI, T1 postcontrast, and rCBV map demonstrates a T2 FLAIR hyperintense lesion within the right hemispheric white matter, which also demonstrates peripheral enhancement and bright signal on DWI, almost similar to the neoplasm from upper row. However, DSC T2* perfusion CBV map showing a very low rCBV of 0.76 to 0.80. At biopsy, this neoplasm was found to be a tumefactive demyelinating lesion. (*Courtesy of* Eytan Raz, MD, NYU.)

been shown to successfully discriminate between high-grade gliomas and TDLs,[27] although this differentiation does not extend to grade II/III gliomas, because these both can demonstrate similar level increases in rCBV.[28]

Differentiating Recurrent Tumor Versus Treatment Effects

One of the predominant roles of perfusion imaging in neuro-oncologic imaging is the accurate differentiation of treatment effects and disease progression, which has important implications for patient care, because correct differentiation can result in changes to a patient's treatment regimen.

Identifying disease progression or response by imaging has relied traditionally on measurement of the contrast-enhancing lesion, using either the RECIST or Macdonald criteria. However, brain tumor enhancement depends on the presence and integrity of the BBB, which can be affected by a number of factors other than disease response or progression, including effects related to particular treatments. Examples of this include both processes that can disrupt the BBB, such as postictal changes, postoperative infarcts, or treatment-related inflammatory processes, as well as those that stabilize the BBB, such as steroids or antiangiogenic therapies. The former, which results in disruption of the BBB, leads to increased enhancement, which mimics disease progression and has been termed 'pseudoprogression.' The latter, which improves the integrity of the BBB resulting in decreased enhancement in the absence of any true treatment response, thereby mimicking disease response, has been termed pseudoresponse (**Fig. 6**).[29,30]

Pseudoprogression

"Pseudoprogression" is the term applied to a treatment-related increase in enhancing lesion size and/or edema without a true increase in tumor burden, which shows either improvement or lack of progression on follow-up imaging. Pseudoprogression generally occurs in the 2- to 6-month period after chemoradiation therapy[31,32] and is believed to result from increased inflammation, edema, and abnormal vessel permeability in the local tissues, which leads to the movement of fluid into the interstitial space and subsequent brain edema.

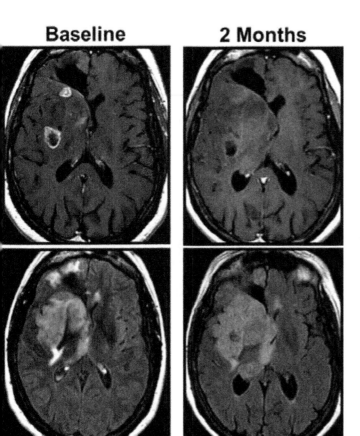

Baseline　　　　**2 Months**

Fig. 6. (*Left column*) Baseline axial postcontrast T1-weighted (*top row*) and axial fluid-attenuated inversion recovery (FLAIR) images demonstrate multiple enhancing lesions with surrounding FLAIR hyperintensity in the region of the right basal ganglia. (*Right column*) After treatment with bevacizumab, the 2-month follow-up demonstrates almost complete resolution of the previously seen enhancing lesions, but the degree of FLAIR hyperintensity has increased. This is consistent with a pseudoresponse owing to the addition of the antiangiogenic agent bevacizumab to the treatment regimen.

Differentiation of pseudoprogression from true tumor progression on MRI alone is not possible because both can demonstrate increased enhancement and edema. However, by evaluating changes occurring on the microvasculature level, perfusion imaging provides a potential tool for differentiating these entities.

Compared with recurrent tumor, enhancing lesions caused by treatment effects (eg, pseudoprogression) lack significant neoangiogenesis, which is the hallmark of recurrent tumor. This lack results in a lower microvascular density and lower vessel leakiness, which manifests as lower blood volume and permeability on perfusion imaging.[33,34]

A study by Mangla and associates[34] found that rCBV at 1 month was able to distinguish pseudoprogression from recurrent progressive disease with a sensitivity of 77% and specificity of 86%. A similar study by Young and colleagues[33] found that pseudoprogression demonstrated a lower median rCBV and permeability. In addition, model-free semiquantitative indices have also been used to differentiate recurrent tumor from treatment effects. By assessing the shape of the uptake and washout of the contrast agent, these semiquantitative methods, provide a more objective means of assessment with Jain and colleagues,[35] showing that pseudoprogression

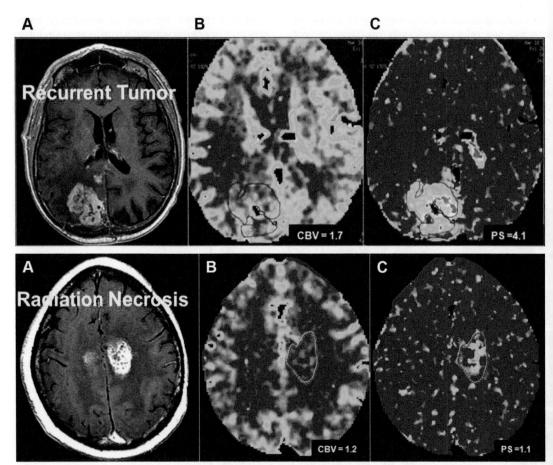

Fig. 7. (*Top row*) A 77-year-old man with initial diagnosis of GBM who underwent gross tumor resection, chemotherapy, and RT (external beam RT, 60 Gy). (*A*) Follow-up MRI shows a recurrent enhancing lesion 26 months after RT in the right parieto-occipital region within the radiation field. (*B, C*) CBV; (*B*) and PS; (*C*) maps show high rCBV and PS, suggesting recurrent progressive tumor, which was confirmed with histopathology. (*Bottom row*) A 41-year-old man with an initial diagnosis of WHO grade II astrocytoma who underwent chemotherapy and RT (intensity modulated RT, 63 Gy). (*A*) Follow-up MRI at 33 months after RT shows development of a recurrent enhancing lesion in the bilateral frontal regions. (*B, C*) CBV (*B*) and PS (*C*) maps show low rCBV and PS, suggesting treatment effects with treatment-induced necrosis suggested by biopsy. (*From* Jain R, Narang J, Schultz L, et al. Permeability estimates in histopathology-proved treatment-induced necrosis using perfusion CT: can these add to other perfusion parameters in differentiating from recurrent/progressive tumors? AJNR Am J Neuroradiol 2011;32:661; with permission.)

demonstrated a lower mean MSIVP, lower nlAUC$_{60}$, and higher nSDEP compared with early tumor progression.

Radiation Necrosis

Radiation necrosis is a delayed effect of radiation injury and is reported to occur in approximately 3% to 24% of patients undergoing standard radiation therapy.[36] Generally occurring between 3 and 12 months after radiation therapy, radiation necrosis most commonly occurs at the site of maximum radiation dose, which is usually in the vicinity of the original tumor and surrounding the surgical cavity.[29]

The clinical manifestations of radiation necrosis, including focal neurologic deficits, seizures, and cognitive dysfunction, as well as symptoms related to increased intracranial pressure and mass effect, are difficult to distinguish from tumor progression, which complicates patient management.[31,37] Similarly, the differentiation of radiation necrosis and recurrent tumor on standard morphologic imaging is also difficult, because both occur in close proximity to the original tumor site, enhance on postcontrast imaging, and demonstrate growth over time, surrounding edema, and mass effect.

As with pseudoprogression, both MR and CT perfusion techniques have shown promise in differentiating delayed radiation necrosis from tumor progression. The most commonly used parameter in this differentiation is relative cerebral blood volume (rCBV), which has been shown to be

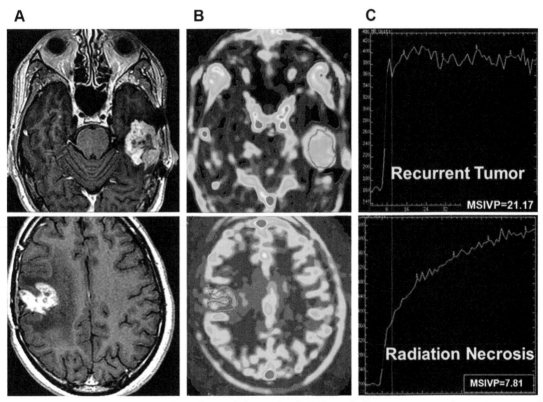

Fig. 8. (*Top Row*) A 40-year-old male with initial diagnosis of WHO grade III astrocytoma underwent gross total resection and received chemotherapy and external-beam radiotherapy (54 Gy). (*A*) Follow-up MRI showed appearance of a recurrent enhancing lesion 19 months postradiotherapy in the right temporal region within the radiation field. (*B*) Maximum slope of enhancement in initial vascular phase (MSIVP) parametric map and (*C*) graph of MSIVP showed high MSIVP, suggesting recurrent/progressive tumor (RPT), which was confirmed by histopathology. (*Bottom Row*) A 19-year-old female with initial diagnosis of GBM underwent chemotherapy and external beam radiotherapy (60 Gy). (*A*) Twelve months after radiotherapy, follow-up MRI showed development of a recurrent enhancing lesion in left parietal region. (*B*) Maximum slope of enhancement in the initial vascular phase (MSIVP) parametric map and (*C*) graph of MSIVP showed low MSIVP, suggesting treatment-induced necrosis, which was confirmed by histopathology. (*From* Narang J, Jain R, Arbab AS, et al. Differentiating treatment-induced necrosis from recurrent/progressive brain tumor using non–model-based semiquantitative indices derived from dynamic contrast-enhanced T1-weighted MR perfusion. Neuro Oncol 2011;13(9):1043; with permission.)

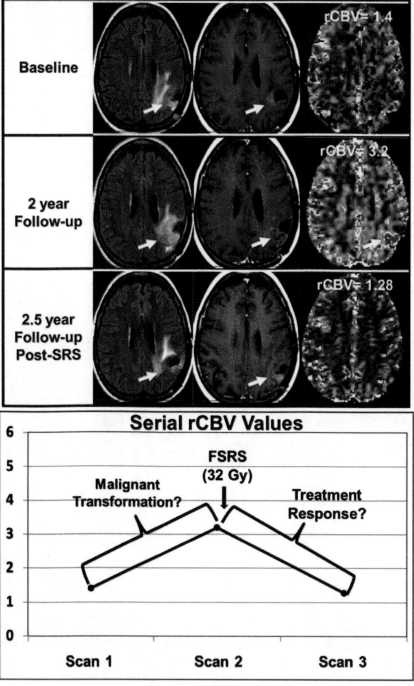

Fig. 9. A 35-year-old female with WHO grade III glioma, previously treated with radiation and temozolomide. Axial T2 FLAIR (*left*), axial T1 postcontrast (*middle*), and rCBV maps (*right*) show interval development of a T2 hyperintense, but predominantly nonenhancing lesion (*arrow*) at the posterior aspect of the surgical resection cavity on the 2-year follow-up study (*middle row*) with mean rCBV of 3.2 compared with 1.4 on the initial follow-up scan (*top row*). Based on an increase in CBV in the follow-up study compared with baseline, the patient underwent additional fractionated stereotactic radiosurgery (FSRS); 32 Gy) to the hot spot using perfusion maps for FSRS planning. At 6 months after FSRS, follow-up imaging (*bottom row*) shows slight improvement in the FLAIR signal, but more importantly marked reduction in rCBV (rCBV = 1.28), suggesting treatment response. A line graph demonstrates nicely this initial increase in rCBV suspicious for recurrent disease followed by a decrease after additional FSRS suggesting treatment response.

increased in the setting of recurrent tumor, whereas it is reduced in the setting of radiation necrosis.[38–40] Estimation of vascular leakiness (K_{trans} with MR perfusion or PS with CT perfusion) has also been used to differentiate tumor progression from treatment effects (eg, radiation necrosis; **Fig. 7**), because blood vessels within previously irradiated tissues tend to maintain an intact BBB versus the leaky BBB seen in recurrent tumor with neoangiogenesis, therefore demonstrating a lower K_{trans}.[41] Similarly, as is the case with pseudoprogression, radiation necrosis and recurrent tumor can also be differentiated using semiquantitative indices with recurrent tumor showing higher MSIVP (**Fig. 8**), nMSIVP, nIAUC$_{60}$, and nIAUC$_{120}$.

Tumor Surveillance

In an attempt to improve accurate tumor surveillance, the Response Assessment in Neuro-Oncology (RANO) working group recently developed new standardized response criteria for clinical trials in brain tumors. In addition to taking into account clinical factors such as patient clinical status and use of steroid, the updated criteria also added assessment of the nonenhancing portion of the tumor based on FLAIR/T2 imaging to assist in the differentiation of pseudoresponse from true treatment response after treatment with antiangiogenic agents.[42] However, although standard imaging provides insight into the gross morphologic changes occurring within and surrounding the tumor, it fails to provide an accurate assessment of the tumor physiology, vascularity, and metabolism.

Perfusion-based quantitative biomarkers, on the other hand, have the potential, when used in conjunction with standard morphologic imaging, to provide early indication of treatment failure or treatment response, which may allow clinicians to either switch a treatment that is not working, or to continue a treatment that may be effective. However, although perfusion imaging has become an important adjunct technique for tumor surveillance in many neuro-oncologic practices, its use at a single time-point limits its effectiveness as an imaging biomarker. One issue in particular has been the difficulty in establishing a definitive cutoff value for effectively distinguishing treatment effects from tumor progression when a new enhancing lesion in identified on follow-up imaging. A potential means to work around this limitation is through the rCBV trends, with a progressively increasing rCBV suggesting tumor progression (**Fig. 9**) and decreasing rCBV, suggesting treatment effects (**Fig. 10**). Evaluating rCBV trends has become possible recently with the increased use of perfusion MR in the routine follow-up imaging of brain tumors.

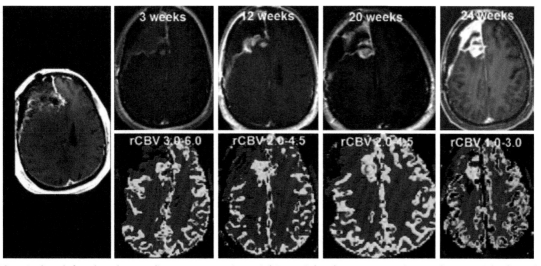

Fig. 10. (*Far left column*) Immediate postoperative axial T1-weighted postcontrast image shows a right frontal resection cavity with residual enhancing resection margins for a GBM. (*Columns 2–4*) Axial T1-weighted postcontrast images redemonstrate the right frontal resection cavity with a progressively increasing focus of nodular enhancement along the posterior aspect of the cavity from the 3 week follow-up scan to the 24 week follow-up scan. However, concurrent rCBV values progressively decreased from a mean of 4.5 at 3 weeks to a mean of 2.0 at 24 weeks. The patient underwent a second surgery and histopathology showed predominantly treatment induced necrosis with no viable tumor.

REFERENCES

1. Konstas AA, Goldmakher GV, Lee TY, et al. Theoretic basis and technical implementations of CT perfusion in acute ischemic stroke, part 1: theoretic basis. AJNR Am J Neuroradiol 2009;30(4):662–8.
2. Endo H, Inoue T, Ogasawara K, et al. Quantitative assessment of cerebral hemodynamics using perfusion-weighted MRI in patients with major cerebral artery occlusive disease: comparison with positron emission tomography. Stroke 2006;37(2):388–92.
3. Rim NJ, Kim HS, Shin YS, et al. Which CT perfusion parameter best reflects cerebrovascular reserve? Correlation of acetazolamide-challenged CT perfusion with single-photon emission CT in Moyamoya patients. AJNR Am J Neuroradiol 2008;29(9):1658–63.
4. Ellika SK, Jain R, Patel SC, et al. Role of perfusion CT in glioma grading and comparison with conventional MR imaging features. AJNR Am J Neuroradiol 2007;28(10):1981–7.
5. Law M, Yang S, Wang H, et al. Glioma grading: sensitivity, specificity, and predictive values of perfusion MR imaging and proton MR spectroscopic imaging compared with conventional MR imaging. AJNR Am J Neuroradiol 2003;24(10):1989–98.
6. Jain R, Griffith B, Narang J, et al. Blood-brain-barrier imaging in brain tumors: concepts and methods. Neurographics 2012;2(2):48–59.
7. Huang AP, Tsai JC, Kuo LT, et al. Clinical application of perfusion computed tomography in neurosurgery. J Neurosurg 2014;120(2):473–88.
8. Jain R. Perfusion CT imaging of brain tumors: an overview. AJNR Am J Neuroradiol 2011;32(9):1570–7.
9. Jain R. Measurements of tumor vascular leakiness using DCE in brain tumors: clinical applications. NMR Biomed 2013;26(8):1042–9.
10. Narang J, Jain R, Scarpace L, et al. Tumor vascular leakiness and blood volume estimates in oligodendrogliomas using perfusion CT: an analysis of perfusion parameters helping further characterize genetic subtypes as well as differentiate from astroglial tumors. J Neurooncol 2011;102(2):287–93.
11. Shiroishi MS, S Lacerda, Tang X, et al. Physical principles of MR perfusion and permeability imaging: gadolinium bolus technique, in functional neuroradiology: principles and clinical applications. In: Faro S, Mohamed FB, Yannes M, et al, editors. 2011.
12. Shiroishi MS, Castellazzi G, Boxerman JL, et al. Principles of T2*-weighted dynamic susceptibility contrast MRI technique in brain tumor imaging. J Magn Reson Imaging 2015;41:296–313.
13. Wolf RL, Detre JA. Clinical neuroimaging using arterial spin-labeled perfusion magnetic resonance imaging. Neurotherapeutics 2007;4(3):346–59.
14. Pollock JM, Tan H, Kraft RA, et al. Arterial spin-labeled MR perfusion imaging: clinical applications. Magn Reson Imaging Clin N Am 2009;17(2):315–38.
15. Watts JM, Whitlow CT, Maldjian JA. Clinical applications of arterial spin labeling. NMR Biomed 2013;26(8):892–900.
16. Essig M, Shiroishi MS, Nguyen TB, et al. Perfusion MRI: the five most frequently asked technical questions. AJR Am J Roentgenol 2013;200(1):24–34.
17. Wu WC, Fernández-Seara M, Detre JA, et al. A theoretical and experimental investigation of the tagging efficiency of pseudocontinuous arterial spin labeling. Magn Reson Med 2007;58(5):1020–7.
18. Folkman J. The role of angiogenesis in tumor growth. Semin Cancer Biol 1992;3(2):65–71.
19. Jackson A, Kassner A, Annesley-Williams D, et al. Abnormalities in the recirculation phase of contrast agent bolus passage in cerebral gliomas: comparison with relative blood volume and tumor grade. AJNR Am J Neuroradiol 2002;23(1):7–14.
20. Provenzale J, Wang GR, Brenner T, et al. Comparison of permeability in high-grade and low-grade brain tumors using dynamic susceptibility contrast MR imaging. AJR Am J Roentgenol 2002;178(3):711–6.
21. Shin JH, Lee HK, Kwun BD, et al. Using relative cerebral blood flow and volume to evaluate the histopathologic grade of cerebral gliomas: preliminary results. AJR Am J Roentgenol 2002;179(3):783–9.
22. Jain R, Ellika SK, Scarpace L, et al. Quantitative estimation of permeability surface-area product in astroglial brain tumors using perfusion CT and correlation with histopathologic grade. AJNR Am J Neuroradiol 2008;29(4):694–700.
23. Lucchinetti CF, Gavrilova RH, Metz I, et al. Clinical and radiographic spectrum of pathologically confirmed tumefactive multiple sclerosis. Brain 2008;131(Pt 7):1759–75.
24. Sugita Y, Terasaki M, Shigemori M, et al. Acute focal demyelinating disease simulating brain tumors: histopathologic guidelines for an accurate diagnosis. Neuropathology 2001;21(1):25–31.
25. Jain R, Ellika S, Lehman NL, et al. Can permeability measurements add to blood volume measurements in differentiating tumefactive demyelinating lesions from high grade gliomas using perfusion CT? J Neurooncol 2010;97(3):383–8.
26. Essig M, Nguyen TB, Shiroishi MS, et al. Perfusion MRI: the five most frequently asked clinical questions. AJR Am J Roentgenol 2013;201(3):W495–510.
27. Hourani R, Brant LJ, Rizk T, et al. Can proton MR spectroscopic and perfusion imaging differentiate between neoplastic and nonneoplastic brain lesions in adults? AJNR Am J Neuroradiol 2008;29(2):366–72.
28. Blasel S, Pfeilschifter W, Jansen V, et al. Metabolism and regional cerebral blood volume in autoimmune

inflammatory demyelinating lesions mimicking malignant gliomas. J Neurol 2011;258(1):113–22.

29. Clarke JL, Chang S. Pseudoprogression and pseudoresponse: challenges in brain tumor imaging. Curr Neurol Neurosci Rep 2009;9(3):241–6.

30. Vogelbaum MA, Jost S, Aghi MK, et al. Application of novel response/progression measures for surgically delivered therapies for gliomas: Response Assessment in Neuro-Oncology (RANO) Working Group. Neurosurgery 2012;70(1):234–43 [discussion: 243–4].

31. Sundgren PC, Cao Y. Brain irradiation: effects on normal brain parenchyma and radiation injury. Neuroimaging Clin N Am 2009;19(4):657–68.

32. Rabin BM, Meyer JR, Berlin JW. Radiation-induced changes in the central nervous system and head and neck. Radiographics 1996;16:1055–72.

33. Young RJ, Gupta A, Shah AD, et al. MRI perfusion in determining pseudoprogression in patients with glioblastoma. Clin Imaging 2013;37(1):41–9.

34. Mangla R, Singh G, Ziegelitz D, et al. Changes in relative cerebral blood volume 1 month after radiation-temozolomide therapy can help predict overall survival in patients with glioblastoma. Radiology 2010;256(2):575–84.

35. Jain R, Narang J, Arbab AS, et al. Role of non-model-based semi-quantitative indices obtained from DCE T1 MR Perfusion in differentiating pseudo-progression from true-progression [meeting abstract]. Neuro Oncol 2011;13:140.

36. Kim JH, Brown SL, Jenrow KA, et al. Mechanisms of radiation-induced brain toxicity and implications for future clinical trials. J Neurooncol 2008;87(3):279–86.

37. Giglio P, Gilbert MR. Cerebral radiation necrosis. Neurologist 2003;9(4):180–8.

38. Hu LS, Baxter LC, Smith KA, et al. Relative cerebral blood volume values to differentiate high-grade glioma recurrence from posttreatment radiation effect: direct correlation between image-guided tissue histopathology and localized dynamic susceptibility-weighted contrast-enhanced perfusion MR imaging measurements. AJNR Am J Neuroradiol 2009;30(3):552–8.

39. Cha S, Lupo JM, Chen MH, et al. Differentiation of glioblastoma multiforme and single brain metastasis by peak height and percentage of signal intensity recovery derived from dynamic susceptibility-weighted contrast-enhanced perfusion MR imaging. AJNR Am J Neuroradiol 2007;28(6):1078–84.

40. Barajas RF, Chang JS, Sneed PK, et al. Distinguishing recurrent intra-axial metastatic tumor from radiation necrosis following gamma knife radiosurgery using dynamic susceptibility-weighted contrast-enhanced perfusion MR imaging. AJNR Am J Neuroradiol 2009;30(2):367–72.

41. Cao Y, Tsien CI, Shen Z, et al. Use of magnetic resonance imaging to assess blood-brain/blood-glioma barrier opening during conformal radiotherapy. J Clin Oncol 2005;23(18):4127–36.

42. Wen PY, Macdonald DR, Reardon DA, et al. Updated response assessment criteria for high-grade gliomas: response assessment in neuro-oncology working group. J Clin Oncol 2010;28(11):1963–72.

Adult Brain Tumors
Clinical Applications of Magnetic Resonance Spectroscopy

Lara A. Brandão, MD[a,b,*], Mauricio Castillo, MD[c]

KEYWORDS

- Proton magnetic resonance spectroscopy (H-MRS) • Adult brain tumors • Tumor histology
- Tumor grade • Tumor extension • Tumor progression • Therapeutic response
- Differential diagnosis

KEY POINTS

- Proton magnetic resonance spectroscopy (H-MRS) may be helpful in suggesting tumor histology and tumor grade and may better define tumor extension and the ideal site for biopsy compared with conventional magnetic resonance imaging.
- Combining H-MRS with other advanced imaging techniques such as diffusion-weighted imaging, perfusion-weighted imaging, and permeability maps improves diagnostic accuracy for intraaxial brain tumors.
- Short echo time allows for recognition of more metabolites than long echo time, which is important for differential diagnosis of brain masses and grading tumors.
- Higher choline (Cho) levels and lower myoinositol (Myo)/creatine (Cr) ratio are seen in more malignant tumors compared with lower-grade tumors.
- Lactate is directly related to tumor grade in adult brain tumors. However, lactate is found in essentially all pediatric brain tumors regardless of histologic grade.
- Gliomas are often invasive and show increased Cho levels in surrounding tissues, which may be used to distinguish these lesions from metastases.
- When lipids and lactate are found in a solid lesion, lymphoma should be suggested.
- A prominent lipid peak is seen in lymphomatosis cerebri, whereas a significant increase in Myo is characteristic of gliomatosis cerebri.
- A significant increase in the Cho peak and the presence of lipids and lactate are commonly seen in pilocytic astrocytoma, a grade I tumor.
- Typically, higher levels of Cho occur in grade III gliomas; whereas, in glioblastoma multiforme, the Cho levels may be much lower as a result of necrosis.
- If the Cho/N-acetylaspartate ratio is increased outside the area of enhancement, tumor infiltration can be diagnosed.
- An increase in Cho-containing compounds after radiation therapy may be seen in radiation necrosis misclassified as tumors.
- H-MRS in specific cases improves the accuracy and level of confidence in differentiating neoplastic from nonneoplastic masses.

This article originally appeared in Neuroimaging Clinics of North America, Volume 23, Issue 3, August 2013.
Funding Sources: None.
Conflict of Interest: L.A. Brandão: None. M. Castillo: Editor in Chief, *American Journal of Neuroradiology*.
[a] Clínica Felippe Mattoso, Av. Das Américas 700, sala 320, Barra da Tijuca, Rio de Janeiro 30112011, Brazil;
[b] Clínica IRM- Ressonância Magnética, Rua Capitão Salomão 44 Humaitá, Rio de Janeiro 22271040, Brazil;
[c] Division of Neuroradiology, Department of Radiology, University of North Carolina School of Medicine, Room 3326, Old Infirmary Building, Manning Drive, Chapel Hill, NC 27599-7510, USA
* Corresponding author. Clínica Felippe Mattoso, Av. Das Américas 700, sala 320, Barra da Tijuca, Rio de Janeiro, CEP 30112011, Brazil.
E-mail address: larabrandao.rad@terra.com.br

Magn Reson Imaging Clin N Am 24 (2016) 781–809
http://dx.doi.org/10.1016/j.mric.2016.07.005

mri.theclinics.com

INTRODUCTION

Localized proton magnetic resonance spectroscopy (H-MRS) of the human brain, first reported more than 20 years ago,[1–3] is a mature methodology used clinically worldwide for evaluation of brain tumors.[4] H-MRS may help with differential diagnosis, histologic grading, degree of infiltration, tumor recurrence, and response to treatment mainly when radiation necrosis develops and is indistinguishable from tumor by conventional magnetic resonance (MR) imaging.[5] Combining H-MRS with other advanced imaging techniques such as diffusion-weighted (DW) imaging, perfusion-weighted (PW) imaging, and permeability maps improves diagnostic accuracy for intraaxial brain tumors.[6–8]

TECHNIQUE
Short Echo Time Versus Long Echo Time

Different H-MRS parameters may be optimized and 1 of the most relevant is echo time (TE).[9] Short TE allows for recognition of more metabolites than long TE, which is important for differential diagnosis of brain masses and grading tumors. For example, myoinositol (Myo), a marker for low-grade gliomas, is only seen on short TE acquisitions.[5]

Multivoxel MRS Versus Single-Voxel MRS

A key consideration for brain tumor evaluations is their metabolic inhomogeneity. Multivoxel (MV) techniques, also called chemical shift imaging (CSI),[10] simultaneously record spectra from multiple regions and therefore map the spatial distribution of metabolites.[11] MV H-MRS provides smaller volumes of interest compared with single-voxel (SV), avoiding sampling error. For these reasons, high-resolution MV MRS such as MRS imaging is often favored for evaluating brain tumors.[5,12] Nevertheless, SV H-MRS has some advantages compared with MV techniques.[13] SV H-MRS is quicker and easier to obtain in standard clinical settings, providing the opportunity to obtain more than 1 spectrum (ie, spectra at 2 different TEs) in a reasonable amount of time. Evaluating spectra at both short and long TE improves the level of accuracy in differentiating focal brain lesions.[13] SV H-MRS provides better quality spectra compared with MRS imaging. The authors recommend that both techniques be used in the evaluation of brain masses (Fig. 1).

SPECTRAL PATTERN OF TUMORS

The spectral pattern of intracranial tumors may vary according to histology and malignancy grade and is discussed here.[14–18]

Reduction in N-Acetylaspartate Levels and in N-Acetylaspartate/Creatine Ratio

Reduction in N-acetylaspartate (NAA) levels and NAA/creatine (Cr) ratio is observed in tumors, indicating decreased viability and number of neurons (see Fig. 1; Fig. 2). The reader should bear in mind that in low-grade gliomas, the spectral pattern might be similar to that of normal brain (Fig. 3).[19] Absence of NAA in an intraaxial tumor generally implies an origin outside the central nervous system (metastasis) (Fig. 4) or a highly malignant tumor that has destroyed all neurons in that location (Fig. 5).[5]

Decreased Cr Levels

Decrease in Cr may occur, representing energy failure in aggressive malignant neoplasms (see Figs. 1 and 2).

Increase in Choline Levels and in Choline/NAA and Choline/Cr Ratios

An increase in choline (Cho) levels is shown by an increase in the Cho/NAA or Cho/Cr ratio, rather than its absolute concentration. Increased Cho is associated with higher turnover in the cell membrane and higher cell density resulting from proliferation of tumor cells (see Figs. 1 and 2).[20,21] In tumors, Cho levels correlate with the degree of malignancy and are linearly correlated with cell density (the inverse of what is seen with the apparent diffusion coefficient [ADC]) instead of the proliferative index. Higher Cho levels are seen in more malignant tumors (see Figs. 1 and 2) and lower levels in lower-grade tumors (see Fig. 3). Cho is usually higher in the center of a solid mass and decreases peripherally. Cho is consistently low in necrotic areas (see Fig. 5).[5]

Myo

Myo is a glial marker because it is primarily synthesized in glial cells, almost only in astrocytes. The Myo/Cr ratio is usually higher in lower-grade (see Fig. 3) than in higher-grade tumors (see Fig. 2).[22]

Lactate Peak

Increased lactate levels are likely the result of anaerobic glycolysis, although they can also be due to insufficient blood flow leading to ischemia or necrosis.[23,24] Lactate is directly related to tumor grade in adult brain tumors, with higher peaks seen in higher-grade tumors (see Fig. 2). However, lactate is found in essentially all pediatric brain tumors regardless of histologic grade.

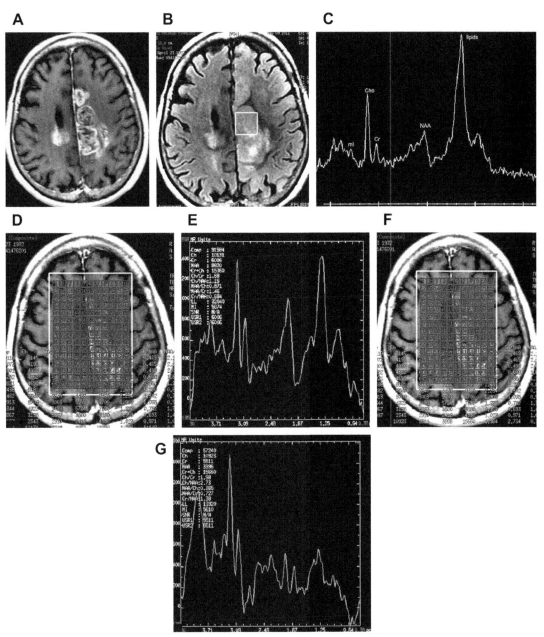

Fig. 1. MV MRS versus SV-MRS. A 79-year-old man presenting with right side hemiparesis of 1 month duration, seizures, and speech difficulties. There is a heterogeneously enhancing mass in the left frontal and parietal lobes, crossing the midline, surrounding the right lateral ventricle posteriorly (A) with extensive necrosis compatible with a GBM. SV-MRS (B, C) provides a good quality spectrum and demonstrates a significant increase of the lipid peak, increase of Cho and reduction of NAA, Cr, and Myo peaks. Spectra obtained from the left parietal region (D, E) demonstrate increased Cho and Cho/Cr and Cho/NAA ratios and a significant increase in the lipid peak compatible with extensive necrosis. MV MRS allows different areas to be evaluated at the same time. In the left frontal region (F, G), the main abnormality is an increase in the Cho peak. Cho, choline; Cho/Cr, choline/creatine; Cho/NAA, choline/N-acetyl-aspartate; Cr, creatine; MV MRS, multivoxel magnetic resonance spectroscopy; Myo, myo-inositol; NAA, N-acetyl-aspartate; SV MRS, single voxel magnetic resonance spectroscopy.

Lipids

Increased levels of lipids are believed to be caused by necrosis and membrane breakdown and are observed in metastasis (see **Fig. 4**),[25–28] aggressive high-grade primary brain tumors such as glioblastoma multiforme (GBM) (see **Figs. 1, 2**, and **5**) and lymphoma (**Fig. 6**), and in nonneoplastic

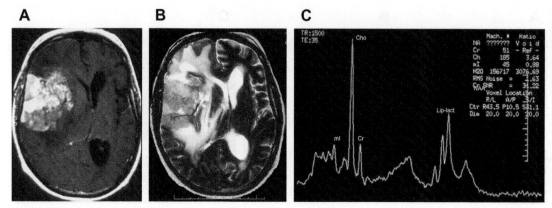

Fig. 2. GBM. There is a right frontal mass presenting with strong enhancement (*A*) and heterogeneous signal intensity on T2 (*B*). H-MRS (*C*) demonstrates significant reduction of NAA, Cr, and Myo. The Myo/Cr ratio is less than 1.0, which is typical for high-grade glioma. Note a significant increase in Cho and the presence of lipids and lactate. Cho, choline; Cr, creatine; H-MRS, proton magnetic resonance spectroscopy; ml, myo-inositol; Myo, myo-inositol; Myo/Cr, myo-inositol/creatine; NAA, N-acetyl-aspartate.

lesions such as inflammatory processes and abscesses. A prominent lipid peak is also characteristic for radiation necrosis.

Alanine

Alanine is an amino acid that has a doublet centered at 1.48 ppm. This peak is located above the baseline in spectra obtained with short or long TE and inverts below the baseline on acquisition using TE of 135 to 144 milliseconds.[5] In tumors, an increased level of alanine is considered specific for meningioma (**Fig. 7**).

Glutamine and Glutamate

Glutamine and glutamate (Glx) and Myo are metabolites better assessed with a TE of 30 milliseconds.[29] Except for meningiomas, in which an increased Glx peak may be seen (see **Fig. 7**), a significant increase in Glx levels should suggest nonneoplastic lesions.[19]

MAIN CLINICAL APPLICATIONS
Suggest Histology

Although conventional MR imaging is a sensitive modality available for detection of brain tumors,

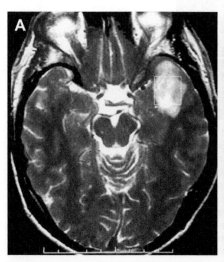
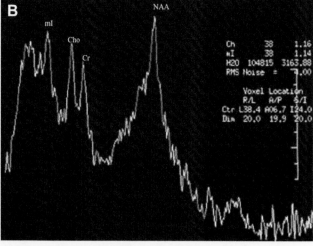

Fig. 3. Low-grade glioma (WHO grade II). A 51-year-old patient presenting with a circumscribed solid lesion in the left temporal lobe (*A*). The spectral pattern (*B*) is nearly normal: there is a discrete reduction in NAA as well a discrete increase in Cho with a Cho/Cr ratio of 1.16. The main abnormality in the curve is an increase in Myo (Myo/Cr 1.14), suggesting a low-grade tumor. Cho, choline; Cho/Cr, choline/creatine; ml, myo-inositol; Myo, myo-inositol; Myo/Cr, myo-inositol/creatine; NAA, N-acetyl-aspartate.

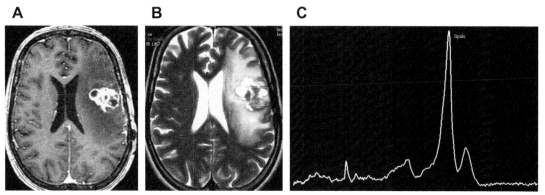

Fig. 4. Metastasis. There is a left frontal metastasis from breast cancer presenting with heterogeneous enhancement (*A*). A prominent lipid peak in the spectra (*B, C*) is related to extensive necrosis. No other metabolites are identified.

its specificity is low, and several tumor types may share a similar MR imaging appearance.[11] On the other hand, some tumors may present with a typical spectral pattern that may help to suggest the histology.

GBM
The spectral pattern of GBM is typical. There is a significant increase in Cho along with reduction of NAA, Cr, and Myo peaks. Increase of lipids and lactate is also common (see **Figs. 1** and **2**). When there is extensive necrosis, no increase in the Cho peak is seen. In this situation, prominent lipid and lactate peaks may be the only spectral abnormality (see **Fig. 5**). An overlap may be seen between the spectral pattern of GBM and metastasis. Although the absence of NAA in an intraaxial tumor generally implies an origin outside the central nervous system (metastasis) (see **Fig. 4**), a highly malignant tumor that has destroyed all neurons in that location may also demonstrate absence of NAA (see **Fig. 5**).[5] On the other hand,

NAA may be present in the spectra of a metastatic lesion if there is a partial volume effect with the adjacent parenchyma. For discriminating solitary metastases from primary high-grade tumors, it has been suggested that investigation of peri-enhancing tumor regions is useful. Metastases are encapsulated and do not show high Cho levels outside the region of enhancement, whereas gliomas are often invasive and show increased Cho in surrounding tissues.[7,30–35] However, if tumor infiltration is not significant, no increase in Cho is seen in the peritumoral area surrounding a GBM (**Fig. 8**).

Meningioma
Meningiomas are readily diagnosed based on conventional imaging features, but the diagnosis may be confirmed by the presence of alanine, which has been reported in many meningiomas.[36,37] A significant increase in Cho along with some increase in the Glx peak and the presence of alanine are common spectral findings (see **Fig. 7**).

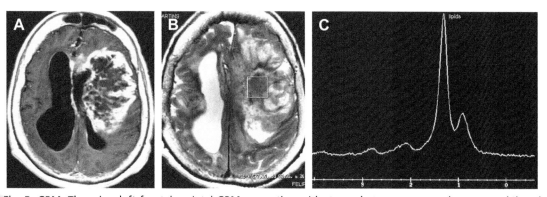

Fig. 5. GBM. There is a left frontal-parietal GBM presenting with strong heterogeneous enhancement (*A*) and heterogeneous signal intensity on T2 (*B*). Spectroscopy (*C*) demonstrates a prominent lipid peak. No other metabolites are identified.

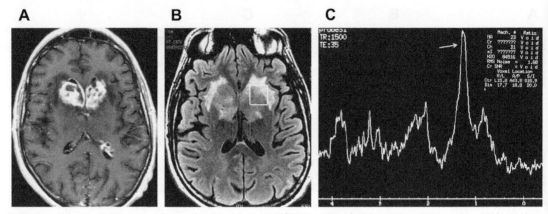

Fig. 6. Lymphoma. A 37-year-old man, human immunodeficiency virus (HIV) positive, diagnosed with brain lymphoma. There is a heterogeneously enhancing mass in the basal ganglia and adjacent to the frontal horns of the lateral ventricles (A). The spectra (B, C) demonstrate significant increase in the lipid peak (arrow).

Increase in Cho is characteristic and should not suggest malignancy. Meningiomas induced by radiation therapy tend to occur in younger patients, with equal frequency in males and females (sometimes more common in males), and present more atypia and higher nuclear/cytoplasm ratios.[38,39] In these cases, a large lipid peak along with reduction of all other metabolites including Cho may be seen. Their spectral pattern is similar to that of dural-based metastasis.

Lymphoma
Lymphomas may present as a solitary or multifocal solid lesion with no macroscopic evidence of necrosis in immunocompetent patients. On DW imaging, lymphoma shows hyperintensity with low ADC reflecting a higher nuclear/cytoplasm ratio.[40] The relative cerebral blood volume (rCBV) of lymphomas may be normal to slightly increased compared with

the rCBV of high-grade gliomas.[41,42] The spectral pattern of lymphomas is similar to that of other malignant tumors[6] and is characterized by increase in Cho, reduction in Myo, and prominent lipids. When lipids and lactate are found in a solid lesion, lymphoma should be suggested.[18,43,44] The spectral pattern described for solitary and multifocal (Fig. 9) lymphomas is similar to that seen in lymphomatosis cerebri (Fig. 10).

Gliomatosis cerebri
Gliomatosis cerebri is a distinct entity of glial tumors characterized by diffuse infiltration of the glial cell neoplasm throughout the brain. The WHO classification denotes grades II, III and IV gliomatosis cerebri.[45] Therefore, patients with this tumor have a variable prognosis. The most common finding in spectroscopy is reduction of NAA. Increase in Myo is characteristic of gliomatosis

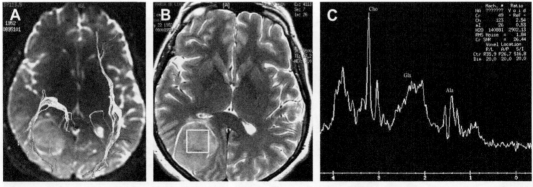

Fig. 7. Meningioma. A 57-year-old woman presenting with memory impairment and headaches. There is a meningioma in the right occipital region, displacing the optic radiations as seen on the diffusion tensor imaging (DTI) tractogram (A). Spectra (B, C) demonstrates elevation of Cho, some elevation of glutamine and glutamate (Glx), and presence of alanine. Ala, alanine; Cho, choline.

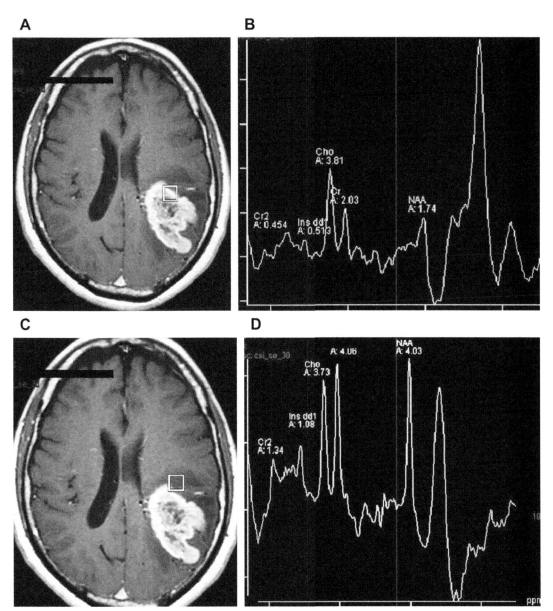

Fig. 8. *GBM*. 50-year-old man diagnosed with GBM. There is a heterogeneously enhancing lesion in the left parietal lobe (*A*). Spectrum from the margins of the lesion (*A, B*) demonstrates a significant increase in the lipid peak along with increases in Cho, Cho/Cr ratio, and Cho/NAA ratio as expected for a GBM. When the voxel is placed within the area of abnormal signal intensity surrounding the area of enhancement (*C*), no increase in the Cho peak, Cho/Cr ratio, or Cho/NAA ratio is demonstrated (*D*). Cho, choline; Cho/Cr, choline/creatine; Cho/NAA, choline/N-acetyl-aspartate; Cr, creatine; GBM, glioblastoma multiforme; Ins, Myo-inositol; NAA, N-acetyl-aspartate.

grade II, especially if there is no increase in Cho (**Fig. 11**).[46–49] Marked increases in Myo and Cr have been found in gliomatosis cerebri and may be attributed to glial activation rather than to glial proliferation because the Cho level is only moderately increased suggesting low glial cell density.[48] Sometimes Cho is reduced (see **Fig. 11**). A prominent lipid peak is seen in lymphomatosis cerebri (see **Fig. 10**), whereas a significant increase in Myo is characteristic of gliomatosis cerebri (see **Fig. 11**). In patients diagnosed with gliomatosis grade III, the Myo peak will be reduced and elevation of the Cho peak will be demonstrated (**Fig. 12**).

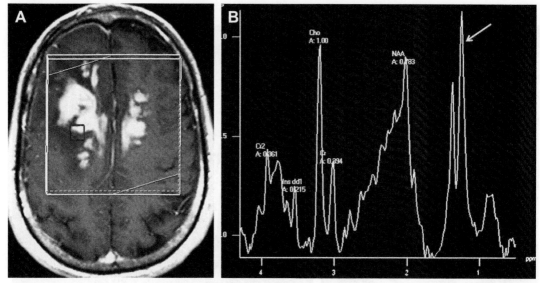

Fig. 9. Multifocal lymphoma. Multifocal solid enhancing nodules (*A*) are demonstrated in the frontal lobes and the cingulate gyri. Spectroscopy (*B*) shows a prominent lipid-lactate peak (*arrow*), increase in Cho, and reduction of Myo. Cho, choline; Cr, creatine; Ins, myo-inositol; Myo, myo-inositol; NAA, N-acetyl-aspartate.

Medulloblastoma

Medulloblastomas are more common in the pediatric population, although they may also present in adults aged 30 to 35 years. They are aggressive tumors (WHO grade IV) with a high propensity to disseminate throughout the cerebral fluid space. Their spectral pattern is characterized by a significant increase in Cho along with a reduction in the NAA and Myo peaks. Some lipids and lactate may be seen. Spectra with short TE show increased taurine at 3.3 ppm in patients.[50–55] Altering the TE can confirm that a

peak at 3.3 ppm corresponds to taurine. At a TE of 30 milliseconds, taurine projects above the baseline, whereas at a TE of 144 milliseconds, the taurine peak is below the baseline.[50] It has been speculated that increased taurine is associated with increased cellular proliferation and tumoral aggressiveness.[50–52,55,56]

Ependymoma

Ependymomas are more common in the pediatric population, although they may also present around the age of 30 to 35 years. They typically

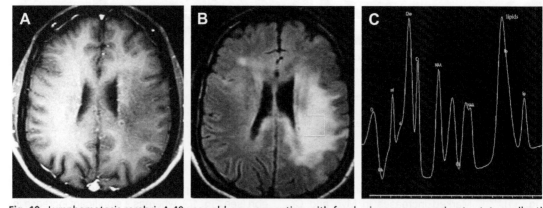

Fig. 10. Lymphomatosis cerebri. A 40-year-old man presenting with focal seizures, progressing to status epilepticus. There is a nonenhancing lesion compromising most of the left hemisphere (*A*), crossing the midline, and presenting with high signal intensity on the fluid attenuated inversion recovery (FLAIR) sequence (*B*). Spectroscopy (*B*, *C*) demonstrates a prominent lipid peak, increase in the Cho peak, and reduction of Myo. Cho, choline; Cr, creatine; ml, myo-inositol; Myo, myo-inositol; NAA, N-acetyl-aspartate. (*Courtesy of* Dr Leonardo Avanza, Espírito Santo, Brazil.)

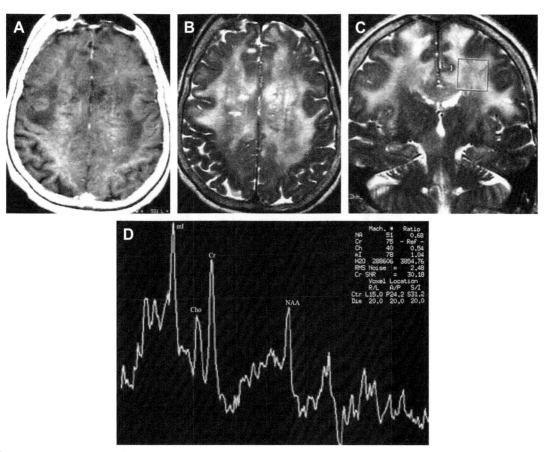

Fig. 11. Gliomatosis cerebri. A 49-year-old woman presenting with a nonenhancing infiltrative lesion (A) with high signal intensity on T2 (B, C) compromising the frontal and parietal lobes bilaterally. Spectroscopy (C, D) demonstrates increased Myo along with a reduction in the Cho and NAA peaks. Cr is also increased. Cho, choline; Cr, creatine; Myo, myo-inositol; NAA, N-acetyl-aspartate.

occur within the fourth ventricle. A most important imaging finding to identify ependymomas is extension of the tumor through the fourth ventricular outflow foramina (Fig. 13).[57–59] On computed tomography, the tumor reveals mixed density with punctate calcification in 50% of cases, with variable enhancement.[57] These tumors are heterogeneous on MR imaging, reflecting a combination of solid

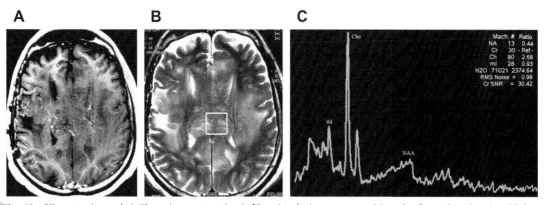

Fig. 12. Gliomatosis cerebri. There is an extensive infiltrating lesion compromising the frontal and parietal lobes, presenting with some tiny areas of discrete irregular enhancement (A) and high signal intensity on T2 (B). Spectroscopy (B, C) demonstrates prominent Cho and reduction in the Myo, Cr, and NAA peaks; a spectral pattern different from that shown in Fig. 11. Cho, choline; Cr, creatine; mI, myo-inositol; Myo, myo-inositol; NAA, N-acetyl-aspartate.

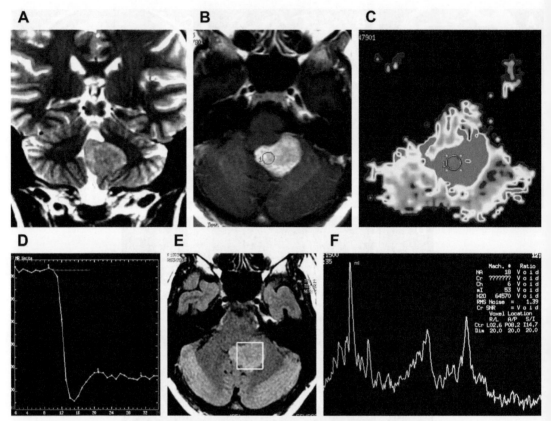

Fig. 13. Ependymoma. A 36-year-old woman presenting with neck pain, gait instability, and dizziness. There is a solid mass within the cavity of the fourth ventricle, isointense on T2 (*A*) with homogeneous enhancement (*B*). The mass extends through the fourth ventricular outflow foramina of Luschka into the left cerebello-pontine angle. A perfusion study (*C, D*) demonstrates a significant increase in rCBV with poor return to baseline indicating leaky tumoral blood vessels (*D*). The main finding on spectroscopy (*E, F*) is increased Myo. No increase in the Cho peak is demonstrated. Cho, choline; ml, myo-inositol; Myo, myo-inositol; rCBV, relative cerebral blood volume.

component, cyst, calcification, necrosis, edema, or hemorrhage.[60] When performed, perfusion MR imaging of ependymoma generally shows markedly increased rCBV and, unlike many other glial neoplasms, poor return to baseline, which may be attributable to fenestrated blood vessels and an incomplete blood-brain barrier (see **Fig. 13**C, D).[61,62] MRS shows considerable heterogeneity.[57] In general, ependymomas have low NAA and moderately increased Cho and Cr.[57] Harris and colleagues[63] stated that the presence of high Myo strongly suggests a diagnosis of ependymoma when short TE (30 milliseconds) is used at 1.5 T (see **Fig. 13**E–F). Another study also demonstrated that high Myo and glycine are found in ependymomas, more significant at short TE.[51] According to these findings, when a mass is found in the fourth ventricle, high Myo and glycine suggest ependymoma, whereas high Cho supports primitive neuroendocrine tumor.[64] Sometimes, no increase in Cho is seen in ependymomas (see **Fig. 13**F).

Suggest Tumor Grade

Differentiation between high-grade and low-grade tumors is important for therapeutic planning and estimating prognosis. H-MRS may indicate the tumor grade with more accuracy than a blind biopsy, because it assesses a larger amount of tissue than what is usually excised at biopsy.[43]

Tumors are commonly heterogeneous, and their spectra may vary depending on the region sampled by MRS.[65,66] Hence, the region of interest chosen for analysis has a large influence on the results, and, as stated earlier, MRS imaging is generally considered preferable because it allows metabolic heterogeneity to be evaluated. One recent MRS imaging study used MR perfusion imaging (arterial spin labeling) to guide the spectral measurement location; in regions with increased flow, Cho was found to be higher in high-grade gliomas compared with low-grade gliomas.[67] No metabolic differences between high-grade and low-grade gliomas were found in normal or hypo-perfused tumor regions.

H-MRS is considered 96% accurate in differentiating low-grade versus high-grade gliomas.[68] H-MRS may be readily integrated into a multimodality MR imaging examination for presurgical evaluation of patients with gliomas.[69–72]

Useful metabolites for suggesting tumor grade
Cho Increased Cho correlates with cellular proliferation and density. There is a high correlation between the in vivo concentration of Cho in brain tumors and in vitro tumor proliferation markers. Statistically significant higher Cho/Cr, Cho/NAA, and rCBV values in high-grade gliomas than in low-grade gliomas have been reported,[42] although threshold values of metabolite ratios for grading of gliomas are not well established. Cho/Cr is the most frequently used ratio. Some institutions use

a threshold value of 2.0 for Cho/Cr to differentiate low-grade from high-grade gliomas; others use a cutoff value of 2.5. Although increased Cho is related to tumor grade (higher Cho is found in higher-grade tumors than in lower-grade tumors), some studies have found grade IV GBM to have lower levels of Cho (see **Fig. 1C**) than grade II or grade III (**Fig. 14**) gliomas.[26] This may be due to the presence of necrosis in high-grade tumors, because necrosis is associated with a prominent lipid peak along with reduction of all other metabolites (see **Fig. 5**).[73]

Lipids and lactate The presence of lipids and lactate correlates with necrosis in high-grade gliomas (see **Figs. 1, 2, and 5**). Di Constanzo and colleagues[69] evaluated 31 patients with either high-grade or low-grade tumors through multimodality 3-T MR imaging (including long TE MRS imaging).

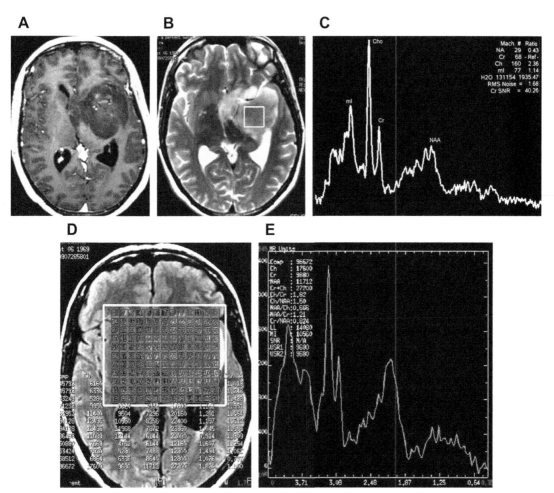

Fig. 14. Grade III glioma. There is a solid mass compromising the left frontal and temporal lobes with tiny foci of enhancement (*A*), isointense on T2 (*B*) suggesting high cell density. SV-MRS (*B, C*) demonstrates a significant increase in Cho along with a reduction in NAA and Cr. MV MRS (*D, E*) demonstrates the same findings. Cho, choline; Cr, creatine; mI, myo-inositol; NAA, N-acetyl-aspartate.

They concluded that high-grade and low-grade tumors and their margins could be differentiated based on the lactate/lipid signal and rCBV. Lipids are also the main spectral finding in metastasis (see **Fig. 4**). When lipids are demonstrated in solid lesions, lymphoma should also be considered (see **Fig. 9**).

Increase in the lipid peak is inversely correlated to survival.[74]

Lipids and lactate, although usually related to high-grade primary brain tumors and metastasis, may also be demonstrated in pilocytic astrocytomas.

Myo Useful information on tumor grade may be acquired by using a short TE (30–35 milliseconds) to assess Myo.[22] In low-grade tumors, the Myo/Cr ratio is typically higher (see **Fig. 3**) than in high-grade tumors (see **Figs. 1** and **2**).[24,26] This may be due to a low mitotic index in low-grade gliomas and, thus, lack of phosphatidylinositol metabolism activation, which results in Myo accumulation. Howe and colleagues[26] concluded that high Myo was characteristic of grade II astrocytomas. Increased levels of Myo have been reported to be useful for identifying low-grade astrocytomas in which the Cho/Cr ratio was not altered.[75,76]

NAA and Cr The greatest reductions in NAA and Cr levels occur in higher-grade tumors (compare **Figs. 1** and **2** with **Fig. 3**).

Glucose Short TE spectra may allow the evaluation of a peak around 3.67 ppm (probably glucose), which is directly related to survival. Tumors with more metabolic activity show low glucose levels in the spectra.[74]

Typical spectral findings in grade II, III, and IV gliomas

Grade II gliomas H-MRS in low-grade gliomas may look similar to normal spectra, demonstrating a discrete reduction in the NAA peak, along with a discrete increase in the Cho peak.[26,50,77] An increase in Myo can be the only finding in the spectra of a grade II astrocytoma (see **Fig. 3**).[13] No lipids or lactate are usually demonstrated. Low-grade glioma was studied in vivo at 4 T in 11 patients using H-MRS (incorporating the direct measurement of macromolecules in the spectrum) and ^{23}Na imaging. The results showed that absolute levels of glutamate and NAA were significantly decreased, whereas levels of Myo and ^{23}Na were significantly increased in low-grade glioma tissue.[78] The observation of decreased NAA levels is consistent with previous studies.[26,50,77–79] The observed decrease in glutamate contradicts a previous study[79] performed at 1.5 T that suggested

that increased Glx maybe characteristic of low-grade gliomas. The discrepancy may be due to the removal of the macromolecule baseline signal intensity in the current study before quantification. The observed increase in Myo is consistent with previous studies.[24,26]

Grade III gliomas In grade III gliomas, there is a significant increase in the Cho peak, which correlates well with high cell density in these tumors.[80] The NAA, Cr, and Myo peaks are reduced (see **Fig. 14**). Metastases and glioblastomas nearly always show increased lipid peaks; thus, if the lesion does not exhibit mobile lipid signals, anaplastic glioma is more likely.[81] In the authors' experience, however, some increase in lipids and lactate may be seen in grade III gliomas (**Fig. 15A, B**).

Grade IV gliomas The spectral pattern of grade IV gliomas is characterized by severe reduction of the NAA, Cr, and Myo peaks. Cho is increased (see **Fig. 1C**), although not as much as in a grade III glioma (see **Fig. 14C**), because a lot of necrosis is usually present in grade IV gliomas, which results in a significant increase in the lipid peak (see **Fig. 1C**). Typically, higher levels of Cho occur in grade III gliomas, whereas, in GBM, the Cho levels may be much lower as a result of necrosis.[82] When the voxel is placed within the necrotic area of a GBM, no Cho is detected and a prominent lipid-lactate peak is the only spectral abnormality (see **Fig. 5**).[82]

Special things to remember

Some overlap in the spectral pattern may be seen between grade II and grade III gliomas (see **Fig. 15A–D**). Evaluation of the spectra along with the information obtained from the other functional studies such as DW imaging, PW imaging, and permeability maps enhance the diagnostic capacity of brain tumors (see **Fig. 15E–J**). Some aggressive tumors, such as metastases, GBM, and gliomatosis cerebri may present with no increase in Cho (see **Figs. 4**, **5**, and **11**). The Cho peak and the Cho/Cr and Cho/NAA ratios may be higher in grade III (see **Fig. 14C**) than in grade IV gliomas (see **Fig. 1C**). Some benign tumors such as meningiomas present with a significant increase in the Cho peak (see **Fig. 7**). Pilocytic astrocytomas usually present with a significant increase in the Cho peak. Some lipids and lactate are also usually seen in these tumors.

Oligodendroglioma This tumor is divided into 2 groups according to the WHO classification: grades II and III.[83] It originates from oligodendrocytes but often contains a mixed population of cells, particularly astrocytes. On dynamic

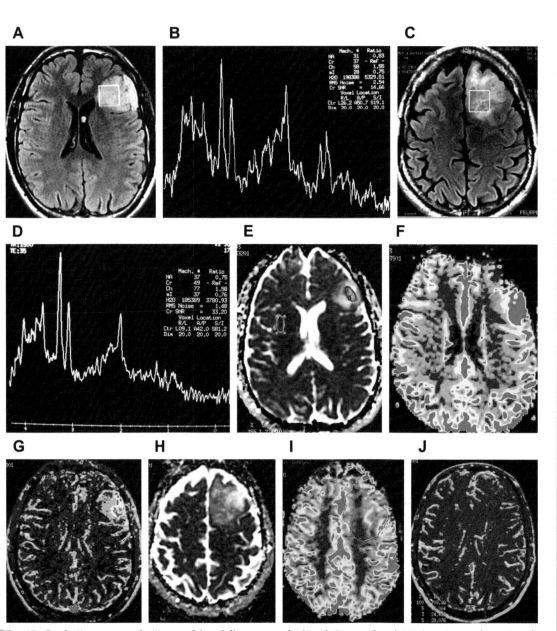

Fig. 15. Grade II versus grade III: a multimodality approach. (*A, B*) Conventional MR imaging and spectra obtained from a grade III glioma and from a grade II oligodendroglial tumor (*C, D*). In both cases there is an increase in the Cho peak. The Cho/Cr ratio is 1.55 in patient 1 (*A, B*) and 1.58 in patient 2 (*C, D*). There is a reduction in Myo in both cases, and the Myo/Cr ratio is 0.75 in patient 1 and 0.76 in patient 2. Despite similarities, some lipids and lactate are seen in the spectrum from patient 1 (*B*), suggesting a higher-grade lesion. In patient 1 (grade III glioma), an area of restricted diffusion is demonstrated within the lesion (*E*, ADC map) indicating high cell density. There is a significant increase in blood volume (*F*, rCBV map) and very high permeability (*G*), once again suggesting a high-grade tumor. In patient 2 (grade II glioma), no areas of restricted diffusion are seen (*H*, ADC map). There is a small area of discrete increased blood volume (*I*, rCBV) and no significant increase in permeability (*J*). ADC map, apparent diffusion coefficient map; Cho, choline; Myo, myo-inositol; rCBV map, relative cerebral blood volume map.

contrast-enhanced MR perfusion, low-grade oligodendrogliomas may demonstrate high rCBV because they contain a dense network of branching capillaries.[84,85] Thus, many oligodendrogliomas can be misinterpreted as high-grade tumors because of their high rCBV.

One study showed that rCBV was not significantly different between low-grade and high-grade oligodendrogliomas.[66] In contrast, another study[86] showed that rCBV was significantly different between low-grade and high-grade oligodendrogliomas. The results of H-MRS studies in oligodendrogliomas are more consistent than those of MR perfusion studies. Similar to astrocytomas, H-MRS of oligodendrogliomas demonstrates significantly higher Cho, Cho/Cr ratio, and a higher incidence of lactate and lipids in high-grade tumors than in low-grade tumors.[79,86,87] Nevertheless, low-grade oligodendrogliomas may show highly increased Cho (see Fig. 15C, D), mimicking high-grade tumors (see Fig. 15A, B), because these low-grade tumors can have high cellular density but absent endothelial proliferation and necrosis.[86] Apart from higher rCBV, the level of Glx is significantly higher in low-grade oligodendrogliomas than in low-grade

astrocytomas and may help to distinguish these tumors from each other.[79]

Assess Tumor Extension

In infiltrative lesions, tumor activity can be demonstrated by H-MRS beyond the enhanced area identified on gadolinium-enhanced conventional MR imaging (Figs. 16 and 17). Comparison of the extent (and location) of active tumor as defined by MR imaging and MRS imaging demonstrates the differences between the 2 techniques.[87] The area of metabolic abnormality as defined by MRS imaging may exceed the area of the abnormal T2-weighted signal.[87–90] H-MRS may better define tumor extension than conventional MR imaging.[91]

Cho has been found to correlate well with the cellular density of the tumor[80] and the degree of

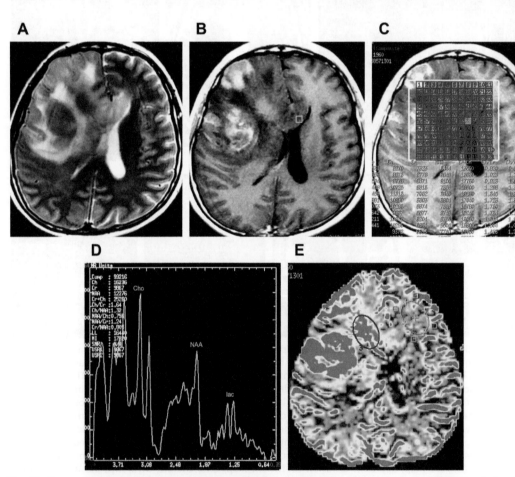

Fig. 16. Tumor extension. A 48-year-old woman diagnosed with GBM. There is a large infiltrative lesion in the right frontal lobe crossing the midline with heterogeneous signal intensity on T2 (A) and areas of contrast enhancement (B). MV MRS (C, D) demonstrates significant increase in Cho and the Cho/Cr and Cho/NAA ratios in the corpus callosum along with the presence of lactate compatible with tumor infiltration beyond the areas of enhancement. There is also an increase in blood volume in the same area (E, rCBV map). Cho, choline; lac, lactate; MV MRS, multivoxel magnetic resonance spectroscopy; NAA, N-acetyl-aspartate; rCBV map, relative cerebral blood volume map.

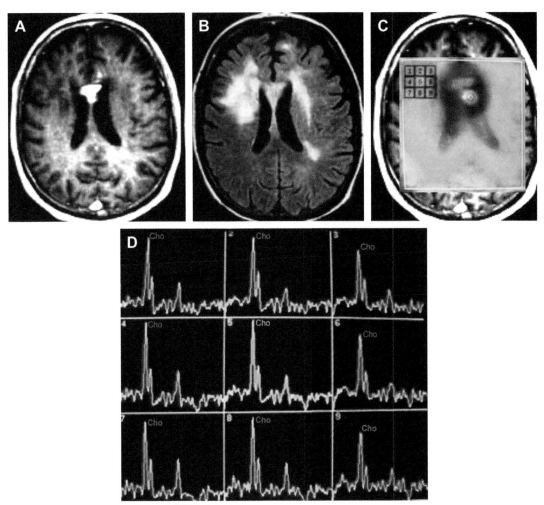

Fig. 17. Tumor extension. A 71-year-old man diagnosed with lymphoma. There is a solid enhancing nodule compromising the corpus callosum (*A*). FLAIR demonstrates an ill-defined high signal intensity abnormality in the frontal lobes surrounding the solid nodule, which could represent vasogenic edema and/or tumor infiltration (*B*). MV MRS (*C, D*) better defines tumor extension, demonstrating a significant increase in Cho, and the Cho/NAA and Cho/Cr ratios in all voxels. Cho, choline; Cho/Cr, choline/creatine; Cho/NAA, choline/N-acetyl-aspartate; MV MRS, multivoxel magnetic resonance spectroscopy.

tumor infiltration into brain tissue.[92] The use of MRS imaging to map Cho levels has been suggested as a method for defining tumor boundaries. To assess the degree of tumor infiltration, MRS imaging data obtained from 7 patients with untreated supratentorial gliomas (WHO grades II and III) were fused with three-dimensional MR imaging data sets and integrated into a frameless stereotactic system for image-guided surgery in an interactive manner.[89] Tissue samples were obtained from 3 regions, defined individually in each patient based on the Cho/NAA ratio: (1) a spectroscopically normal region, (2) a transitional region, and (3) a region with maximum spectroscopic abnormality. In all cases, the highest Cho/NAA ratios were obtained in the tumor center, and intermediate values in the regions of low tumor invasion. In 4 patients, however, biopsies sampled in regions with normal Cho/NAA ratio showed tumor infiltration. One of the reasons may be the low resolution of MRS imaging with respect to glioma borders.[89] Based on this observation, it can be concluded that if the Cho/NAA ratio is increased outside the area of enhancement, tumor infiltration can be diagnosed. On the other hand, if no increase in the Cho/NAA ratio is demonstrated, tumor infiltration cannot be ruled out. The reason for this is probably the fact that increases in the Cho/Cr and Cho/NAA ratios are related to the number of neoplastic cells that have infiltrated outside the enhancing lesion. A retrospective study performed on 10 gliomas examined the relationship between metabolite levels and histopathologic parameters in the border zone of gliomas.[93] A strong negative correlation was detected between NAA concentration and both absolute and relative measures of tumor infiltration; no correlation for Cho was detected. The study concluded that NAA concentration is the most significant parameter for the detection of low levels of tumor cell infiltration.[93] MRS may demonstrate tumor infiltration not only in the area of vasogenic edema but also in the normal-appearing white matter (NAWM) contralateral to the affected hemisphere. Kallenberg and colleagues[94] have shown that, in patients with histopathologically confirmed primary GBM, H-MRS of the NAWM contralateral to the affected hemisphere revealed an increase in the concentrations

of Myo and glutamine but otherwise normal metabolite levels. These results indicate increased density of cells of astrocytic origin in the NAWM of patients with GBM in the presence of still normal neuroaxonal tissue, as indicated by the absence of changes in the major metabolites. This observation may, in turn, be taken as a potential indicator of the presence of tumor cells in NAWM, representing an early sign of neoplastic infiltration, suggesting a new role for H-MRS in the treatment of patients with brain tumors.[94]

The results from this study are in agreement with findings observed in previous reports on H-MRS and conventional MR imaging of glioma infiltration in inconspicuous brain parenchyma remote from the tumor.[95–98]

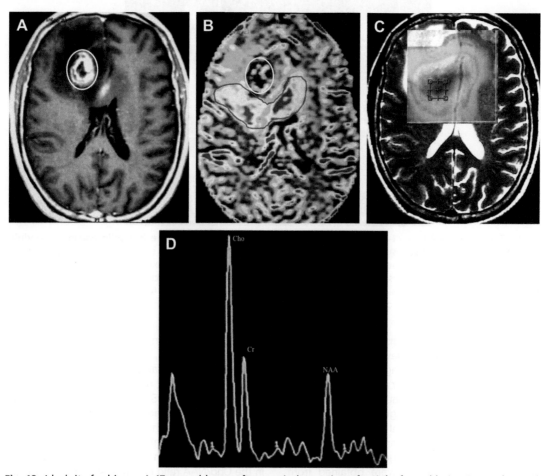

Fig. 18. Ideal site for biopsy. A 47-year-old man after surgical resection of a right frontal lesion 3 months previously; pathology was negative. The area that enhances (*circle A*) presents with low capillary density seen as low perfusion (*B*, rCBV map) and thus is not the ideal site for biopsy. Surrounding the area of enhancement posteriorly, there is an area of high capillary density (*B, red circle*) seen as high perfusion and high cell density (*C, D*) presenting with high Cho and high Cho/Cr and Cho/NAA ratios. This area is the best site for biopsy. Cho, choline; Cho/Cr, choline/creatine; Cho/NAA, choline/N-acetyl-aspartate; Cr, creatine; NAA, N-acetyl-aspartate; rCBV map, relative cerebral blood volume map.

Indicate the Ideal Site for Biopsy

Biopsy is not always performed in the area of the tumor with greatest cellularity so it may underestimate the pathology of the lesion.[43] By evaluating metabolic abnormalities, H-MRS may better define the ideal site for biopsy than conventional MR imaging.[42] Stereotactic brain biopsy is usually performed based on the anatomic appearance of the lesion or enhancement characteristics.[99] The area of enhancement does not necessarily represent the area of greater tumor activity. In high-grade heterogeneous tumors, there is a possibility that unspecific or lower-grade tumor tissue is sampled or that important functional tracts are damaged. Ideally, regions of increased angiogenesis, vascular permeability, and high metabolic activity should be sampled.[100] The role of H-MRS in biopsy guidance is to recognize regions of high metabolic activity: regions of increased Cho levels (and low NAA levels) indicating tumor tissue are a good target for biopsy (Fig. 18).[99,101–104] Regions with low Cho and NAA levels may indicate radiation necrosis, astrogliosis, macrophage infiltration, or mixed tissue.

Follow Tumor Progression

Serial H-MRS examinations may be used to follow the progression of gliomas.[105,106] Anaplastic degeneration can be demonstrated early with H-MRS and perfusion mapping compared with conventional MR imaging. Tumor progression is characterized by increased Cho levels in serial examinations (Fig. 19).[105] Tedeschi and colleagues[105] demonstrated that interval percentage changes in Cho intensity in stable gliomas and progressive gliomas (malignant degeneration or recurrent disease) is less than 35 and more than 45, respectively. Interval increased Cho/Cr or Cho/NAA is suggestive of malignant progression.

Predict Prognosis and Survival

Histopathology remains the gold standard for prognostic assessment, providing insights into

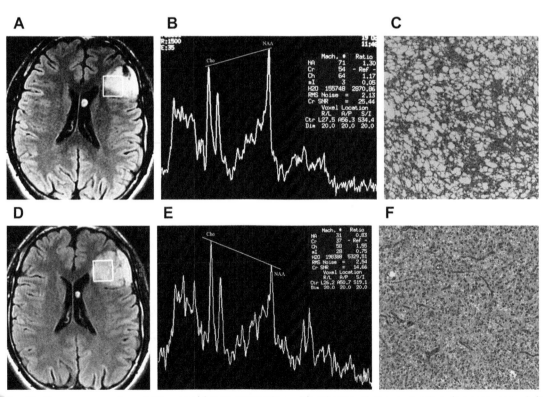

Fig. 19. Tumor progression. A 27-year-old man presenting with seizures. First examination demonstrates a left frontal lesion with high signal intensity on the FLAIR sequence (A). Spectroscopy demonstrates that the NAA peak is higher than the Cho peak (B). Biopsy results were compatible with a grade II glioma (C). Nine months later, (D, E) Cho is higher than NAA indicating higher cell density and suggesting anaplastic transformation. The lesion was resected and pathology demonstrated a high cell density and highly vascular lesion, compatible with grade III glioma (F), as suggested by the MRS study. Cho, choline; MRS, magnetic resonance spectroscopy; NAA, N-acetyl-aspartate. ([C, E] Courtesy of Dr Leila Chimelli, Rio de Janeiro, Brazil.)

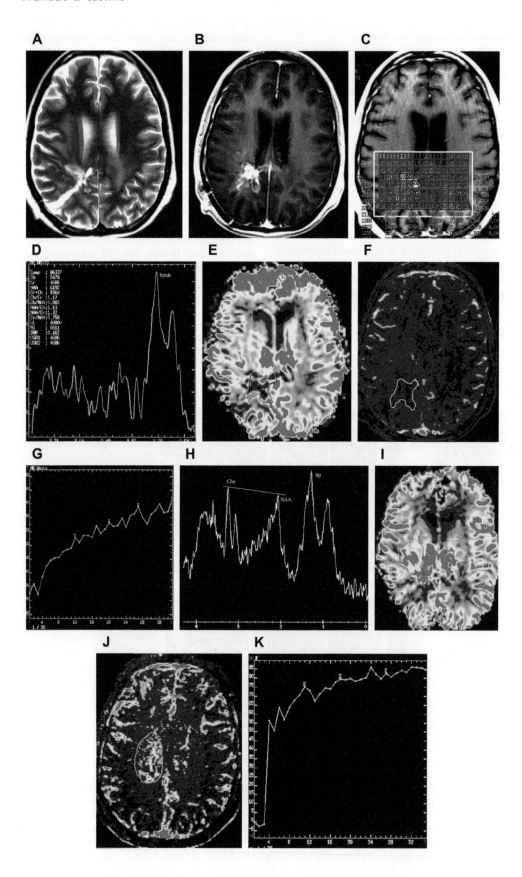

the morphologic cytostructure of the tumor. However, histopathology has limitations in providing prognostic value.[74] DW imaging, PW imaging, and H-MRS yield structural and metabolic information that may provide better insight into tumor functionality and improve the prognostic stratification of brain tumors.[74]

A pretreatment H-MRS study of 187 patients with high-grade astrocytomas produced 180 spectra at short TE (30 milliseconds) and 182 at long TE (136 milliseconds).[74] The study demonstrated that a high-intensity value of the peaks at 0.98 and 1.25 ppm, attributed to lipids, correlated with tumoral necrosis and with low survival. More interesting was the finding that another region of the short TE spectrum, around 3.67 ppm, showed a direct correlation with patient survival. This peak probably represents glucose. High metabolic activity and consequently poor prognosis correlate with depletion of glucose in the extracellular compartment and, accordingly, with low intensity of the resonances that represent this compound in the spectra, centered at 3.67 ppm. The investigators found that H-MRS could be used to stratify prognostic groups in high-grade gliomas and that this prognostic assessment could be made by evaluating the intensity values of 2 points on the spectrum at short TE (0.98 and 3.67 ppm) and another 2 at long TE (0.98 and 1.25 ppm). Short TE H-MRS may be considered somewhat superior to long TE H-MRS for prognostic assessment of high-grade gliomas. Nevertheless, spectra at both TEs may provide relevant information.[74]

Oh and colleagues[107] found a significantly shorter median survival time for patients with a large volume of metabolic abnormality, measured by H-MRS. Additional studies have evaluated some particular resonances of the spectrum such as Cho-containing compounds, NAA, Cr, lipids, and lactate, and have found them to be useful for predicting patient outcome in gliomas.[108,109] A series of articles have evaluated the role of MRS imaging in predicting survival of patients with GBM.[108,110–113] In a recent study, conventional MR imaging, MRS imaging, DW imaging, and perfusion MR imaging were used in a group of grade IV gliomas (examined before surgery and treatment). Survival was relatively poor in patients with lesions exhibiting large areas of contrast enhancement, abnormal metabolism, or restricted diffusion. Specifically, of the H-MRS parameters, high relative volumes of regions with increased Cho/NAA index were negatively associated with survival. Survival time was also negatively associated with high lactate and lipid levels (see **Fig. 1**) and the ADC within the enhancing volume.

Not all studies have found associations between metabolic indices and prognosis; for instance, in 16 patients with a B-cell lymphoma, the presence of lactate and lipids in the spectra collected before treatment was not associated with overall survival.[114] In another prospective H-MRS study, 50 patients with newly diagnosed low-grade gliomas (WHO grade II) evaluated before surgery showed no relationship between Cho and Cr levels in the tumor and survival.[115] Despite the few studies mentioned here,[114,115] most of the studies published in the literature agree that H-MRS is helpful for predicting the prognosis of brain tumors.

Assess Therapeutic Response

An important issue about postradiation therapy in patients with brain tumors is differentiation between recurrent brain tumor and radiation injury/change, particularly when new contrast-enhancing lesions are seen in previously operated and/or irradiated regions.[116–120] Typical conventional MR imaging appearance of radiation necrosis is a T2 hyperintense signal and enhancement after contrast administration, which is difficult to distinguish from tumor progression or pseudoprogression (a transient increase in edema, mass effect, and contrast enhancement that resolves over time).[115] Differentiating residual or recurrent tumors from treatment-related changes is limited on conventional MR imaging as well as on histologic examination; areas of T1 contrast enhancement after radiation

Fig. 20. Radiation necrosis versus tumor recurrence. A 24-year-old woman diagnosed with GBM after surgical resection, radiation therapy, chemotherapy, and steroids. A surgical cavity is seen in the right parietal lobe (A) with some irregular enhancement in the surrounding parenchyma (B). MV MRS (C, D) demonstrates a significant reduction in the NAA, Cho, and Cr peaks along with a prominent lipid peak consistent with radiation necrosis. Perfusion is reduced in the surgical bed (E, rCBV map) and there is no increase in permeability (F, G) also indicating therapeutic response rather than tumor. Four months later, H-MRS shows an increase in Cho and the Cho/NAA ratio indicating tumor cell proliferation (H). A perfusion study (I) demonstrates high capillary density and there is increased permeability (J, K) in the same area. Results from H-MRS, perfusion, and permeability studies are compatible with tumor recurrence. Cho, choline; Cho/NAA, choline/N-acetyl-aspartate; Cr, creatine; H-MRS, proton magnetic resonance spectroscopy; lip, lipids; MV MRS, multivoxel magnetic resonance spectroscopy; NAA, N-acetyl-aspartate; rCBV map, relative cerebral blood volume map.

treatment often contain both residual and recurrent tumor and tissue affected by therapy-related changes. In addition, the heterogeneity of gliomas before and after therapy and the inaccuracy of biopsy sampling pose another challenge in the histologic differentiation of tumors from necrosis.[121] On conventional MR imaging, the evaluation of treatment response and categorization as stable disease, responder (partial remission), and nonresponder (progression) are based predominantly on changes in tumor volumes.[122] MRS imaging may distinguish metabolic changes in the tumor before any change in volume. H-MRS has been applied to differentiate between radiation-induced tissue injury and tumor recurrence in adult and pediatric patients with brain tumors after radiation, gamma knife radiosurgery, and brachytherapy.[123] Significantly reduced Cho and Cr levels suggest radiation necrosis.[73,75,124–129] Necrotic regions may also show increased lipid and lactate signals (**Fig. 20A–G**).[75,130,131] On the other hand, increased Cho (evaluated as Cho levels relative to the Cho signal in normal-appearing tissue, Cho/Cr, or Cho/NAA ratios) suggests recurrence (see **Fig. 20H–K**).[112,125,128,129] Many studies have found that Cho/Cr and/or Cho/NAA ratios are significantly higher in recurrent tumor (or predominantly tumor) than in radiation injury.[117–120] In a retrospective MRS imaging study of 33 tumors using an intermediate TE of 144 milliseconds, Smith and colleagues[118] demonstrated that higher Cho/Cr and Cho/NAA ratios and a lower NAA/Cr ratio suggest recurrence compared with radiation change. According to this study, the Cho/NAA ratio demonstrated the best confidence interval to distinguish between tumor recurrence and radiation change. The distinction between recurrent tumor and radiation necrosis using the Cho/NAA ratio could be made with 85% sensitivity and 69% specificity.[118] According to Elias and colleagues,[132] the Cho/NAA and NAA/Cr ratios best differentiated recurrent brain tumor from radiation injury using H-MRS in previously treated patients diagnosed with primary intracranial neoplasm. Comparison with biopsy specimens revealed that MRS imaging cannot reliably differentiate between tissue containing mixed tumor/radiation necrosis and either tumor or radiation necrosis, although it did achieve good separation between pure necrosis and pure tumor.[75]

H-MRS is a promising, noninvasive tool for predicting and monitoring the clinical response to temozolamide in patients with low-grade gliomas.[133] In these patients, the H-MRS profile changes more widely and rapidly than tumor volume during relapse and represents an early predictive factor of outcome over 14 months of follow-up.

Tumor recurrence may be detected by H-MRS in a site remote from the irradiated area. In some cases, the development of a spectral abnormality may precede a coincident increase in contrast enhancement by 1 to 2 months.[126,134]

Some overlap may be seen in the H-MRS of tumors and radiation change. An increase in Cho-containing compounds after radiation therapy as a result of cell damage and astrogliosis may be seen in radiation necrosis misclassified as tumors.[135] In addition, both tumors and necrotic tissue have low levels of NAA, consistent with neuronal damage. Also, residual tumor may be present along with some radiation changes in the same patient. If the spectrum is indeterminate (ie, indicating the presence of both residual tumor and radiation change), repeated examination is suggested after an interval of 6 to 8 weeks.[130] If the increase in Cho is related to radiation change, it will normalize with time. Additional information from the perfusion and permeability studies may also help to correctly differentiate between tumors and radiation necrosis. Recurrent tumors have a higher rCBV (see **Fig. 20I**) and higher permeability (see **Fig. 20J, K**) compared with radiation necrosis (see **Fig. 20E–G**).[10,94]

A discrete and isolated increase in Cho in serial examinations should not be considered evidence of tumor recurrence. Interval increased Cho/Cr or Cho/NAA is suggestive of malignant progression/tumor recurrence if the percentage change in Cho is more than 45% and/or is associated with increased blood volume and permeability indicating vascular proliferation and significant compromise of the blood-brain barrier, respectively.

H-MRS is able to detect the effects of radiation on normal brain. The most commonly reported changes after radiation are decreases in NAA,[136] which can be detected 1 to 4 months after radiation in nontumoral regions receiving between 20 and 50 Gy[137] and decreases in Cho levels.[123] Radiation therapies may result in a decrease in whole-brain NAA with no corresponding changes in the mental status.

DIFFERENTIAL DIAGNOSIS BETWEEN LESIONS THAT LOOK ALIKE

In many cases, reliable differentiation of neoplastic from nonneoplastic brain masses is difficult or even impossible with conventional MR imaging.[137–147] Use of contrast agent may also not increase diagnostic specificity because various nonneoplastic processes are often associated with disruption of the blood-brain barrier and not all tumors enhance.[135] Studies have shown that the use of H-MRS in specific cases improves the accuracy and level of confidence in differentiating neoplastic from nonneoplastic masses.[13,15,135,138,148–150] The differential diagnosis of a brain mass varies depending on its solid or necrotic aspect.[13] When a necrotic mass is encountered in the brain, the main diagnoses include aggressive brain tumors, abscess, tuberculous granuloma, parasitic infection, or radiation necrosis. On the other hand, when the lesion is solid, the main diagnoses include tumors without necrosis, lymphoma, and pseudotumoral demyelinating disease. Hourani and colleagues,[135] using cutoff points of NAA/Cho equal to or less than 0.61 and rCBV equal to or greater than 1.50 (corresponding to diagnosis of the tumors), achieved a sensitivity of 72.2% and specificity of 91.7% in differentiating tumors from nonneoplastic lesions. Although studies have shown that perfusion MR imaging and the combination of H-MRS imaging and perfusion MR imaging had were comparable with MRS imaging alone in differentiating tumors from nonneoplastic lesions, in the authors' experience, a multifunctional approach with DW imaging, PW imaging, permeability mapping, and H-MRS is the most accurate way to make a precise diagnosis.

Tumor Versus Stroke

Differentiation between a glioma and a vascular lesion may be difficult or impossible using conventional MR imaging. In these cases, increased Cho makes the diagnosis of neoplasm more likely, whereas no increase in Cho makes the diagnosis of tumor less likely. Increased lipids along with reduction of all other metabolites is characteristic of infarcts but these findings may also be present in tumors with extensive necrosis (see **Fig. 5**). On the other hand, increased Cho may be seen in infarction especially in the subacute stage, mimicking tumor (**Fig. 21**). In this situation, the clinical history and a multifunctional approach with DW imaging and perfusion mapping help in making the correct diagnosis.

Tumor Versus Demyelination

Differentiation between high-grade gliomas and some acute demyelinating lesions based on H-MRS alone may be difficult because of histopathologic similarities, which include hypercellularity, reactive astrocytes, mitotic figures, and areas of necrosis.[121,125,138,149] Both entities typically present with increased Cho and decreased NAA, and lactate and lipids are often increased (**Fig. 22**).[148–153]

In the acute stage of a demyelinating disease, increased lactate reflects the metabolism of inflammatory cells.[148–150]

Majós and colleagues[13] found that the increase in Cho and decrease in NAA at long TE are even higher in tumors and that these metabolites can discriminate between tumors and pseudotumoral lesions. However, in the authors' experience, a significant increase in Cho along with significant reduction of NAA may be demonstrated in acute demyelinating plaques (see **Fig. 22**). According to Cianfoni and colleagues,[150] increase in Glx helps differentiate demyelinating tumefactive lesions from neoplastic masses, avoiding unnecessary biopsy and potentially harmful surgery, as well as providing a more specific diagnosis during the initial MR examination, allowing the earlier institution of appropriate therapy.

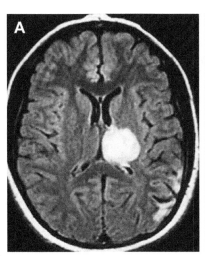
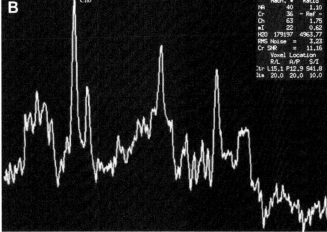

Fig. 21. Infarct with high Cho in the spectrum. A significant increase in the Cho peak is demonstrated in the spectrum from a left thalamic infarct. The spectral pattern resembles that of a brain tumor. Cho, choline.

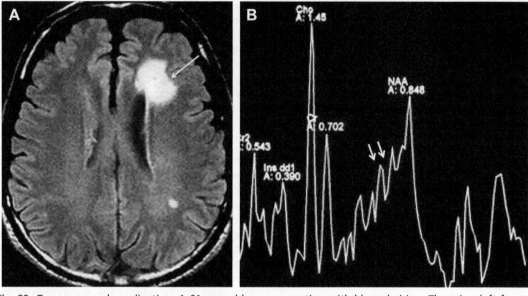

Fig. 22. Tumor versus demyelination. A 61-year-old man presenting with blurred vision. There is a left frontal lesion hyperintense on FLAIR (*A*) that shows a significant increase in Cho and the Cho/NAA and Cho/Cr ratios along with a reduction in NAA (*B*). A diagnosis of tumor was suggested and a stereotactic biopsy showed findings consistent with demyelination. A close inspection of the spectrum shows a high Glx peak (*B*, *arrows*), more consistent with demyelination than high-grade glioma. Cho, choline; Cho/Cr, choline/creatine; Cho/NAA, choline/N-acetyl-aspartate; Cr, creatine; Glx, glutamine and glutamate; Ins, myo-inositol; NAA, N-acetyl-aspartate.

Tumor Versus Focal Cortical Dysplasia

In some cases of focal cortical dysplasia, Cho may be moderately increased probably as a result of intrinsic epileptic ictal activity.[154]

Tumor Versus Abscess

The differential diagnosis between brain abscess and neoplasms (primary and secondary) is a challenge. Both appear as cystic lesions with rim enhancement on conventional MR imaging. Pyogenic abscesses have high signal intensity on DW imaging, which is usually not seen in tumors. Nevertheless, some neoplasms may occasionally have restricted diffusion and biopsy is inevitable. H-MRS may help to establish a diagnosis. In the case of a rim-enhancing lesion, to differentiate between a necrotic tumor and an abscess, the voxel should be placed within the cystic-necrotic area.[155] Abscesses and tumors both demonstrate high lactate peaks. Nonetheless, the presence of acetate, succinate, and amino acids such as valine, alanine, and leucine in the core of the lesion has high sensitivity for pyogenic abscess (**Fig. 23**).[82,155,156] To demonstrate the typical spectral abnormalities in the abscess cavity, an intermediate (144 milliseconds) or high (270 milliseconds) TE should be used.[155]

Typical spectra of anaerobic bacterial abscesses (acetate, succinate, and amino acids) do not exist in abscesses caused by *Staphylococcal aureus*, which are aerobic bacterial abscesses.[156] In this situation, lipids and lactate may be the only spectral findings and the spectrum is similar to that of a necrotic brain lesion.[155] Also, the resonances of acetate, succinate, and amino acids may disappear with effective antibiotic therapy. A high Cho peak and high Cho/NAA and Cho/Cr ratios may be seen in infection and should not be considered as evidence of tumor.

Tumor Versus Encephalitis

Among the encephalitis, herpes simplex encephalitis has a typical distribution of brain involvement at the hippocampus and cortex of the temporal, frontobasal, and insular lobes.[157] H-MRS shows marked reduction of NAA and the NAA/Cr ratio, and increase in Cho and the Cho/Cr ratio at the involved region, which reflect neuronal loss and gliosis and correlate with histopathologic findings. H-MRS findings may resemble those of brain tumors. However, increase in the Glx peak should favor encephalitis over tumor.

A practical MRI-based algorithm, including the results from postcontrast MR imaging, DW imaging, perfusion MR imaging, and MRS imaging, allowed the classification of tumors and nonneoplastic lesions with accuracy, sensitivity, and specificity of 90%, 97%, and 67%, respectively.[7,8]

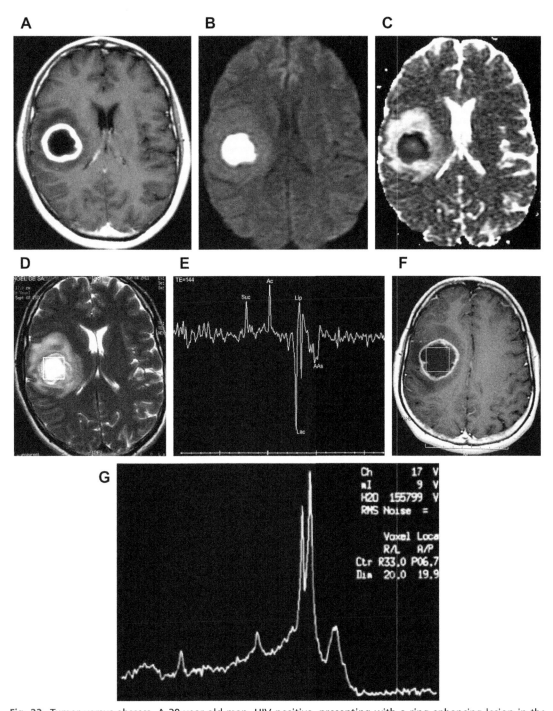

Fig. 23. Tumor versus abscess. A 39-year-old man, HIV positive, presenting with a ring-enhancing lesion in the right frontal lobe (*A*). There is restricted diffusion (high signal intensity on DW imaging (*B*) and low signal intensity on the ADC map (*C*)), compatible with the diagnosis of pyogenic abscess. Spectra from the abscess cavity performed with intermediate TE (144 milliseconds) (*D, E*) demonstrates lipids and lactate, which can also be seen in the necrotic core of a GBM (*F, G*) in the study obtained with low TE (30 milliseconds). However, amino acids (0.9 ppm), acetate (1.9 ppm), and succinate (2.4 ppm) are also seen in the abscess cavity (*E*). These findings have high sensitivity for the diagnosis of pyogenic abscesses and are not demonstrated within the necrotic core of a GBM. AAS, aminoacids; Ac, acetate; ADC, apparent diffusion coefficient; DW, diffusion weighted; GBM, glioblastoma multiforme; lac, lactate; lip, lipids; Suc, succinate; TE, echo time.

These results suggest that integration of advanced imaging techniques with conventional MR imaging may help to improve the reliability of the diagnosis and classification of brain lesions.[158]

SUMMARY

H-MRS may be helpful in suggesting tumor histology and tumor grade and may better define tumor extension and the ideal site for biopsy compared with conventional MR imaging. A multifunctional approach with DW imaging, PW imaging and permeability mapping, along with H-MRS, may enhance the accuracy of the diagnosis and characterization of brain tumors and estimation of therapeutic response. Also, integration of advanced imaging techniques with conventional MR imaging and the clinical history helps to improve the accuracy, sensitivity, and specificity in differentiating between tumors and nonneoplastic lesions.

REFERENCES

1. Bottomley PA, Edelstein WA, Foster TH, et al. In vivo solvent suppressed localized hydrogen nuclear magnetic resonance spectroscopy: a window to metabolism? Proc Natl Acad Sci U S A 1985;82: 2148–52.
2. Hanstock CC, Rothman DL, Prichard JW, et al. Spatially localized ^{1}H NMR spectra of metabolites in the human brain. Proc Natl Acad Sci U S A 1988;85:1821–5.
3. Frahm J, Bruhn H, Gynell ML, et al. Localized high resolution proton NMR spectroscopy using stimulated echoes: initial applications to human brain in vivo. Magn Reson Med 1989;9:79–93.
4. Bruhn H, Frahm J, Gynell ML, et al. Noninvasive differentiation of tumors with use of localized H-1 MR spectroscopy in vivo: initial experience in patients with cerebral tumors. Radiology 1989;172:541–8.
5. Bertholdo D, Watcharakorn A, Castillo M. Magnetic resonance spectroscopy: introduction and overview. Neuroimaging Clin North Am, in press.
6. Morita N, Harada M, Otsuka H, et al. Clinical application of MR spectroscopy and imaging of brain tumor. Magn Reson Med Sci 2010;9(4):167–75.
7. Al-Okaili RN, Krejza J, Wang S, et al. Advanced MR imaging techniques in the diagnosis of intraaxial brain tumors in adults. Radiographics 2006;26: 173–89.
8. Al-Okaili RN, Krejza J, Woo JH, et al. Intraaxial brain masses: MR-imaging-based diagnostic strategy–initial experience. Radiology 2007;243:539–50.
9. Majós C, Julià-Sapé M, Alonso J, et al. Brain tumor classification by proton MR spectroscopy: comparison of diagnostic accuracy at short and long TE. AJNR Am J Neuroradiol 2004;25:1696–704.
10. Brown TR, Kinkaid BM, Ugurbil K. NMR chemical shift imaging in three dimensions. Proc Natl Acad Sci U S A 1982;79:3523–6.
11. Horska A, Baker PB. Imaging of brain tumors: MR spectroscopy and metabolic imaging. Neuroimaging Clin N Am 2010;20:293–310.
12. Hourani R, Horska A, Albayram S, et al. Proton magnetic resonance spectroscopic imaging to differentiate between non neoplastic lesions and brain tumors in children. J Magn Reson Imaging 2006;23:99–107.
13. Majós C, Aguilera C, Alonso J, et al. Proton MR spectroscopy improves discrimination between tumor and pseudotumoral lesion in solid brain masses. AJNR Am J Neuroradiol 2009;30:544–51.
14. Tzika AA, Vajapeyam S, Barnes PD. Multivoxel proton MR spectroscopy and hemodynamic MR imaging of childhood brain tumors: preliminary observations. AJNR Am J Neuroradiol 1997;18: 203–18.
15. Butzen J, Prost R, Chetty V, et al. Discrimination between neoplastic and non neoplastic brain lesions by use of proton MR spectroscopy. The limits of accuracy with a logistic regression model. AJNR Am J Neuroradiol 2000;21:1213–9.
16. Voge TJ, Jassoy A, Söllner O, et al. The proton MR spectroscopy of intracranial tumors. The differential diagnostic aspects for gliomas, metastases and meningeomas. Rofo 1992;157:371–7 [in German].
17. Kinoshita Y, Yokota A. Absolute concentrations of metabolites in human brain tumors using in vitro proton magnetic resonance spectroscopy. NMR Biomed 1997;10:2–12.
18. Castillo M. Proton MR spectroscopy of the brain. Neuroimaging Clin N Am 1998;8(4):733–52.
19. Rand SD. MR spectroscopy: single voxel. Presented at the 39th Annual Meeting of the American Society of Neuroradiology. Boston, April, 2001.
20. Michaelis T, Merboldt KD, Bruhn H, et al. Absolute concentrations of metabolites in the adult human brain in vivo: quantification of localized proton MR spectra. Neuroradiology 1993;187:219–27.
21. Herminghaus S, Pilatus U, Raab P, et al. Impact of in vivo proton MR spectroscopy for the assessment of the proliferative activity in viable and partly necrotic brain tumor tissue. Presented at the 39th Annual Meeting of the American Society of Neuroradiology. Boston, April, 2001.
22. Palasis S. Utility of short TE MR spectroscopy in determination of histology, grade and behavior of pediatric brain tumors. Presented at the 39th Annual Meeting of the American Society of Neuroradiology. Boston, April, 2001.
23. Herholz K, Heindel W, Luyten PR, et al. In vivo imaging of glucose consumption and lactate concentration in human gliomas. Ann Neurol 1992;31: 319–27.

24. Castillo M, Smith JK, Kwock L. Correlation of myo-inositol levels and grading of cerebral astrocytomas. AJNR Am J Neuroradiol 2000;21: 1645–9.

25. Pilatus U, Reichel C, Raab P, et al. ERM detectable lipid signal in low- and high-grade glioma, recurrent gliomas, metastases, lymphomas and abscesses. Presented at the 39th Annual Meeting of the American Society of Neuroradiology. Boston, April, 2001.

26. Howe FA, Barton SJ, Cudlip SA, et al. Metabolic profiles of human brain tumors using quantitative in vivo ^{1}H magnetic resonance spectroscopy. Magn Reson Med 2003;49:223–32.

27. Kuesel AC, Sutherland GR, Halliday W, et al. ^{1}H MRS of high-grade astrocytomas: mobile lipid accumulation in necrotic tissue. NMR Biomed 1994;7:149–55.

28. Di Costanzo A, Scarabino T, Trojsi F, et al. Proton MR spectroscopy of cerebral gliomas at 3 T: spatial heterogeneity, and tumour grade and extent. Eur Radiol 2008;18:1727–35.

29. Hawley J, Pennizi A, Paul C, et al. Clinical evaluation of ultrashort TE proton spectroscopy imaging of the brain. Presented at the 39th Annual Meeting of the American Society of Neuroradiology. Boston, April, 2001.

30. Fan G, Sun B, Wu Z, et al. In vivo single-voxel proton MR spectroscopy in the differentiation of high-grade gliomas and solitary metastases. Clin Radiol 2004;59:77–85.

31. Law M, Cha S, Knopp EA, et al. High-grade gliomas and solitary metastases: differentiation by using perfusion and proton spectroscopic MR imaging. Radiology 2002;222:715–21.

32. Chiang IC, Kuo YT, Lu CY, et al. Distinction between high-grade gliomas and solitary metastases using peritumoral 3-T magnetic resonance spectroscopy, diffusion, and perfusion imagings. Neuroradiology 2004;46:619–27.

33. Ricci R, Bacci A, Tugnoli V, et al. Metabolic findings on 3T H-MR spectroscopy in peritumoral brain edema. AJNR Am J Neuroradiol 2007;28: 1287–91.

34. Burtscher IM, Skagerberg G, Geijer B, et al. Proton MR spectroscopy and preoperative diagnostic accuracy: an evaluation of intracranial mass lesions characterized by stereotactic biopsy findings. AJNR Am J Neuroradiol 2000;21:84–93.

35. Weber MA, Zoubaa S, Schlieter M, et al. Diagnostic performance of spectroscopic and perfusion MR for distinction of brain tumors. Neurology 2006;66: 1899–906.

36. Demir MK, Iplikcioglu AC, Dincer A, et al. Single voxel proton MR spectroscopy findings of typical and atypical intracranial meningiomas. Eur J Radiol 2006;60:48–55.

37. Bulakbasi N, Kocaoglu M, Örs F, et al. Combination of single-voxel proton MR spectroscopy and apparent diffusion coefficient calculation in the evaluation of common brain tumors. AJNR Am J Neuroradiol 2003;24:225–33.

38. Rabin RM, Meyer JR, Derlin JW, et al. Radiation-induced changes in the central nervous system and head and neck. Radiographics 1996;16: 1055–72.

39. Kado H, Ogawa T, Hatazawa J, et al. Radiation-induced meningioma evaluated with positron emission tomography with fludeoxyglucose F 18. AJNR Am J Neuroradiol 1996;17:937–8.

40. Zacharia TT, Law M, Naidich TP, et al. Central nervous system lymphoma characterization by diffusion-weighted imaging and MR spectroscopy. J Neuroimaging 2008;18:411–7.

41. Hakyemez B, Erdogan C, Bolca N, et al. Evaluation of different cerebral mass lesions by perfusion-weighted MR imaging. J Magn Reson Imaging 2006;24:817–24.

42. Law M, Yang S, Wang H, et al. Glioma grading: sensitivity, specificity, and predictive values of perfusion MR imaging and proton MR spectroscopic imaging compared with conventional MR imaging. AJNR Am J Neuroradiol 2003;24: 1989–98.

43. Brandão L, Domingues R. Intracranial neoplasms. In: McAllister L, Lazar T, Cook RE, editors. MR spectroscopy of the brain. Philadelphia: Lippincott Williams & Wilkins; 2002. p. 130–67.

44. Knopp EA. Advanced MR imaging of tumors: using spectroscopy and perfusion. Presented at the 39th Annual Meeting of the American Society of Neuroradiology. Boston, April, 2001.

45. Taillibert S, Chodkiewicz C, Laigle-Donadey F, et al. Gliomatosis cerebri: a review of 296 cases from the ANOCEF database and the literature. J Neurooncol 2006;76:201–5.

46. Mohana-Borges AV, Imbesi SG, Dietrich R, et al. Role of proton magnetic resonance spectroscopy in the diagnosis of gliomatosis cerebri. J Comput Assist Tomogr 2004;28(1):103–5.

47. Sarafi-Lavi E, Bowen BC, Pattany PM, et al. Proton MR spectroscopy of gliomatosis cerebri: case report of elevated myoinositol with normal choline levels. AJNR Am J Neuroradiol 2003;24:946–51.

48. Guzmán-de-Villoria JA, Sánchez-González J, Muñoz L, et al. ^{1}H MR spectroscopy in the assessment of gliomatosis cerebri. AJR Am J Roentgenol 2007;188:710–4.

49. Galanaud D, Chinot O, Nicoli F, et al. Use of proton magnetic resonance spectroscopy of the brain to differentiate gliomatosis cerebri from low-grade glioma. J Neurosurg 2003;98:269–76.

50. Tong Z, Yamaki T, Harada K, et al. In vivo quantification of the metabolites in normal brain and brain

tumors by proton MR spectroscopy using water as an internal standard. Magn Reson Imaging 2004; 22:1017–24.

51. Panigrahy A, Krieger MD, Gonzalez-Gomes I, et al. Quantitative short echo time ^{1}H-MR spectroscopy of untreated pediatric brain tumors: preoperative diagnosis and characterization. AJNR Am J Neuroradiol 2006;27:560–72.

52. Schneider JF, Gouny C, Viola A, et al. Multiparametric differentiation of posterior fossa tumors in children using diffusion-weighted imaging and short echo-time ^{1}H-MR spectroscopy. J Magn Reson Imaging 2007;26:1390–8.

53. Majós C, Aguilera C, Cós M, et al. In vivo proton magnetic resonance spectroscopy of intraventricular tumors of the brain. Eur Radiol 2009;19: 2049–59.

54. Jouanneau E, Tovar RA, Desuzinges C. Very late frontal relapse of medulloblastoma mimicking a meningioma in an adult. Usefulness of ^{1}H magnetic resonance spectroscopy and diffusion-perfusion magnetic resonance imaging for preoperative diagnosis: case report. Neurosurgery 2006;58(4): E789.

55. Yamasaki F, Kurisu K, Satoh K, et al. Apparent diffusion coefficient of human brain tumors at MR imaging. Radiology 2005;235:985–91.

56. Peeling J, Sutherland G. High-resolution ^{1}H NMR spectroscopy studies of extracts of human cerebral neoplasms. Magn Reson Med 1992;24:123–6.

57. Raybaud C, Barkovich AJ. Intracranial, orbital and neck masses of childhood. In: Barkovich AJ, Raybaud C, editors. Pediatric neuroimaging. 5th edition. Philadelphia: Lippincott Williams & Wilkins; 2012. p. 637–711.

58. Barkovich A. Intracranial, orbital and neck masses of childhood. In: Barkovich AJ, Raybaud C, editors. Pediatric neuroimaging. 5th edition. Philadelphia: Lippincott Williams & Wilkins; 2005. p. 637–750.

59. Blaser SI, Harwood-Nash DC. Neuroradiology of pediatric posterior fossa medulloblastoma. J Neurooncol 1996;29:23–34.

60. Kleihues P, Cavenee WK. World Health Organization classification of tumors: pathology and genetics of tumors of the central nervous system. Lyon (France): IARC Press; 2000.

61. Yuh EL, Barkovich AJ, Gupta N. Imaging of ependymomas: MRI and CT. Childs Nerv Syst 2009; 25:1203–13.

62. Uematsu Y, Hirano A, Llena JF. Electron microscopic observations of blood vessels in ependymoma. No Shinkei Geka 1988;16:1235–42 [in Japanese].

63. Harris L, Davies N, MacPherson L, et al. The use of short-echo time ^{1}H MRS for childhood cerebellar tumors prior to histopathological diagnosis. Pediatr Radiol 2007;37:1101–9.

64. Bourgouin PM, Tampieri D, Grahovac SZ, et al. CT and MR imaging findings in adults with cerebellar medulloblastoma: comparison with findings in children. AJR Am J Roentgenol 1992; 159:609–12.

65. Movsas B, Li BS, Babb JS. Quantifying radiation therapy–induced brain injury with whole-brain proton MR spectroscopy: initial observations. Radiology 2001;221:327–31.

66. Ricci PE, Pitt A, Keller PJ, et al. Effect of voxel position on single-voxel MR spectroscopy findings. AJNR Am J Neuroradiol 2000;21:367–74.

67. Chawla S, Wang S, Wolf RL, et al. Arterial spin labeling and MR spectroscopy in the differentiation of gliomas. AJNR Am J Neuroradiol 2007;28: 1683–9.

68. Hollingworth W, Medina LS, Lenkinski RE, et al. A systematic literature review of magnetic resonance spectroscopy for the characterization of brain tumors. AJNR Am J Neuroradiol 2006;27: 1404–11.

69. Di Costanzo A, Scarabino T, Trojsi F, et al. Multiparametric 3T MR approach to the assessment of cerebral gliomas: tumor extent and malignancy. Neuroradiology 2006;48:622–31.

70. Chang SM, Nelson S, Vandenberg S, et al. Integration of preoperative anatomic and metabolic physiologic imaging of newly diagnosed glioma. J Neurooncol 2009;92:401–15.

71. Arnold DL, Shoubridge EA, Villemure JG, et al. Proton and phosphorus magnetic resonance spectroscopy of human astrocytomas in vivo. Preliminary observations on tumor grading. NMR Biomed 1990;3:184–9.

72. Gill SS, Thomas DG, Van Bruggen N, et al. Proton MR spectroscopy of intracranial tumours: in vivo and in vitro studies. J Comput Assist Tomogr 1990;14:497–504.

73. Preul MC, Leblanc R, Caramanos Z, et al. Magnetic resonance spectroscopy guided brain tumor resection: differentiation between recurrent glioma and radiation change in two diagnostically difficult cases. Can J Neurol Sci 1998;25:13–22.

74. Majós C, Bruna J, Julià-Sapé M, et al. Proton MR spectroscopy provides relevant prognostic information in high-grade astrocytomas. AJNR Am J Neuroradiol 2011;32:74–80.

75. Rock JP, Hearshen D, Scarpace L, et al. Correlations between magnetic resonance spectroscopy and image-guided histopathology, with special attention to radiation necrosis. Neurosurgery 2002;51:912–9.

76. Covarrubias DJ, Rosen BR, Lev MH. Dynamic magnetic resonance perfusion imaging of brain tumors. Oncologist 2004;9:528–37.

77. Isobe T, Matsumura A, Anno I, et al. Quantification of cerebral metabolites in glioma patients with

proton MR spectroscopy using T2 relaxation time correction. Magn Reson Imaging 2002;20:343–9.

78. Bartha R, Megyesi JF, Watling CJ, et al. Low-grade glioma: correlation of short echo time ^{1}H-MR spectroscopy with ^{23}Na MR imaging. AJNR Am J Neuroradiol 2008;29:464–70.

79. Rijpkema M, Schuuring J, van der Meulen Y, et al. Characterization of oligo-dendrogliomas using short echo time ^{1}H MR spectroscopic imaging. NMR Biomed 2003;16:12–8.

80. Gupta RK, Cloughesy TF, Sinha U, et al. Relationships between choline magnetic resonance spectroscopy, apparent diffusion coefficient and quantitative histopathology in human glioma. J Neurooncol 2000;50:215–26.

81. Ishimaru H, Morikawa M, Iwanaga S, et al. Differentiation between high-grade glioma and metastatic brain tumor using single-voxel proton MR spectroscopy. Eur Radiol 2001;11:1784–91.

82. Grand S, Passaro C, Ziegler A, et al. Necrotic tumor versus brain abscess: importance of aminoacids detected at ^{1}H MR spectroscopy–initial results. Radiology 1999;213:785–93.

83. Louis DN, Ohgaki H, Wiestler OD, editors. WHO classification of tumours of the central nervous system. Lyon (France): IARC; 2007. 978-92-832-2430-2.

84. Lev MH, Ozsunar Y, Henson JW, et al. Glial tumor grading and outcome prediction using dynamic spin-echo MR susceptibility mapping compared with conventional contrast-enhanced MR: confounding effect of elevated rCBV of oligodendrogliomas [corrected]. AJNR Am J Neuroradiol 2004;25:214–21.

85. Cha S, Tihan T, Crawford F, et al. Differentiation of low-grade oligodendrogliomas from low-grade astrocytomas by using quantitative blood-volume measurements derived from dynamic susceptibility contrast-enhanced MR imaging. AJNR Am J Neuroradiol 2005;26:266–73.

86. Spampinato MV, Smith JK, Kwock L, et al. Cerebral blood volume measurements and proton MR spectroscopy in grading of oligodendroglial tumors. AJR Am J Roentgenol 2007;188:204–12.

87. Xu M, See SJ, Ng WH, et al. Comparison of magnetic resonance spectroscopy and perfusion-weighted imaging in presurgical grading of oligodendroglial tumors. Neurosurgery 2005;56:919–26.

88. Pirzkall A, McKnight TR, Graves EE, et al. MR-spectroscopy guided target delineation for high-grade gliomas. Int J Radiat Oncol Biol Phys 2001; 50:915–28.

89. Ganslandt O, Stadlbauer A, Fahlbusch R, et al. Proton magnetic resonance spectroscopic imaging integrated into image-guided surgery: correlation to standard magnetic resonance imaging and tumor cell density. Neurosurgery 2005;56:291–8.

90. McKnight TR, Von Dem Bussche MH, Vigneron DB, et al. Histopathological validation of a three-dimensional magnetic resonance spectroscopy index as a predictor of tumor presence. J Neurosurg 2002;97:794–802.

91. Poussaint TY. Pediatric brain tumors. In: Newton HB, Jolesz FA, editors. Handbook of neuro-oncology neuroimaging. New York: Academic Press; 2008. p. 469–84.

92. Croteau D, Scarpace L, Hearshen D, et al. Correlation between magnetic resonance spectroscopy imaging and image-guided biopsies: semiquantitative and qualitative histopathological analyses of patients with untreated glioma. Neurosurgery 2001;49:823–9.

93. Stadlbauer A, Nimsky C, Buslei R, et al. Proton magnetic resonance spectroscopic imaging in the border zone of gliomas: correlation of metabolic and histological changes at low tumor infiltration-initial results. Invest Radiol 2007;42:218–23.

94. Kallenberg K, Bock HC, Helms G. Untreated glioblastoma multiforme: increased myo-inositol and glutamine levels in the contralateral cerebral hemisphere at proton MR spectroscopy. Radiology 2009;253(3):805–12.

95. Luyten PR, Marien AJ, Heindel W, et al. Metabolic imaging of patients with intracranial tumors: H-1 MR spectroscopic imaging and PET. Radiology 1990;176:791–9.

96. McBride DQ, Miller BL, Nikas DL, et al. Analysis of brain tumors using ^{1}H magnetic resonance spectroscopy. Surg Neurol 1995;44:137–44.

97. Nelson SJ, Huhn S, Vigneron DB, et al. Volume MRI and MRSI techniques for the quantitation of treatment response in brain tumors: presentation of a detailed case study. J Magn Reson Imaging 1997;7:1146–52.

98. Kelly PJ, Daumas-Duport C, Scheithauer BW, et al. Stereotactic histologic correlations of computed tomography- and magnetic resonance imaging-defined abnormalities in patients with glial neoplasms. Mayo Clin Proc 1987;62:450–9.

99. Martin AJ, Liu H, Hall WA, et al. Preliminary assessment of turbo spectroscopic imaging for targeting in brain biopsy. AJNR Am J Neuroradiol 2001;22:959–68.

100. Klingebiel R, Bohner G. Neuroimaging. Recent Results Cancer Res 2009;171:175–90.

101. Dowling C, Bollen AW, Noworolski SM, et al. Preoperative proton MR spectroscopic imaging of brain tumors: correlation with histopathologic analysis of resection specimens. AJNR Am J Neuroradiol 2001;22:604–12.

102. Hall WA, Martin A, Liu H, et al. Improving diagnostic yield in brain biopsy: coupling spectroscopic targeting with real-time needle placement. J Magn Reson Imaging 2001;13:12–5.

103. Hall WA, Galicich W, Bergman T, et al. 3-Tesla intraoperative MR imaging for neurosurgery. J Neurooncol 2006;77:297–303.

104. Hermann EJ, Hattingen E, Krauss JK, et al. Stereotactic biopsy in gliomas guided by 3-Tesla ^{1}H-chemical-shift imaging of choline. Stereotact Funct Neurosurg 2008;86:300–7.

105. Tedeschi G, Lundbom N, Ramon R, et al. Increased choline signal coinciding with malignant degeneration of cerebral gliomas: a serial proton magnetic resonance spectroscopy imaging study. J Neurosurg 1997;87:516–24.

106. Castillo M, Kwock L. Proton MR spectroscopy of common brain tumors. Neuroimaging Clin N Am 1998;8:733–52.

107. Oh J, Henry RG, Pirzkall A, et al. Survival analysis in patients with glioblastoma multiforme: predictive value of choline-to-N-acetylaspartate index, apparent diffusion coefficient, and relative cerebral blood volume. J Magn Reson Imaging 2004;19:546–54.

108. Kuznetsov YE, Caramanos Z, Antel SB, et al. Proton magnetic resonance spectroscopic imaging can predict length of survival in patients with supratentorial gliomas. Neurosurgery 2003;53: 565–74 [discussion: 574–76].

109. Li X, Jin H, Lu Y, et al. Identification of MRI and ^{1}H MRSI parameters that may predict survival for patients with malignant gliomas. NMR Biomed 2004; 17:10–20.

110. Saraswathy S, Crawford FW, Lamborn KR, et al. Evaluation of MR markers that predict survival in patients with newly diagnosed GBM prior to adjuvant therapy. J Neurooncol 2009;91:69–81.

111. Crawford FW, Khayal IS, McGue C, et al. Relationship of pre-surgery metabolic and physiological MR imaging parameters to survival for patients with untreated GBM. J Neurooncol 2009;91:337–51.

112. Arslanoglu A, Bonekamp D, Barker PB, et al. Quantitative proton MR spectroscopic imaging of the mesial temporal lobe. J Magn Reson Imaging 2004;20:772–8.

113. Chan AA, Lau A, Pirzkall A, et al. Proton magnetic resonance spectroscopy imaging in the evaluation of patients undergoing gamma knife surgery for Grade IV glioma. J Neurosurg 2004;101:467–75.

114. Raizer JJ, Koutcher JA, Abrey LE, et al. Proton magnetic resonance spectroscopy in immunocompetent patients with primary central nervous system lymphoma. J Neurooncol 2005;71:173–80.

115. Hattingen E, Raab P, Franz K, et al. Prognostic value of choline and creatine in WHO grade II gliomas. Neuroradiology 2008;50:759–67.

116. Yang I, Aghi MK. New advances that enable identification of glioblastoma recurrence. Nat Rev Clin Oncol 2009;6:648–57.

117. Rabinov JD, Lee PL, Barker FG, et al. In vivo 3-T MR spectroscopy in the distinction of recurrent glioma versus radiation effects: initial experience. Radiology 2002;225:871–9.

118. Smith EA, Carlos RC, Junck LR, et al. Developing a clinical decision model: MR spectroscopy to differentiate between recurrent tumor and radiation change in patients with new contrast-enhancing lesions. AJR Am J Roentgenol 2009; 192:W45–52.

119. Weybright P, Sundgren PC, Maly P, et al. Differentiation between brain tumor recurrence and radiation injury using MR spectroscopy. AJR Am J Roentgenol 2005;185:1471–6.

120. Zeng QS, Li CF, Liu H, et al. Distinction between recurrent glioma and radiation injury using magnetic resonance spectroscopy in combination with diffusion-weighted imaging. Int J Radiat Oncol Biol Phys 2007;68:151–8.

121. Cha S. Update on brain tumor imaging: from anatomy to physiology. AJNR Am J Neuroradiol 2006; 27:475–87.

122. Weber MA, Giesel FL, Stieltjes B. MRI for identification of progression in brain tumors: from morphology to function. Expert Rev Neurother 2008;8:1507–25.

123. Sundgren PC. MR spectroscopy in radiation injury. AJNR Am J Neuroradiol 2009;30:1469–76.

124. Nelson SJ, Graves E, Pirzkall A, et al. In vivo molecular imaging for planning radiation therapy of gliomas: an application of ^{1}H MRSI. J Magn Reson Imaging 2002;16:464–76.

125. Taylor JS, Langston JW, Reddick WE, et al. Clinical value of proton magnetic resonance spectroscopy for differentiating recurrent or residual brain tumor from delayed cerebral necrosis. Int J Radiat Oncol Biol Phys 1996;36:1251–61.

126. Graves EE, Nelson SJ, Vigneron DB, et al. Serial proton MR spectroscopic imaging of recurrent malignant gliomas after gamma knife radiosurgery. AJNR Am J Neuroradiol 2001;22:613–24.

127. Lichy MP, Plathow C, Schulz-Ertner D, et al. Follow-up gliomas after radiotherapy: ^{1}H MR spectroscopic imaging for increasing diagnostic accuracy. Neuroradiology 2005;47:826–34.

128. Wald LL, Nelson SJ, Day MR, et al. Serial proton magnetic resonance spectroscopy imaging of glioblastoma multiforme after brachytherapy. J Neurosurg 1997;87:525–34.

129. Chernov MF, Hayashi M, Izawa M, et al. Multivoxel proton MRS for differentiation of radiation-induced necrosis and tumor recurrence after gamma knife radiosurgery for brain metastases. Brain Tumor Pathol 2006;23:19–27.

130. Law M. MR spectroscopy of brain tumors. Top Magn Reson Imaging 2004;15:291–313.

131. Li X, Vigneron DB, Cha S, et al. Relationship of MR-derived lactate, mobile lipids, and relative blood volume for gliomas in vivo. AJNR Am J Neuroradiol 2005;26:760–9.

132. Elias AE, Carlos RC, Smith EA, et al. MR spectroscopy using normalized and non-normalized metabolite ratios for differentiating recurrent brain tumor from radiation injury. Acad Radiol 2011;18:1101–8.

133. Murphy PS, Viviers L, Abson C, et al. Monitoring temozolomide treatment of low-grade glioma with proton magnetic resonance spectroscopy. Br J Cancer 2004;90:781–6.

134. Lewin JS. Percutaneous MR image-guided procedures in neuroradiology. Presented at the 39th Annual Meeting of the American Society of Neuroradiology. Boston, April, 2001.

135. Hourani R, Brant LS, Rizk T, et al. Can proton MR spectroscopic and Perfusion Imaging Differentiate Between Neoplastic and Nonneoplastic Brain Lesions in Adults? AJNR Am J Neuroradiol 2008;29: 366–72.

136. Sundgren PC, Nagesh V, Elias A, et al. Metabolic alterations: a biomarker for radiation-induced normal brain injury–an MR spectroscopy study. J Magn Reson Imaging 2009;29:291–7.

137. Esteve F, Rubin C, Grand S, et al. Transient metabolic changes observed with proton MR spectroscopy in normal human brain after radiation therapy. Int J Radiat Oncol Biol Phys 1998;40:279–86.

138. Rand SD, Prost R, Haughton V, et al. Accuracy of single-voxel proton MR spectroscopy in distinguishing neoplastic from non neoplastic brain lesions. AJNR Am J Neuroradiol 1997;18:1695–704.

139. Paley RJ, Persing JA, Doctor A, et al. Multiple sclerosis and brain tumor: a diagnostic challenge. J Emerg Med 1989;7:241–4.

140. Giang DW, Poduri KR, Eskin TA, et al. Multiple sclerosis masquerading as a mass lesion. Neuroradiology 1992;34:150–4.

141. Hunter SB, Ballinger WE Jr, Rubin JJ. Multiple sclerosis mimicking primary brain tumor. Arch Pathol Lab Med 1987;111:464–8.

142. Kurihara N, Takahashi S, Furuta A, et al. MR imaging of multiple sclerosis simulating brain tumor. Clin Imaging 1996;20:171–7.

143. Mastrostefano R, Occhipinti E, Bigotti G, et al. Multiple sclerosis plaque simulating cerebral tumor: case report and review of the literature. Neurosurgery 1987;21:244–6.

144. Silva HC, Callegaro D, Marchiori PE, et al. Magnetic resonance imaging in five patients with a tumefactive demyelinating lesion in the central nervous system. Arq Neuropsiquiatr 1999;57:921–6.

145. Tate AR, Underwood J, Acosta D, et al. Development of a decision support system for diagnosis and grading of brain tumours using in vivo magnetic resonance single voxel spectra. NMR Biomed 2006;19:411–34.

146. Preul MC, Caramanos Z, Collins DL, et al. Accurate, noninvasive diagnosis of human brain tumors by using proton magnetic resonance spectroscopy. Nat Med 1996;2:323–5.

147. Majós C, Alonso J, Aguilera C, et al. Proton magnetic resonance spectroscopy (^{1}H MRS) of human brain tumors: assessment of differences between tumour types and its applicability in brain tumour categorization. Eur Radiol 2003;13:582–91.

148. De Stefano N, Caramanos Z, Preul MC, et al. In vivo differentiation of astrocytic brain tumors and isolated demyelinating lesions of the type seen in multiple sclerosis using ^{1}H magnetic resonance spectroscopic imaging. Ann Neurol 1998;44:273–8.

149. Saindane AM, Cha S, Law M, et al. Proton MR spectroscopy of tumefactive demyelinating lesions. AJNR Am J Neuroradiol 2002;23:1378–86.

150. Cianfoni A, Niku S, Imbesi SG, et al. Metabolite findings in tumefactive demyelinating lesions utilizing short echo time proton magnetic resonance spectroscopy. AJNR Am J Neuroradiol 2007;28:272–7.

151. Srinivasan R, Sailasuta N, Hurd R, et al. Evidence of elevated glutamate in multiple sclerosis using magnetic resonance spectroscopy at 3 T. Brain 2005;128:1016–25.

152. Bitsch A, Bruhn H, Vougioukas V, et al. Inflammatory CNS demyelination: histopathologic correlation with in vivo quantitative proton MR spectroscopy. AJNR Am J Neuroradiol 1999;20:1619–27.

153. Fernando KT, McLean MA, Chard DT, et al. Elevated white matter myo-inositol in clinically isolated syndromes suggestive of multiple sclerosis. Brain 2004;127:1361–9.

154. Vuori K, Kankaanranta L, Häkkinen AM, et al. Low-grade gliomas and focal cortical developmental malformations: differentiation with proton MR spectroscopy. Radiology 2004;230(3):703–8.

155. Pal D, Bhattacharyya A, Husain M, et al. In vivo proton MR spectroscopy evaluation of pyogenic brain abscesses: a report of 194 cases. AJNR Am J Neuroradiol 2010;31:360–6.

156. Lai PH, Ho JT, Chen WL, et al. Brain abscess and necrotic brain tumor: discrimination with proton MR spectroscopy and diffusion-weighted imaging. AJNR Am J Neuroradiol 2002;23(8):1369–77.

157. Samann PG, Schlegel J, Muller G, et al. Serial proton MR spectroscopy and diffusion imaging findings in HIV-related herpes simplex encephalitis. AJNR Am J Neuroradiol 2003;24:2015–9.

158. Law M, Hamburger M, Johnson G, et al. Differentiating surgical from non-surgical lesions using perfusion MR imaging and proton MR spectroscopic imaging. Technol Cancer Res Treat 2004; 3:557–65.

Pediatric Cerebellar Tumors

Emerging Imaging Techniques and Advances in Understanding of Genetic Features

Asim F. Choudhri, MD[a,b,c,d,*], Adeel Siddiqui, MD[a,d],
Paul Klimo Jr, MD, MPH[b,d,e,f]

KEYWORDS

- Pediatric radiology • Neuroradiology • Brain tumor • Cerebellum • Medulloblastoma
- Pilocytic astrocytoma • Ependymoma

KEY POINTS

- Cerebellar tumors are the most common solid neoplasms in children, with the 3 most common entities including pilocytic astrocytoma, medulloblastoma, and ependymoma.
- Diffusion-weighted/tensor imaging plays a key role in preoperative characterization of pediatric cerebellar tumors, with lower apparent diffusion coefficient values correlating with higher-grade tumors.
- Genetic characterization is resulting in new understanding of medulloblastoma.
- The previous 4 histologic categories are in the process of being supplanted with 4 genetic groupings, in particular based on analysis of the WNT and Sonic Hedgehog pathway genes.
- This genetic characterization has allowed therapeutic options targeted to the specific tumor and improved prediction of tumor aggressiveness compared with histologic categorization.

INTRODUCTION

Cerebellar tumors are among the most common central nervous system (CNS) neoplasms, not to mention solid neoplasms, in children.[1] These tumors include benign and malignant entities, tumors that have slow local spread, and others with leptomeningeal dissemination. Although there are a small number of tumor types that account for most of these tumors, recent work on the genetic origins of these lesions has created an understanding of a much broader landscape of tumors.[2]

The newer understanding of genetic origins has the potential for targeted therapy, and imaging features that may help determine the tumor type (or even subtype) take on an increasingly critical role.

TUMOR TYPES

Pediatric cerebellar tumors most commonly involve four entities. Pilocytic astrocytomas (PAs), ependymomas, and medulloblastomas are the key players, with atypical teratoid rhabdoid tumor (ATRT)

This article originally appeared in Neuroimaging Clinics of North America, Volume 26, Issue 3, August 2016.
Disclosures: none.
[a] Department of Radiology, University of Tennessee Health Science Center, 848 Adams Ave, Memphis, TN 38103, USA; [b] Department of Neurosurgery, University of Tennessee Health Science Center, 847 Monroe Avenue, Memphis, TN 38163, USA; [c] Department of Ophthalmology, University of Tennessee Health Science Center, 930 Madison Avenue, Memphis, TN 38163, USA; [d] Le Bonheur Neuroscience Institute, Le Bonheur Children's Hospital, 848 Adams Avenue, Memphis, TN 38103, USA; [e] Division of Neurosurgery, St. Jude's Children's Hospital, 262 Danny Thomas Place, Memphis, TN 38105, USA; [f] Semmes Murphey Neurologic & Spine Institute, 6325 Humphreys Boulevard, Memphis, TN 38120, USA
* Corresponding author. Department of Radiology, Le Bonheur Children's Hospital, 848 Adams Avenue–G216, Memphis, TN 38103.
E-mail address: achoudhri@uthsc.edu

mri.theclinics.com

representing a high-grade embryonal tumor most common in the first year or two of life. Initial clinical presentation for all of these lesions is typically due to mass effect, including headaches, nausea and emesis, cranial neuropathies, and obstructive hydrocephalus.

PILOCYTIC ASTROCYTOMA

PAs, sometimes referred to as juvenile PAs, are benign neoplasms, classified as World Health Organization (WHO) grade I tumors. They account for more than two-thirds of all cerebellar astrocytomas and can be seen from birth to about 15 years of age. Other more aggressive astrocytomas, such

as anaplastic astrocytomas and glioblastomas, are rare and usually seen in older children. There is an equal incidence of PA in boys and girls. PA of the cerebellum can arise from nearly any location in the cerebellum, including the hemispheres and vermis. PA of the cerebellum most classically has an imaging appearance of a cystic lesion with a mural nodule (**Fig. 1**). The solid portions of the tumor have a large volume of interstitial space with a high water content, which results in a somewhat hyperintense appearance on T2-weighted (T2W) imaging, and results in facilitated diffusion. The solid portion of PAs typically has diffusion characteristics of greater than 1300×10^{-6} mm^2/s (or 1.3×10^{-3} mm^2/s).[3] The solid portions will

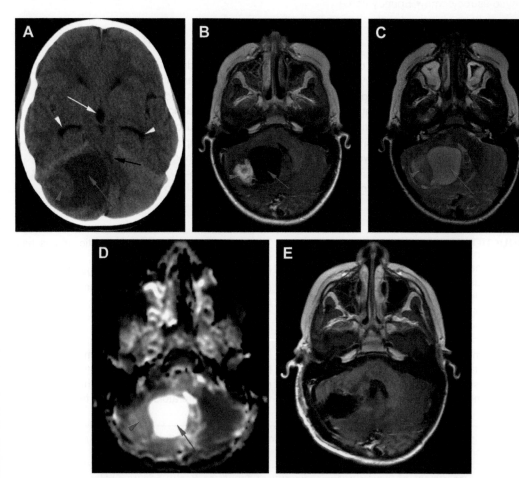

Fig. 1. PA. (*A*) Axial–computed tomography image in a 6-year-old boy shows a mass in the right cerebellar hemisphere that has a cystic component (*red arrow*) and a solid component (*red arrowhead*). There is near-complete effacement of the fourth ventricle (*black arrow*) with signs of obstructive hydrocephalus in the third ventricle (*white arrow*) and temporal horns of the lateral ventricles (*white arrowheads*). (*B*) Axial T1W + C image shows enhancement of the solid nodule (*red arrowhead*) but not of the cystic component (*red arrow*). (*C*) Axial T2W image shows intermediate hyperintense signal for the solid nodule (*red arrowhead*), suggesting a high water content, and fluidlike signal in the cystic component (*red arrow*). (*D*) ADC map shows facilitated diffusion in the solid nodule (*red arrowhead*), with diffusion characteristics of 1570×10^{-6} mm^2/s. The diffusion characteristics of the cystic component (*red arrow*) were greater than 3000×10^{-6} mm^2/s. (*E*) Axial T1W + C MR imaging after surgical resection shows gross total resection. This lesion was confirmed to be a PA. T1W + C, T1 + contrast.

usually enhance after contrast administration because of leaky capillaries. Accordingly, there is delayed accumulation of gadolinium within the interstitial space, and the lesions will enhance more on delayed imaging. The contrast enhancement is *not* due to increased vascularity, as would be the case for a hemangioblastoma.

The cyst walls of a PA may or may not enhance. If the enhancement is thin and smooth, this is likely due to leaky capillaries as a result of the pressure from the cyst and not due to neoplasm. If the enhancement is irregular and nodular, then neoplasm is more likely. Inspection of the inside of the cyst under microscopic magnification and illumination will usually allow the surgeon to distinguish whether the wall of the cyst is neoplastic or not. Many PAs are amenable to gross-total resection (GTR) with appropriate surgical planning, but these can be challenging lesions. These tumors can be difficult to distinguish from normal adjacent cerebral tissue, and there can be a transition zone of tumor infiltration. When GTR is achieved, no adjuvant chemotherapy or radiation is typically indicated and patients will undergo imaging surveillance. A recurrence along the margins of the resection cavity may undergo continued surveillance, repeat surgical resection, or (if not amenable to resection) focal irradiation. If surgery is performed and there is a small focus of residual tumor, the neuro-oncologic team may still advocate for observation over radiation, especially if patients are young. Chemotherapy is typically reserved for young children with unresectable residual or recurrent disease, although it is less effective at achieving local disease control than radiation.

PAs tend to have local growth, both of the initial lesion and recurrences. Distant cerebral spinal fluid (CSF) dissemination of the disease, either intracranially or to the spine, is much less common than the other lesions discussed, seen in as little as 2% of these lesions.[4] The 25-year survival rate of cerebellar PA is greater than 90%, and the 25-year survival rate of solid cerebellar astrocytomas is approximately 40%[4,5] but may be improved with more recent therapy.

Recent work has shown that mutations in the BRAF gene are present in some PAs.[6–8] The BRAF proto-oncogene makes a protein called B-Raf that is involved in the mitogen-activated protein kinase (MAPK)/Extracellular signal regulated kinases signaling pathway, which affects cell division and differentiation. BRAF alterations may be a point mutation (V600E) or various fusions (KIAA 1549); the pattern of such genetic alterations may be tumor location specific.[9–11] MAPK (eg, trametinib) and BRAF inhibitors (eg, dabrafenib and vemurafinib in patients who are V600E positive) are under investigation as a treatment option for PA. Interestingly, the initial studies with these inhibitors were done in patients with melanoma.[12]

MEDULLOBLASTOMA

Medulloblastoma is a malignant tumor classified as WHO grade IV, which most commonly arises from the superior medullary velum in young children and cerebellar hemispheres in adolescents. Medulloblastomas are the most common posterior fossa tumor and the most common brain tumor overall in the 6- to 11-year age group. The median age at diagnosis is 6 years, and boys are affected more than girls. This highly cellular tumor is a small, round, blue cell tumor with 4 histologic subtypes, as defined by the 2007 WHO criteria: classic medulloblastoma, large cell, anaplastic, and nodular desmoplastic[13] (**Fig. 2**). Nodular desmoplastic medulloblastomas tend to occur in older patients, adolescents, and young adults and occur in the cerebellar hemispheres[14] (**Fig. 3**). Based on histologic criteria, medulloblastoma has been considered to be a subtype of a primitive neuroectodermal tumor (PNET) and is sometimes referred to as medulloblastoma-PNET to reflect this relationship.

Beyond histologic characteristics, molecular analysis has given rise to 4 subtypes.[15,16] The Sonic Hedgehog pathway (SHH) and WNT pathway, in particular, correlate with the site of origin of these tumors, and importantly with treatment response and outcome. WNT medulloblastomas are thought to arise from the lower rhombic lip of the brainstem, whereas SHH tumors arise from the external granular layer and are found within the cerebellar hemispheres (overlapping with the histologic category of nodular desmoplastic). Given the different genetic origins and biological behavior, different therapeutic options exist for these tumors. Accordingly, active investigations are underway to determine clinical and imaging biomarkers to help stratify these tumors.[17–19]

Because of the highly cellular nature of these tumors, there are low apparent diffusion coefficient (ADC) values, typically lower than 800×10^{-6} mm^2/s.[3] ADC has not yet been shown to correspond to the genetic subtype of medulloblastoma or treatment responsiveness. Medulloblastomas usually demonstrate postcontrast enhancement, and approximately half of lesions show signs of calcification. The high nuclear to cytoplasmic ratio results in a high-density appearance on computed tomography (CT), even in the absence of calcifications, and a relative hypointense appearance on T2W imaging. Unlike ependymomas,

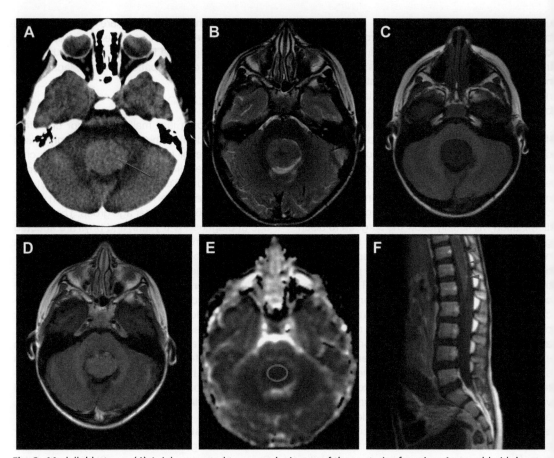

Fig. 2. Medulloblastoma. (*A*) Axial–computed tomography image of the posterior fossa in a 4-year-old girl shows a high-density lesion within the fourth ventricle (*red arrow*). (*B*) Axial T2W image shows the lesion demonstrates intermediate hypointense signal characteristics. (*C*) Axial T1W image shows the lesion demonstrates intermediate signal characteristics. (*D*) Axial T1W + C image shows the lesion demonstrates diffuse postcontrast enhancement. (*E*) Apparent diffusion coefficient maps show the lesion demonstrates restricted diffusion, with diffusivity of 655×10^{-6} mm^2/s as measured within the red oval region of interest. (*F*) Sagittal T1W + C image of the lumbar spine shows irregular enhancement along the posterior aspect of the conus medullaris and thoracolumbar cord (*red arrowheads*), consistent with leptomeningeal metastatic deposits. This lesion was confirmed to be medulloblastoma with intracranial and spinal metastatic disease.

medulloblastomas tend to displace rather than conform to margins and are described as being more spherical. This feature also explains why patients with medulloblastoma have a relatively short clinical history and come to medical attention more quickly than their ependymoma counterparts. Spinal metastatic disease is more common with medulloblastoma than ependymoma.

Like ependymoma, optimal management is multimodal, including maximal cytoreductive surgery in nonmetastatic patients, followed by chemotherapy and depending, on the extent of disease and age of patients, radiation.

EPENDYMOMA

Ependymomas are of 2 types: well differentiated (WHO grade II) and anaplastic (WHO grade III).

Anatomically, posterior fossa ependymomas can be thought of as either midline or lateral in origin (**Fig. 4**). They have a bimodal age distribution, the first between 1 and 5 years of age and the second much later during the fourth decade of life. They account for up to one-fifth of the posterior fossa tumors in children with a slight increase incidence in boys.

Ependymomas are histologically defined by perivascular and ependymal pseudorosettes, among other features.[20] Recent work suggests that the exact cell of origin of ependymoma and genetic origin may vary in lesions of different locations.[21–25] The tumors that are predominantly midline, typically filling the fourth ventricle, represent the most commonly described location for posterior fossa ependymomas. Lateral ependymomas arise from the inferior margin of the middle

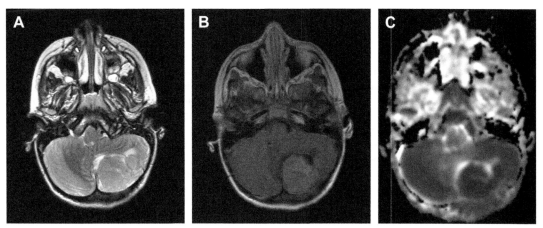

Fig. 3. Hemispheric medulloblastoma. (*A*) Axial T2W image in an 8-year-old boy shows a predominantly solid lesion in the periphery of the left cerebellar hemisphere, with smaller cystic components. The lesion is intermediate hypointense on T2W images. (*B*) Axial T1W + C image shows mild heterogeneous enhancement of the solid component of the tumor. (*C*) Apparent diffusion coefficient map shows the solid portion demonstrates restricted diffusion, with a diffusivity of 655×10^{-6} mm^2/s. This lesion was a nodular-desmoplastic medulloblastoma.

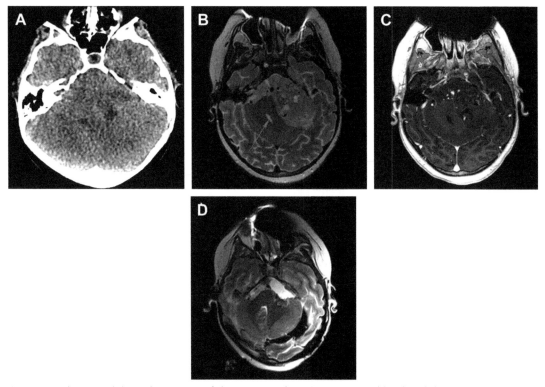

Fig. 4. Ependymoma. (*A*) Axial CT image of the posterior fossa in a 10-year-old girl with headaches and altered mental status shows a paucity of CSF space as well as rightward and posterior displacement of the fourth ventricle (*red arrow*) and internal cystic areas (*red arrowhead*) within a suspected mass. (*B*) Axial T2W image shows a mass in the left cerebellopontine angle with internal cystic changes pushing on the left middle cerebellar peduncle, reconfirmation of the mass effect on the fourth ventricle (*red arrow*). There is extension across midline in the prepontine cistern and encasement of vascular structures including the basilar artery (*red arrowhead*). (*C*) Axial T1W + C image shows only minimal heterogeneous enhancement within the lesion. (*D*) Axial T2W image from intraoperative MR imaging shows resection of this component of the lesion and significantly decreased mass effect on the brainstem. This lesion was confirmed to be an ependymoma.

cerebellar peduncle and can project into the cerebellopontine and medullary angles as well as through the foramen of Luschka into the fourth ventricle. Lateral ependymomas have a higher incidence of recurrence owing to the increased difficulty of achieving a gross total resection.[24]

Ependymomas have a tendency to spread along subarachnoid planes, such as the foramina of Luschka and Magendie around the brainstem and into the cervical spine, encasing vessels and cranial nerves thereby earning the title of "plastic ependymoma."[26] This pattern of growth explains why ependymoma patients typically have a long clinical history of vague symptoms before coming to clinical attention.

Ependymomas have intermediate diffusion characteristics in the range of approximately 1000 to 1300 $\times$ 10^{-6} mm^2/sec, with ADC values lower than that of PAs but higher than that of medulloblastomas. Ependymomas may not enhance, complicating evaluation of metastatic deposits. Small internal cystic components are common, and approximately half of all lesions show signs of calcification.

Outcomes from ependymoma are best when a gross total resection is achieved. Therefore, characterization of metastatic deposits and tumor extent is critical. Ependymomas are not typically responsive to chemotherapy; radiation is critical in achieving long-term local disease control.

ATYPICAL TERATOID RHABDOID TUMOR

ATRT is a malignant tumor classified as WHO grade IV, which can be located in the fourth ventricle, cerebellum, basal cisterns (cerebellopontine and medullary cisterns), and, rarely, in the brainstem. This tumor is primarily identified in the first year or two of life, with the median age at diagnosis being 2 to 4 years. However, ATRT can be seen throughout early childhood. This tumor is another small, blue, cell embryonal tumor and on imaging follows many features of medulloblastoma. ATRT is a highly cellular tumor with low ADC values, typically lower than 700 $\times$ 10^{-6} mm^2/s. ATRT may present with obstructive hydrocephalus and is prone to CSF dissemination of disease. Unlike medulloblastomas, ATRT does not usually respond to chemotherapy and, therefore, overall has a poorer prognosis.

OTHER ENTITIES
Ganglioglioma

Gangliogliomas can occur in the cerebellum as well as within the brainstem with extension into the cerebellum. Cerebellar gangliogliomas accounted for less than 1% of cerebellar tumors in a large series.[27] Cerebellar, brainstem, and cervicomedullary junction gangliogliomas tend to be more infiltrating and less discrete than supratentorial gangliogliomas.[28] The cerebellar component is often within the middle and inferior cerebellar peduncles and the region of the dentate nuclei. They are often calcified, with indistinct margins and a characteristic flame-shape enhancement pattern. Although these lesions may not be amenable to gross total resection because of their infiltrating nature and involvement of more central structures, as opposed to the more peripheral nature of most of the other cerebellar tumors, the unresectable components may be well controlled by adjunct therapy in many cases.

Infiltrating Glioma

Infiltrating gliomas, including fibrillary astrocytomas, anaplastic astrocytoma, and glioblastoma, can occur in the cerebellum. The imaging appearance matches that of their supratentorial counterparts, including expansile areas of T2 hyperintense signal. More high-grade lesions have variable heterogeneous areas of enhancement, diffusion restriction, cystic changes, and hemorrhagic changes. When these lesions are encountered, careful analysis of the clinical history and imaging features are required to differentiate from inflammatory processes such as acute disseminated encephalomyelitis (ADEM), vasculitis, and rhombencephalitis. Advanced imaging techniques, such as diffusion-weighted imaging (DWI) and diffusion tensor imaging (DTI), perfusion imaging, and spectroscopy, can be used; however, lumbar puncture analysis and short-term follow-up imaging may be the most helpful.

Radiation-Induced Glioma

In patients with a history of a radiation therapy to the posterior cranial fossa, radiation-induced gliomas may occur, most commonly at least 5 years after treatment.[29] These lesions will appear ill defined and infiltrating and will not have the same imaging appearance of the original tumor. Differentiating radiation-induced glioma from late radiation necrosis may be aided by PET scan, perfusion imaging, and magnetic resonance (MR) spectroscopy[30–32]; however, ultimately biopsy may be required (Fig. 5). In patients with a tumor predisposition condition, a secondary glioma may be a part of the underlying disease process and may or may not be solely related to radiation.

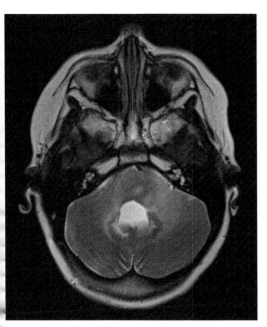

Fig. 5. Secondary glioma. Axial T2W image in a 7-year-old girl with a history of fourth ventricular ependymoma shows an infiltrating slightly expansile lesion in the brainstem as well as the middle cerebellar peduncles and deep cerebellar white matter, left greater than right. This finding did not match the appearance of her original tumor, and biopsy was performed to differentiate an infiltrating glioma versus late radiation necrosis. Biopsy confirmed this to be an infiltrating high-grade glioma without any features to suggest ependymoma.

Metastatic Disease

Intracranial metastatic disease from extracranial primary tumors is exceedingly rare in children, which is very different compared with adults. This disease may be considered in children with known primary tumors, other sites of metastatic disease, and a new cerebellar lesion. This finding is a diagnosis of exclusion and may require biopsy for confirmation. Cerebellar leptomeningeal metastatic disease from known intracranial tumors is a common occurrence.

Syndromic-Associated Tumors

Syndromic-associated cerebellar tumors in children are rare; however, of these, the most common is PA with neurofibromatosis type I (von Recklinghausen disease).[33] Hemangioblastomas are cystic lesions with enhancing nodules that have imaging overlap with PA and are located in the cerebellar hemispheres. Hemangioblastomas in children and adolescents are rarely found without von Hippel Lindau syndrome. A rare but characteristic posterior fossa lesion is dysplastic

gangliocytoma, also known as Lhermitte-Duclos disease, a nonenhancing hamartomatous lesion that has a "cerebellum within a cerebellum" appearance. Dysplastic gangliocytomas are commonly associated with Cowden syndrome, which is a syndrome resulting in development of multiple tumors and hamartomas due to mutations in the *PTEN* gene.[34] Medulloblastomas may occur in association with 2 different inherited cancer syndromes: Gorlin and Turcot, the latter also known as nevoid basal cell carcinoma syndrome.

Tumor Mimicking Conditions

An enhancing and/or edematous lesion in the cerebellum does not always represent tumor. Infectious rhombencephalitis can look like a tumor. In the developed world, the most common infectious rhombencephalitis is related to Listeria, however globally it is due to tuberculosis. Noninfectious inflammatory conditions, such as ADEM, vasculitis, and multiple sclerosis all can overlap with tumors. Radiation necrosis and treatment induced so-called pseudoprogression can also have an aggressive appearance, including changes after proton beam therapy.[35] Appropriate recognition of potential mimicking conditions can help direct prompt and appropriate therapy, and may help prevent unnecessary surgery.

Imaging Considerations

For any patient with a known posterior fossa mass, the MR imaging protocol should be carefully prescribed. Thin-slice T2W and T1-weighted imaging should be performed to rule out foraminal or internal auditory canal invasion, including evaluation in multiple planes. Cranial nerve and vessel involvement may be misleading on sequences with greater than a 2-mm slice thickness. Volumetric image acquisition allows images to be reformatted into any imaging plane, including oblique planes.

Staging requires imaging of the entire neural axis, the brain, and complete spine. Spine imaging should extend to include the caudal most aspect of the thecal sac, often at approximately the S2 level, as CSF dissemination of disease can result in metastatic deposits in the dependent-most portion of the thecal sac. This point is important to be aware of because adult degenerative spine imaging protocols do not always extend below the superior end plate of S1 and could miss metastatic deposits. This point is most important for ependymomas, medulloblastomas, and ATRT, whereas leptomeningeal metastatic disease is less common in PAs. When possible, the spine imaging should take place before surgical resection of the primary lesion to prevent postoperative changes, namely, blood products, confounding the imaging. Postcontrast T2–fluid-attenuated inversion recovery imaging of the brain may provide increased sensitivity to detect leptomeningeal metastatic deposits, however, is subject to artifact and false-positive findings as well.[36]

DWI plays a critical role in characterization of pediatric brain tumors. In particular, quantitative analysis of ADC maps can aid in prediction of tumor cellularity and in conjunction with morphologic features can help predict tumor histology.[3,37] Lower ADC values correspond to more cellular tumors, typically more aggressive. Tumors with ADC values less than 1000×10^{-6} mm^2/s tend to be high grade.

Research has shown that medulloblastomas are more likely to have identification of taurine on MR spectroscopy versus other lesions.[17] Spectroscopy can help differentiate an enhancing edematous demyelinating lesion from a high-grade tumor; however, low-grade tumors and demyelinating lesions can have similar spectroscopic profiles. For practical reasons, MR spectroscopy does not typically play a significant role in the primary characterization of cerebellar tumors.

Advanced physiologic imaging techniques have advanced diagnosis and surgical planning in supratentorial tumors,[38] which have some applicability to cerebellar tumors as well. DTI can evaluate the location of key white matter fiber bundles.[39] Diffusion tensor fiber tracking has been shown to be able to aid differentiation between discrete lesions, which splay white matter fibers and are, thus, more amenable to resection, and infiltrating lesions, which may not be able to be resected without disruption of the encompassed fiber pathways. Perfusion imaging, including dynamic susceptibility of contrast perfusion and arterial spin labeling perfusion, can show increased blood flow and blood volume within high-grade tumors.[40] Dynamic contrast-enhanced (DCE) perfusion can document signs of neovascularity and capillary leakage. DCE perfusion can also show differences in enhancement between the otherwise structurally similar PA and hemangioblastoma, with slow progressive enhancement in PA and rapid arterial enhancement in hemangioblastoma. Task-based functional MR imaging (fMR imaging) and resting-state fMR imaging do not currently play a significant role in diagnosis or surgical planning of cerebellar tumors. Susceptibility-weighted imaging (SWI) is an imaging sequence that is highly sensitive to magnetic field heterogeneity due to diamagnetic and/or paramagnetic substances, such as calcium and some blood products, respectively. This imaging can provide visualization of calcifications, which

may be present in prior stroke, infections, and some syndromic conditions as well as within many cerebellar tumors. Identification of hemorrhagic changes on SWI can be a biomarker indicating an aggressive tumor. SWI has also been shown to be helpful in evaluation of vascularity, including characterization of altered perfusion patterns after stroke.[41,42]

PET with fludeoxyglucose F 18 is not widely used in the primary characterization of pediatric cerebellar tumors; however, 11-C-methionine PET has more recently been shown to be a way of differentiating low-grade from high-grade tumors.[43,44] PET and perfusion imaging have been shown to have a role in differentiating posttreatment tumor recurrence versus radiation necrosis or pseudoprogression.[30,45–47] These techniques have been more widely studied in adult supratentorial gliomas than pediatric cerebellar tumors.

Intraoperative MR Imaging

Intraoperative MR imaging (iMR imaging) is a technology that allows immediate imaging evaluation of a resection cavity while patients are in the operating room.[48,49] This technology is especially suited for the evaluation of pediatric brain tumors, whereby gross-total resection (GTR) is the most important determinant of local control and survival in many tumors. In cases whereby the preoperative surgical goal is a GTR, rates of up to 95% have been achieved with the iMR imaging.[48] Recent advances have allowed iMR imaging to be performed in children as young as 4 months of age.[50] Studies to date have not shown MR imaging–related complications or increased infection rates in patients undergoing iMR imaging–guided surgery. Like other new technologies, iMR imaging does have its challenges, including image interpretation and spatial distortion.[51]

TREATMENT AND MANAGEMENT CONSIDERATIONS
Radiation

Radiation therapy, photons or protons, is commonly performed for ependymoma, medulloblastoma, and ATRT and can serve as an excellent alternative for PA. Depending on the type of tumor and the presence or absence of metastatic disease, local radiation to the surgical bed only with a margin may be appropriate. With metastatic disease or with more aggressive tumors, such as medulloblastoma, more extensive treatment, such as whole-brain irradiation or craniospinal irradiation, may be warranted. Adjunct radiation is avoided, when possible, in children younger than 3 years of age because of the profound detrimental effects on neural development.

Posterior Fossa Syndrome

The resection of any midline/fourth ventricular tumor may lead to a constellation of symptoms known as posterior fossa syndrome (PFS). This syndrome typically occurs several days after surgical resection. The sine qua non of PFS is an inability of the child to speak but still able to comprehend (cerebellar mutism). Additional features of PFS include emotional lability, hypotonia, and ataxia.[52] Large tumors within the fourth ventricle, splaying of the peduncles or invasion into the region of the dentate nuclei, obstructive hydrocephalus, young age, male sex, and medulloblastoma tumor are all risk factors for PFS. PFS may be the result of injury to the efferent cerebellar pathway bilaterally, with resultant imaging and physiologic features, including components of bilateral cerebellar diaschisis and bilateral hypertrophic olivary degeneration.[53,54]

SUMMARY

Cerebellar tumors are the most commonly encountered pediatric CNS neoplasms. We have moved well beyond the days of providing the standard 3-part differential: medulloblastoma, ependymoma, and PA. Advanced imaging techniques, in particular quantitative diffusion analysis, in conjunction with morphologic features and location, combined with knowledge of advances in genetic subtyping of these tumors, can maximize the information provided to the neurosurgical and neuro-oncologic teams. Effective use of advanced imaging, including iMR imaging when available, can maximize the possibility of adequate tumor characterization and GTR, which translates to optimal patient outcomes.

REFERENCES

1. Poussaint Tina Y, Panigrahy A, Huisman TA. Pediatric brain tumors. Pediatr Radiol 2015;45(S3):443–53.
2. Gajjar A, Bowers DC, Karajannis MA, et al. Pediatric brain tumors: innovative genomic information is transforming the diagnostic and clinical landscape. J Clin Oncol 2015;33(27):2986–98.
3. Rumboldt Z, Camacho DLA, Lake D, et al. Apparent diffusion coefficients for differentiation of cerebellar tumors in children. AJNR Am J Neuroradiol 2006; 27(6):1362–9.
4. Koeller Kelly K, Rushing Elisabeth J. From the archives of the AFIP. Radiographics 2004;24(6): 1693–708.
5. Gjerris F, Klinken L. Long-term prognosis in children with benign cerebellar astrocytoma. J Neurosurg 1978;49(2):179–84.
6. Jones DT, Kocialkowski S, Liu L, et al. Tandem duplication producing a novel oncogenic BRAF fusion gene defines the majority of pilocytic astrocytomas. Cancer Res 2008;68(21):8673–7.
7. Jones David TW, Gronych J, Lichter P, et al. MAPK pathway activation in pilocytic astrocytoma. Cell Mol Life Sci 2012;69(11):1799–811.
8. Raabe Eric H, Lim KS, Kim JM, et al. BRAF activation induces transformation and then senescence in human neural stem cells: a pilocytic astrocytoma model. Clin Cancer Res 2011;17(11):3590–9.
9. Gierke M, Sperveslage J, Schwab D, et al. Analysis of IDH1-R132 mutation, BRAF V600 mutation and KIAA1549-BRAF fusion transcript status in central nervous system tumors supports pediatric tumor classification. J Cancer Res Clin Oncol 2016; 142(1):89–100.
10. Bergthold G, Bandopadhayay P, Hoshida Y, et al. Expression profiles of 151 pediatric low-grade gliomas reveal molecular differences associated with location and histological subtype. Neuro Oncol 2015;17(11):1486–96.
11. Faulkner C, Ellis HP, Shaw A, et al. BRAF fusion analysis in pilocytic astrocytomas: KIAA1549-BRAF 15-9 fusions are more frequent in the midline than within the cerebellum. J Neuropathol Exp Neurol 2015; 74(9):867–72.
12. Vennepureddy A, Thumallapally N, Motilal Nehru V, et al. Novel drugs and combination therapies for the treatment of metastatic melanoma. J Clin Med Res 2016;8(2):63–75.
13. Louis David N, Ohgaki H, Wiestler Otmar D, et al. The 2007 WHO classification of tumours of the central nervous system. Acta Neuropathol 2007;114(2): 97–109.
14. Levy RA, Blaivas M, Muraszko K, et al. Desmoplastic medulloblastoma: MR findings. AJNR Am J Neuroradiol 1997;18(7):1364–6.
15. Gibson P, Tong Y, Robinson G, et al. Subtypes of medulloblastoma have distinct developmental origins. Nature 2010;468(7327):1095–9.
16. Taylor MD, Northcott PA, Korshunov A, et al. Molecular subgroups of medulloblastoma: the current consensus. Acta Neuropathol 2011;123(4): 465–72.
17. Panigrahy A, Krieger MD, Gonzalez-Gomez I, et al. Quantitative short echo time 1H-MR spectroscopy of untreated pediatric brain tumors: preoperative diagnosis and characterization. AJNR Am J Neuroradiol 2006;27(3):560–72.
18. Patay Z, DeSain LA, Hwang SN, et al. MR imaging characteristics of wingless-type-subgroup pediatric medulloblastoma. AJNR Am J Neuroradiol 2015; 36(12):2386–93.

19. Perreault S, Ramaswamy V, Achrol AS, et al. MRI surrogates for molecular subgroups of medulloblastoma. AJNR Am J Neuroradiol 2014;35(7): 1263–9.

20. Nobuyuki K, Yagishita S, Hara M, et al. Pathologic features of ependymoma: histologic patterns and a review of the literature. Neuropathology 1998; 18(1):1–12.

21. Johnson Robert A, Wright Karen D, Poppleton H, et al. Cross-species genomics matches driver mutations and cell compartments to model ependymoma. Nature 2010;466(7306):632–6.

22. Taylor Michael D, Poppleton H, Fuller C, et al. Radial glia cells are candidate stem cells of ependymoma. Cancer Cell 2005;8(4):323–35.

23. Pajtler Kristian W, Witt H, Sill M, et al. Molecular classification of ependymal tumors across all CNS compartments, histopathological grades, and age groups. Cancer Cell 2015;27(5):728–43.

24. Hendrik W, Mack Stephen C, Ryzhova M, et al. Delineation of two clinically and molecularly distinct subgroups of posterior fossa ependymoma. Cancer Cell 2011;20(2):143–57.

25. Raghunathan A, Wani K, Armstrong Terri S, et al. Histological predictors of outcome in ependymoma are dependent on anatomic site within the central nervous system. Brain Pathol 2013;23(5):584–94.

26. Courville CB, Broussalian SL. Plastic ependymomas of the lateral recess. Report of eight verified cases. J Neurosurg 1961;18:792–9.

27. Chang T, Teng MM, Lirng JF. Posterior cranial fossa tumours in childhood. Neuroradiology 1993;35(4): 274–8.

28. McAbee JH, Modica J, Thompson CJ, et al. Cervicomedullary tumors in children. J Neurosurg Pediatr 2015;16(4):357–66.

29. Klimo P Jr, Nesvick CL, Broniscer A, et al. Malignant brainstem tumors in children, excluding diffuse intrinsic pontine gliomas. J Neurosurg Pediatr 2015;17(1):57–65.

30. Shah R, Vattoth S, Jacob R, et al. Radiation necrosis in the brain: imaging features and differentiation from tumor recurrence. Radiographics 2012;32(5): 1343–59.

31. Kralik SF, Ho CY, Finke W, et al. Radiation necrosis in pediatric patients with brain tumors treated with proton radiotherapy. AJNR Am J Neuroradiol 2015; 36(8):1572–8.

32. Sundgren PC. MR spectroscopy in radiation injury. AJNR Am J Neuroradiol 2009;30(8):1469–76.

33. Collins VP, Jones DTW, Giannini C. Pilocytic astrocytoma: pathology, molecular mechanisms and markers. Acta Neuropathol 2015;129(6):775–88.

34. Pilarski R, Burt R, Kohlman W, et al. Cowden syndrome and the PTEN hamartoma tumor syndrome: systematic review and revised diagnostic criteria. J Natl Cancer Inst 2013;105(21):1607–16.

35. Sabin ND, Merchant TE, Harreld JH, et al. Imaging changes in very young children with brain tumors treated with proton therapy and chemotherapy. AJNR Am J Neuroradiol 2013; 34(2):446–50.

36. Fukuoka H, Hirai T, Okuda T, et al. Comparison of the added value of contrast-enhanced 3D fluid-attenuated inversion recovery and magnetization-prepared rapid acquisition of gradient echo sequences in relation to conventional postcontrast T1-weighted images for the evaluation of leptomeningeal diseases at 3T. AJNR Am J Neuroradiol 2010;31(5):868–73.

37. Poretti A, Meoded A, Cohen KJ, et al. Apparent diffusion coefficient of pediatric cerebellar tumors: a biomarker of tumor grade? Pediatr Blood Cancer 2013;60(12):2036–41.

38. Pillai JJ, Zaca D, Choudhri AF. Clinical impact of integrated physiologic brain tumor imaging. Technol Cancer Res Treat 2010;9(4):359–80.

39. Choudhri AF, Chin EM, Blitz AM, et al. Diffusion tensor imaging of cerebral white matter. Radiol Clin North Am 2014;52(2):413–25.

40. Yeom KW, Mitchell LA, Lober RM, et al. Arterial spin-labeled perfusion of pediatric brain tumors. AJNR Am J Neuroradiol 2014;35(2):395–401.

41. Bosemani T, Poretti A, Huisman TA. Susceptibility-weighted imaging in pediatric neuroimaging. J Magn Reson Imaging 2014;40(3):530–44.

42. Bosemani T, Poretti A, Orman G, et al. Pediatric cerebral stroke: susceptibility-weighted imaging may predict post-ischemic malignant edema. Neuroradiol J 2013;26(5):579–83.

43. Ogawa T, Inugami A, Hatazawa J, et al. Clinical positron emission tomography for brain tumors: comparison of fludeoxyglucose F 18 and L-methyl-11C-methionine. AJNR Am J Neuroradiol 1996; 17(2):345–53.

44. Kato T, Shinoda J, Oka N, et al. Analysis of 11C-methionine uptake in low-grade gliomas and correlation with proliferative activity. AJNR Am J Neuroradiol 2008;29(10):1867–71.

45. Hustinx R, Pourdehnad M, Kaschten B, et al. PET imaging for differentiating recurrent brain tumor from radiation necrosis. Radiol Clin North Am 2005;43(1):35–47.

46. Fatterpekar GM, Galheigo D, Narayana A, et al. Treatment-related change versus tumor recurrence in high-grade gliomas: a diagnostic conundrum—use of dynamic susceptibility contrast-enhanced (DSC) perfusion MRI. Am J Roentgenol 2012; 198(1):19–26.

47. Zach L, Guez D, Last D, et al. Delayed contrast extravasation MRI: a new paradigm in neuro-oncology. Neuro Oncol 2015;17(3):457–65.

48. Choudhri AF, Klimo P, Auschwitz TS, et al. 3T intraoperative MRI for management of pediatric CNS

neoplasms. AJNR Am J Neuroradiol 2014;35(12): 2382–7.

49. Choudhri AF, Siddiqui A, Klimo P Jr, et al. Intraoperative MRI in pediatric brain tumors. Pediatr Radiol 2015;45(3):397–405.

50. Boop FA, Bate B, Choudhri AF, et al. Preliminary experience with an intraoperative MRI-compatible infant headholder: technical note. J Neurosurg Pediatr 2015;15(5):539–43.

51. Choudhri AF, Chin EM, Klimo P, et al. Spatial distortion due to field inhomogeneity in 3.0 Tesla intraoperative MRI. Neuroradiol J 2014;27(4):387–92.

52. Turgut M. Cerebellar mutism. J Neurosurg Pediatr 2008;1(3):262.

53. Miller NG, Reddick WE, Kocak M, et al. Cerebellocerebral diaschisis is the likely mechanism of postsurgical posterior fossa syndrome in pediatric patients with midline cerebellar tumors. AJNR Am J Neuroradiol 2010;31(2):288–94.

54. Patay Z, Enterkin J, Harreld JH, et al. MR imaging evaluation of inferior olivary nuclei: comparison of postoperative subjects with and without posterior fossa syndrome. AJNR Am J Neuroradiol 2014; 35(4):797–802.

Index

Note: Page numbers of article titles are in **boldface** type.

A

Abscess, brain tumors versus, 802, 803

Acetate, 1-^{13}C, metabolized, 692–693

Acetate metabolism, in brain, 692

Adenocarcinoma, metastatic, 672–673, 677

Alanine, spectral pattern of, in intracranial tumors, 784, 786

Amide proton transfer, 696–697

Anaplastic astrocytomas, WHO classification of, 744

Antiangiogenic treatment, advanced imaging and, 710–711

    magnetic resonance-perfusion-weighted imaging in, 711

    tissue classification in, multimodality parametric approach to, 711–712

Arterial spin labeling, to measure blood flow, 769–771

Astrocytoma(s), pilocytic, juvenile, 812–813

    resection of, radiation necrosis following, 775–777

    WHO classification of, 744

B

Bevacizumab, in gliomas, 654, 656, 657, 658

Brain, acetate metabolism in, 692

    hyperpolarized Xenon imaging in, 697–698

    inflammation in, imaging in, 694–695

Brain cancer, cell lines, hyperpolarized MR spectroscopy in, 693–694

    chemical exchange saturation transfer imaging in, 695–697

    gas chromatography/mass spectrometry-based metabolomics of, 689–691

    hypolarized MR imaging and metabolic imaging in, 688

    interrogating metabolism in, **687–703**

        for prediction of outcome or response to therapy, 689

        for tumor characterization, 689

Brain lesions, that look alike, differential diagnosis of, 800–804

Brain metastases, response assessment in neuro-oncology, 713

Brain tumor(s), adult, MR spectroscopy in, **781–809**

    DSC-MR imaging in, for distinquishing tumor from nontumor, 650–651, 652

    imaging of, metabolites evaluated with, 671, 672

        nonliposomal nanoparticles for, 756–757

    molecular imaging of, 752–753

        barriers to nanoparticles in, 752–753

        liposomal contrast agents for, 753–756

        probe classification of nanoparticles for, 753

        signal amplification in, 753

        using liposomal contrast agents and nonoparticles, **751–763**

    perfusion imaging for grading, 771, 772

    radiomics in, **719–729**

    versus abscess, 802, 803

    versus demyelination, 801, 802

    versus encephalitis, 802–804

    versus focal cortical dysplasia, 802

    versus stroke, 801

C

Central nervous system tumors, World Health Organization Classification (2016) of, 742

Cerebellar tumors, pediatric, **811–821**

    imaging considerations in, 817–818

    intraoperative MR imaging in, 818

    metastatic, 817

    radiation therapy in, 818–891

    resection of, posterior fossa syndrome following, 819

    treatment and management considerations in, 818–819

    types of, 811–812

Chemical exchange saturation transfer imaging, in brain cancer, 695–697

Children, cerebrellar tumors in. See *Cerebellar tumors, pediatric.*

Computed tomography perfusion, to measure blood flow, 766, 767

Creatine chemical exchange saturation transfer, 696

D

Demyelinating lesions, brain tumors versus, 801, 802

Dendritic cell vaccine therapy, 662, 663

Dynamic contrast enhanced-T1 imaging, to measure blood flow, 767–769

Dynamic susceptibility contrast MR imaging, applications to brain tumors. See *specific tumors.*

    basic principles of, 649–650

    protocols, 664–665

Dynamic susceptibility contrast T2* imaging, to measure blood flow, 769, 770

Magn Reson Imaging Clin N Am 24 (2016) 823–826

http://dx.doi.org/10.1016/S1064-9689(16)30080-0

1064-9689/16/$ – see front matter

UNITED STATES POSTAL SERVICE ®
Statement of Ownership, Management, and Circulation
(All Periodicals Publications Except Requester Publications)

1. Publication Title	2. Publication Number	3. Filing Date
MAGNETIC RESONANCE IMAGING CLINICS OF NORTH AMERICA	011 – 909	9/18/2016

4. Issue Frequency	5. Number of Issues Published Annually	6. Annual Subscription Price
FEB, MAY, AUG, NOV	4	$375.00

7. Complete Mailing Address of Known Office of Publication (Not printer) (Street, city, county, state, and ZIP+4®)

ELSEVIER INC.
360 PARK AVENUE SOUTH
NEW YORK, NY 10010-1710

Contact Person: STEPHEN R. BUSHING
Telephone (Include area code): 215-239-3688

8. Complete Mailing Address of Headquarters or General Business Office of Publisher (Not printer)

ELSEVIER INC.
360 PARK AVENUE SOUTH
NEW YORK, NY 10010-1710

9. Full Names and Complete Mailing Addresses of Publisher, Editor, and Managing Editor (Do not leave blank)

Publisher (Name and complete mailing address)
ADRIANNE BRIGIDO, ELSEVIER INC.
1600 JOHN F KENNEDY BLVD. SUITE 1800
PHILADELPHIA, PA 19103-2899

Editor (Name and complete mailing address)
JOHN VASSALLO, ELSEVIER INC.
1600 JOHN F KENNEDY BLVD. SUITE 1800
PHILADELPHIA, PA 19103-2899

Managing Editor (Name and complete mailing address)
PATRICK MANLEY, ELSEVIER INC.
1600 JOHN F KENNEDY BLVD. SUITE 1800
PHILADELPHIA, PA 19103-2899

10. Owner (Do not leave blank. If the publication is owned by a corporation, give the name and address of the corporation immediately followed by the names and addresses of all stockholders owning or holding 1 percent or more of the total amount of stock. If not owned by a corporation, give the names and addresses of the individual owners. If owned by a partnership or other unincorporated firm, give its name and address as well as those of each individual owner. If the publication is published by a nonprofit organization, give its name and address.)

Full Name	Complete Mailing Address
WHOLLY OWNED SUBSIDIARY OF REED/ELSEVIER, US HOLDINGS	1600 JOHN F KENNEDY BLVD. SUITE 1800 PHILADELPHIA, PA 19103-2899

11. Known Bondholders, Mortgagees, and Other Security Holders Owning or Holding 1 Percent or More of Total Amount of Bonds, Mortgages, or Other Securities. If none, check box ▶ ☐ None

Full Name	Complete Mailing Address
N/A	

12. Tax Status (For completion by nonprofit organizations authorized to mail at nonprofit rates) (Check one)
The purpose, function, and nonprofit status of this organization and the exempt status for federal income tax purposes:
☐ Has Not Changed During Preceding 12 Months
☐ Has Changed During Preceding 12 Months (Publisher must submit explanation of change with this statement)

PS Form 3526, July 2014 [Page 1 of 4 (see instructions page 4)] PSN: 7530-01-000-9931   PRIVACY NOTICE: See our privacy policy on www.usps.com

13. Publication Title	14. Issue Date for Circulation Data Below
MAGNETIC RESONANCE IMAGING CLINICS OF NORTH AMERICA	AUGUST 2016

15. Extent and Nature of Circulation		Average No. Copies Each Issue During Preceding 12 Months	No. Copies of Single Issue Published Nearest to Filing Date
a. Total Number of Copies (Net press run)		691	835
b. Paid Circulation (By Mail and Outside the Mail)	(1) Mailed Outside-County Paid Subscriptions Stated on PS Form 3541 (Include paid distribution above nominal rate, advertiser's proof copies, and exchange copies)	407	493
	(2) Mailed In-County Paid Subscriptions Stated on PS Form 3541 (Include paid distribution above nominal rate, advertiser's proof copies, and exchange copies)	0	0
	(3) Paid Distribution Outside the Mails Including Sales Through Dealers and Carriers, Street Vendors, Counter Sales, and Other Paid Distribution Outside USPS®	125	152
	(4) Paid Distribution by Other Classes of Mail Through the USPS (e.g. First-Class Mail®)	0	0
c. Total Paid Distribution (Sum of 15b (1), (2), (3), and (4))		532	645
d. Free or Nominal Rate Distribution (By Mail and Outside the Mail)	(1) Free or Nominal Rate Outside-County Copies included on PS Form 3541	51	75
	(2) Free or Nominal Rate In-County Copies Included on PS Form 3541	0	0
	(3) Free or Nominal Rate Copies Mailed at Other Classes Through the USPS (e.g. First-Class Mail)	0	0
	(4) Free or Nominal Rate Distribution Outside the Mail (Carriers or other means)	0	0
e. Total Free or Nominal Rate Distribution (Sum of 15d (1), (2), (3) and (4))		51	75
f. Total Distribution (Sum of 15c and 15e)		583	720
g. Copies not Distributed (See Instructions to Publishers #4 (page #3))		108	115
h. Total (Sum of 15f and g)		691	835
i. Percent Paid (15c divided by 15f times 100)		91%	90%

PS Form 3526, July 2014 (Page 2 of 4)

16. Electronic Copy Circulation	Average No. Copies Each Issue During Preceding 12 Months	No. Copies of Single Issue Published Nearest to Filing Date
a. Paid Electronic Copies ▶	0	0
b. Total Paid Print Copies (Line 15c) + Paid Electronic Copies (Line 16a) ▶	532	645
c. Total Print Distribution (Line 15f) + Paid Electronic Copies (Line 16a) ▶	583	720
d. Percent Paid (Both Print & Electronic Copies) (16b divided by 16c × 100) ▶	91%	90%

☒ I certify that 50% of all my distributed copies (electronic and print) are paid above a nominal price.

17. Publication of Statement of Ownership
☒ If the publication is a general publication, publication of this statement is required. Will be printed in the NOVEMBER 2016 issue of this publication.   ☐ Publication not required.

18. Signature and Title of Editor, Publisher, Business Manager, or Owner

STEPHEN R. BUSHING – INVENTORY DISTRIBUTION CONTROL MANAGER   Date 9/18/2016

I certify that all information furnished on this form is true and complete. I understand that anyone who furnishes false or misleading information on this form or who omits material or information requested on the form may be subject to criminal sanctions (including fines and imprisonment) and/or civil sanctions (including civil penalties).

PS Form 3526, July 2014 (Page 3 of 4)   PRIVACY NOTICE: See our privacy policy on www.usps.com

Moving?

Make sure your subscription moves with you!

To notify us of your new address, find your **Clinics Account Number** (located on your mailing label above your name), and contact customer service at:

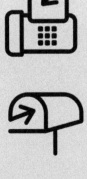

Email: journalscustomerservice-usa@elsevier.com

800-654-2452 (subscribers in the U.S. & Canada)
314-447-8871 (subscribers outside of the U.S. & Canada)

Fax number: 314-447-8029

Elsevier Health Sciences Division
Subscription Customer Service
3251 Riverport Lane
Maryland Heights, MO 63043

Printed and bound by CPI Group (UK) Ltd, Croydon, CR0 4YY

08/05/2025

01864686-0018